D1587553

COLORECTAL SURGERY

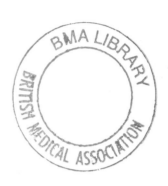

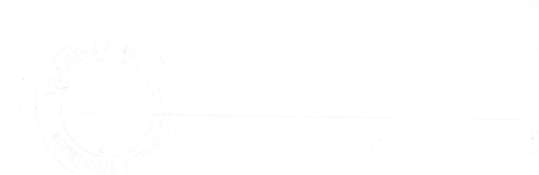

A Companion to Specialist Surgical Practice

Series Editors

O. James Garden
Simon Paterson-Brown

COLORECTAL SURGERY

SIXTH EDITION

Edited by

Sue Clark

MA MD FRCS(Gen Surg) EBSQ(Coloproctology)

Consultant Colorectal Surgeon, St Mark's Hospital, Harrow;
Adjunct Professor of Surgery, Imperial College, London, UK

For additional online content visit ExpertConsult.com

ELSEVIER Edinburgh London New York Oxford Philadelphia St Louis Sydney 2019

ELSEVIER

First edition 1997
Second edition 2001
Third edition 2005
Fourth edition 2009
Fifth edition 2014
Sixth edition 2019

Notice

Practitioners and researchers must always rely on their own experience and knowledge in evaluating and using any information, methods, compounds or experiments described herein. Because of rapid advances in the medical sciences, in particular, independent verification of diagnoses and drug dosages should be made. To the fullest extent of the law, no responsibility is assumed by Elsevier, authors, editors or contributors for any injury and/or damage to persons or property as a matter of products liability, negligence or otherwise, or from any use or operation of any methods, products, instructions, or ideas contained in the material herein.

ISBN: 978-0-7020-7243-7

Printed in China
Last digit is the print number: 9   8   7   6   5   4   3   2   1

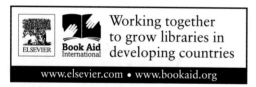

Working together
to grow libraries in
developing countries

www.elsevier.com • www.bookaid.org

Content Strategist: Laurence Hunter
Content Development Specialist: Lynn Watt
Project Manager: Umarani Natarajan
Design: Miles Hitchen
Illustration Manager: Nichole Beard
Illustrator: MPS North America LLC

Contents

Contents

Series Editors' preface

The *Companion to Specialist Surgical Practice* series has now come of age. This Sixth Edition takes the series to a different level since it was first published in 1997. The intention from the outset was to ensure that we could support the educational needs of those in the later years of specialist surgical training and of consultant surgeons in independent practice who wished for contemporary, evidence-based information on the subspecialist areas relevant to their general surgical practice. Although there still seems to be a role for larger reference surgical textbooks, and having contributed to many of these, we appreciate that it is difficult for them to keep pace with changing surgical practice.

This Sixth Edition continues to keep abreast of the increasing specialisation in general surgery. The rise of minimal access surgery and therapy, and the desire of some subspecialities, such as breast and vascular surgery, to separate away from 'general surgery' may have proved challenging in some countries. However, they also underline the importance for all surgeons of being aware of current developments in their surgical field. This series as a consequence continues to place emphasis on the need for surgeons to deliver a high-quality emergency surgical practice. The importance of evidence-based practice remains throughout, and authors have provided recommendations and highlighted key resources within each chapter. The ebook version of the textbook has also enabled improved access to the reference abstracts and links to video content relevant to many of the chapters.

We have recognised in this Sixth Edition that new blood is required to maintain the vitality of content. We are indebted to the volume editors, and contributors, who have stood down since the last edition and welcome the new leadership on several volumes. The contents have been comprehensively updated by our contributors and editorial team. We remain grateful for the support and encouragement of Laurence Hunter and Lynn Watt at Elsevier. We trust that our original vision of delivering an up-to-date affordable text has been met and that readers, whether in training or independent practice, will find this Sixth Edition an invaluable resource.

O. James Garden, CBE, BSc, MBChB, MD, FRCS (Glas), FRCS(Ed), FRCP(Ed), FRACS(Hon), FRCSC (Hon), FACS(Hon), FCSHK(Hon), FRCSI(Hon), FRCS(Engl)(Hon), FRSE
Regius Professor of Clinical Surgery, Clinical Surgery, The University of Edinburgh and Honorary Consultant Surgeon, Royal Infirmary of Edinburgh, Edinburgh, UK

Simon Paterson-Brown, MBBS, MPhil, MS, FRCS(Ed), FRCS(Engl), FCSHK, FFST(RCSEd)
Honorary Clinical Senior Lecturer, Clinical Surgery, The University of Edinburgh and Consultant General and Upper Gastrointestinal Surgeon, Royal Infirmary of Edinburgh, Edinburgh, UK

Editors' preface

Colorectal surgery continues to evolve, as has this Sixth Edition. In particular, minimally invasive techniques are now part of the repertoire of the majority of colorectal surgeons; rather than being covered in a distinct chapter, this aspect of surgery is now incorporated in the relevant chapters, mirroring the development of surgical practice.

The running order has been changed to provide a more logical flow, and separate chapters have been introduced on colon cancer and on advanced and recurrent colorectal cancer. New techniques, including complete mesocolic excision, transanal TME, TAMIS and LIFT, are covered. Links to videos of procedures have been added for the first time, and will complement the written descriptions and diagrams.

A number of new authors have joined the team, and have helped to ensure that the content is up to date. The aim has been to be clear, concise, authoritative and contemporary, and to emphasise the underlying evidence base. This is achieved using clearly signposted 'expert opinion' (one tick) and 'strong recommendation' (two tick) panels, together with brief descriptions of the key papers.

This volume provides more than enough information for those preparing for general and colorectal surgical examinations, and to support those in consultant practice. Each print volume has access to the accompanying ebook version which should enhance the overall experience, and ensure that it is enjoyable to read and to use.

Acknowledgements

The editor would like to acknowledge and offer grateful thanks for the input of all previous editions' contributors, without whom this new edition would not have been possible. Grateful thanks also to the retiring volume editor of all the previous editions, Robin K.S. Phillips, who did a superb job in developing this volume to its current standard.

Sue Clark
Harrow, Middlesex

Evidence-based practice in surgery

Critical appraisal for developing evidence-based practice can be obtained from a number of sources, the most reliable being randomised controlled clinical trials, systematic literature reviews, meta-analyses and observational studies. For practical purposes three grades of evidence can be used, analogous to the levels of 'proof' required in a court of law:

1. **Beyond all reasonable doubt.** Such evidence is likely to have arisen from high-quality randomised controlled trials, systematic reviews or high-quality synthesised evidence such as decision analysis, cost-effectiveness analysis or large observational datasets. The studies need to be directly applicable to the population of concern and have clear results. The grade is analogous to burden of proof within a criminal court and may be thought of as corresponding to the usual standard of 'proof' within the medical literature (i.e. $P < 0.05$).

2. **On the balance of probabilities.** In many cases a high-quality review of literature may fail to reach firm conclusions due to conflicting or inconclusive results, trials of poor methodological quality or the lack of evidence in the population to which the guidelines apply. In such cases it may still be possible to make a statement as to the best treatment on the 'balance of probabilities'. This is analogous to the decision in a civil court where all the available evidence will be weighed up and the verdict will depend upon the balance of probabilities.

3. **Not proven.** Insufficient evidence upon which to base a decision, or contradictory evidence.

Depending on the information available, three grades of recommendation can be used:

a. Strong recommendation, which should be followed unless there are compelling reasons to act otherwise.

b. A recommendation based on evidence of effectiveness, but where there may be other factors to take into account in decision-making, for example the user of the guidelines may be expected to take into account patient preferences, local facilities, local audit results or available resources.

c. A recommendation made where there is no adequate evidence as to the most effective practice, although there may be reasons for making a recommendation in order to minimise cost or reduce the chance of error through a locally agreed protocol.

✔✔ Evidence where a conclusion can be reached **'beyond all reasonable doubt'** and therefore where a **strong recommendation** can be given. This will normally be based on evidence levels:
- Ia. Meta-analysis of randomised controlled trials
- Ib. Evidence from at least one randomised controlled trial
- IIa. Evidence from at least one controlled study without randomisation
- IIb. Evidence from at least one other type of quasi-experimental study.

✔ Evidence where a conclusion might be reached **'on the balance of probabilities'** and where there may be other factors involved which influence the recommendation given. This will normally be based on less conclusive evidence than that represented by the double tick icons:
- III. Evidence from non-experimental descriptive studies, such as comparative studies and case–control studies
- IV. Evidence from expert committee reports or opinions or clinical experience of respected authorities, or both.

Evidence that is associated with either a **strong recommendation** or **expert opinion** is highlighted in the text in panels such as those shown above, and is distinguished by either a double or single tick icon, respectively. The references associated with double-tick evidence are listed as Key References at the end of each chapter, along with a short summary of the paper's conclusions where applicable. The full reference list for each chapter is available in the ebook.

The reader is referred to Chapter 1, 'Evaluation of surgical evidence' in the volume *Core Topics in General and Emergency Surgery* of this series, for a more detailed description of this topic.

Contributors

Omer Aziz, MBBS, BSc(Hons), DIC, PhD, FRCS
Consultant Colorectal, General, and Laparoscopic Surgeon, Colorectal and Peritoneal Oncology Centre; Honorary Senior Lecturer, The University of Manchester, Manchester, UK

John Bunni, MBChB(Hons), DipLapSurg, FRCS [ASGBI Medal]
Consultant Colorectal and General Surgeon, Royal United Hospitals Bath NHS Foundation Trust, Bath; Honorary Lecturer, Cardiff University, Cardiff, UK

Sue Clark, MA, MD, FRCS(Gen Surg), EBSQ(Coloproctology)
Consultant Colorectal Surgeon, St Mark's Hospital, Harrow; Adjunct Professor of Surgery, Imperial College, London, UK

Eric J. Dozois, MD, FACS, FACRS
Colon and Rectal Surgery, Mayo Clinic, Rochester, MN, USA

Anton V. Emmanuel, BSc, MD, FRCP
Department of Gastroenterology (GI Physiology), University College London, UK

Nicola S. Fearnhead, BMBCh, FRCS, DM
Consultant Colorectal Surgeon, Department of Colorectal Surgery, Addenbrooke's Hospital, Cambridge, UK

Pasquale Giordano, MD, FRCS
Consultant Surgeon, Department of Colorectal Surgery, Royal London Hospital; Honorary Senior Lecturer Queen Mary University London, London, UK

Simon Gollins, BMBCh, MA, DPhil, MRCP, FRCR
Consultant Clinical Oncologist and Oncology Clinical Director, North Wales Cancer Treatment Centre, Rhyl, UK

Gianpiero Gravante, MBBS, MD, PhD
Surgical Registrar, Colorectal Surgery, Leicester Royal Infirmary, Leicester, UK

Adam Haycock, MBBS, MRCP, BSc, MD
Wolfson Unit for Endoscopy, St Mark's Hospital, London, UK

David J. Humes, BSc, MSc, MBBS, PhD, FRCS
Associate Professor of Surgery, Nottingham Digestive Diseases Biomedical Research Centre, University of Nottingham, Nottingham, UK

Scott R. Kelley, MD, FACS, FASCRS
Assistant Professor of Surgery, Colon and Rectal Surgery, Mayo Clinic, Rochester, MN, USA

Robin Kennedy, MS, FRCS
Consultant Colorectal Surgeon, St Mark's Hospital, Harrow; Adjunct Professor of Surgery and Cancer, Imperial College, London, UK

Andrew Latchford, BSc(Hons), MBBS, FRCP, MD
Consultant Gastroenterologist, St Mark's Hospital, Harrow, UK

Paul-Antoine Lehur, MD, PhD
Professor, Digestive and Endocrine Surgery, University Hospital, Nantes, France

Brendan J. Moran, MBBCh, FRCS, FRCSI, MCh
Consultant Colorectal Surgeon, Hampshire Hospitals Foundation Trust, Basingstoke, UK

Robin K.S. Phillips, MBBS, MS, FRCS
Professor of Colorectal Surgery, Imperial College London; Consultant Colorectal Surgeon, St Mark's Hospital, Harrow, UK

Eanna Ryan, MBBCh, BAO, MD Candidate
Surgical Professorial Unit, St Vincent's University Hospital, Dublin, Ireland

Alexis M.P. Schizas, BSc, MBBS, MSc, MD, FRCS(Gen Surg)
Consultant Colorectal Surgeon, Guy's and St Thomas' Hospitals, London, UK

Contributors

John H. Scholefield, MBChB, FRCS, ChM (Distinction)
Professor of Surgery, Head of Division, Division of GI Surgery, University Hospital, Nottingham, UK

David Sebag-Montefiore, MBBS, FRCP, FRCR
Professor of Clinical Oncology, University of Leeds and Leeds Cancer Centre, St James's University Hospital, Leeds, UK

Robert J.C. Steele, MD, FRCSEd, FRCSEng, FCSHK, FRCPE, MFPH(Hon), FRSE
Professor of Surgery, Head of Department of Surgery, University of Dundee Medical School, Ninewells Hospital, Dundee, UK

Gregory P. Thomas, MBBS, BSc, FRCS, MD
Resident Surgical Officer, St Mark's Hospital, Harrow, UK

Siwan Thomas-Gibson, MD, FRCP
Consultant Gastroenterologist, Wolfson Unit for Endoscopy, St Mark's Hospital, Harrow; Honorary Senior Lecturer, Surgery, Imperial College, London, UK

Mark W. Thompson-Fawcett, MBChB, MD, FRACS
Associate Professor, Department of Surgical Sciences, University of Otago, Dunedin, New Zealand

Phil Tozer, MBBS, FRCS, MD(Res)
Consultant Colorectal Surgeon, and Lead, Robin Phillips Fistula Research Unit, St Mark's Hospital, Harrow, UK

Carolynne Vaizey, MBChB, MD, FRCS(Gen), FCS(SA)
Consultant Colorectal Surgeon, St Mark's Hospital, Harrow, UK

Janindra Warusavitarne, BMed, FRACS, PhD
Consultant Colorectal Surgeon, St Mark's Hospital, Harrow, UK

Des Winter, MB, FRCSI, MD, FRCS(Gen)
Consultant Surgeon, Centre for Colorectal Disease, St Vincent's University Hospital and University College, Dublin, Ireland

Andrew B. Williams, MBBS, BSc, MS, FRCS
Consultant Colorectal Surgeon, Director Pelvic Floor Unit, Colorectal Surgery, Guy's and St Thomas' Hospitals, London, UK

1

Anorectal investigation

Alexis M.P. Schizas
Andrew B. Williams

Introduction

Many tests are available to investigate anorectal disorders, each only providing part of a patient's assessment, so results should be considered together and alongside the clinical picture derived from a careful history and physical examination.

Investigations provide information about structure alone, function alone, or both, and have been directed to five general areas of interest: faecal incontinence, constipation (including Hirschsprung's disease), anorectal sepsis, rectal prolapse (including solitary rectal ulcer syndrome) and anorectal malignancy.

Anatomy and physiology of the anal canal

The adult anal canal is approximately 4 cm long and begins as the rectum narrows, passing backwards between the levator ani muscles. There is in fact wide variation in length between the sexes, particularly anteriorly, and between individuals of the same sex. The canal has an upper limit at the pelvic floor and a lower limit at the anal opening. The proximal canal is lined by simple columnar epithelium, changing to stratified squamous epithelium lower in the canal via an intermediate transition zone just above the dentate line. Beneath the mucosa is the subepithelial tissue, composed of connective tissue and smooth muscle. This layer increases in thickness throughout life and forms the basis of the vascular cushions thought to aid continence.

Outside the subepithelial layer the caudal continuation of the circular smooth muscle of the rectum forms the internal anal sphincter, which terminates distally with a well-defined border at a variable distance from the anal verge. Continuous with the outer layer of the rectum, the longitudinal layer of the anal canal lies between the internal and external anal sphincters and forms the medial edge of the intersphincteric space. The longitudinal muscle comprises smooth muscle cells from the rectal wall, augmented with striated muscle from a variety of sources, including the levator ani, puborectalis and pubococcygeus muscles. Fibres from this layer traverse the external anal sphincter forming septa that insert into the skin of the lower anal canal and adjacent perineum as the corrugator cutis ani muscle.

The striated muscle of the external sphincter surrounds the longitudinal muscle and between these lies the intersphincteric space. The external sphincter is arranged as a tripartite structure, classically described by Holl and Thompson and later adopted by Gorsch and by Milligan and Morgan. In this system, the external sphincter is divided into deep, superficial and subcutaneous portions, with the deep and subcutaneous sphincter forming rings of muscle and, between them, the elliptical fibres of the superficial sphincter running anteriorly from the perineal body to the coccyx posteriorly. Some consider the external sphincter to be a single muscle contiguous with the puborectalis muscle, while others have adopted a two-part model. The latter proposes a deep anal sphincter and a superficial anal sphincter, corresponding to the puborectalis and deep external anal sphincter combined, as well as the fused superficial and subcutaneous sphincter of the tripartite model. Anal endosonography (AES) and magnetic resonance imaging (MRI) have not resolved the dilemma, although most authors report a three-part sphincter where the puborectalis muscle is fused with the deep sphincter.[1,2] The external anal sphincter is innervated by the pudendal nerve (S2–S4), which leaves the pelvis through the lower part of the greater sciatic notch, where it passes under the pyriformis muscle. It then crosses the ischial spine and sacrospinous ligament to enter the ischiorectal fossa through the lesser sciatic notch or foramen via the pudendal (or Alcock's) canal.

The pudendal nerve has two branches: the inferior rectal nerve, which supplies the external anal sphincter and sensation to the perianal skin; and the perineal nerve, which innervates the anterior perineal muscles together with the sphincter urethrae and forms the dorsal nerve of the clitoris (or penis). Although the puborectalis receives its main innervation from a direct branch of the fourth sacral nerve root, it may derive some innervation from the pudendal nerve.

The autonomic supply to the anal canal and pelvic floor comes from two sources. The fifth lumbar nerve root sends sympathetic fibres to the superior and inferior hypogastric plexuses, and the parasympathetic supply is from the second to fourth sacral nerve roots through the nervi erigentes. Fibres of both systems pass obliquely across the lateral surface of the lower rectum to reach the region of the perineal body.

The internal anal sphincter has an intrinsic nerve supply from the myenteric plexus together with an additional supply from both the sympathetic and parasympathetic nervous systems. Sympathetic nervous activity is thought to enhance and parasympathetic activity to reduce internal sphincter contraction. Relaxation of the internal anal sphincter may be mediated by non-adrenergic, non-cholinergic nerve activity via the neural transmitter nitric oxide.

Anorectal physiological studies alone cannot separate the different structures of the anal canal; instead, they provide measurements of the resting and squeeze pressures along the canal. Between 60% and 85% of resting anal pressure can be attributed to the action of the internal anal sphincter.[3] The external anal sphincter and the puborectalis muscle generate the maximal squeeze pressure.[3] Symptoms of passive anal leakage (where the patient is unaware that episodes are happening) are attributed to internal sphincter dysfunction, whereas urge symptoms and frank incontinence of faeces are due to external sphincter problems.[4]

Faecal continence is maintained by the complex interaction of many different variables. Stool must be delivered at a manageable rate from the colon into a compliant rectum of adequate volume. The consistency of this stool should be appropriate and accurately sensed by the sampling mechanism. Sphincters should be intact and able to contract adequately to produce pressures sufficient to prevent leakage of flatus, liquid and solid stool. For effective defecation there needs to be coordinated relaxation of the striated muscle components with an increase in intra-abdominal pressure to expel the rectal contents. The structure of the anorectal region should prevent herniation or prolapse of elements of the anal canal and rectum during defecation.

Because of the complex interplay between the factors involved in continence and faecal evacuation, a wide range of investigations is needed for full assessment. A defect in any one element of the system in isolation is unlikely to have great functional significance and so in most clinical situations there is more than one contributing factor.

Rectoanal inhibitory reflex

Increasing rectal distension is associated with transient reflex relaxation of the internal anal sphincter and contraction of the external anal sphincter, known as the rectoanal inhibitory reflex (**Fig. 1.1**). The exact neurological pathway for this reflex is unknown, although it may be mediated via the myenteric plexus and stretch receptors in the pelvic floor. Patients with rectal hyposensitivity have higher thresholds for rectoanal inhibitory reflex; it is absent in patients with Hirschsprung's disease, progressive systemic sclerosis, Chagas' disease, and initially absent after a coloanal anastomosis, although it rapidly recovers.

✔ The rectoanal inhibitory reflex may enable rectal contents to be sampled by the transition zone mucosa to allow discrimination between solid, liquid and flatus. The rate of recovery of sphincter tone after this relaxation differs between the proximal and distal canal, which may be important in maintaining continence.[5]

Further studies investigating the role of the rectoanal inhibitory reflex in incontinent patients show that as rectal volume increases, greater sphincter relaxation is seen, whereas constipated patients have a greater recovery velocity of the resting anal pressure in the proximal anal canal. There is a longer recovery time back to resting pressure in patients with faecal incontinence.[6]

Manometry

A variety of different catheter systems can be used to measure anal pressure and it is important to note that measurements differ depending on which is employed. Systems include microballoons filled with air or water, microtransducers and water-perfused

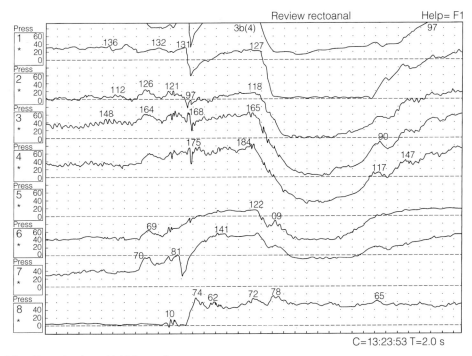

C=13:23:53 T=2.0 s

Figure 1.1 • Normal rectoanal inhibitory reflex.

catheters. These may be hand-held or automated. Hand-held systems are withdrawn in a measured stepwise fashion with recordings made after each step (usually of 0.5–1.0-cm intervals); this is called a station pull-through. Automated withdrawal devices allow continuous data recording (vector manometry).

Water-perfused catheters use hydraulic capillary infusers to perfuse catheter channels, which are arranged either radially or obliquely staggered. Each catheter channel is then linked to a pressure transducer (**Fig. 1.2**). Infusion rates of perfusate (sterile water) vary between 0.25 and 0.5 mL/min per channel. Systems need to be free from air bubbles, which may lead to inaccurate recordings, and must avoid leakage of perfusate onto the perianal skin, which may lead to falsely high resting pressures due to reflex external sphincter action. Perfusion rates should remain constant, because faster rates are associated with higher resting pressures, while larger diameter catheters lead to greater recorded pressure.[7]

Balloon systems may be used to overcome some of these problems and may be more representative of pressure generated within a hollow viscus than recordings using a perfusion system. They are not subject to the same problems as a perfusion system when canal pressures are radially asymmetrical.[7] Balloons can be filled with either air or water. Over the range of balloon sizes used (diameter 2–10 mm), diameter appears to have less of an effect on the

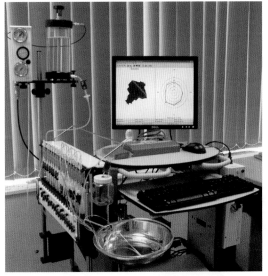

Figure 1.2 • Perfusion system used for anorectal manometry. Standard water perfusion set-up plus computer interface for anorectal manometry. The screen shows a vector volume profile.

pressures recorded than it does with water-perfused catheter systems.

Microtransducers that can accurately measure canal pressure continue to be developed, but they are expensive and fragile.

High-resolution anal manometry uses the same catheters as standard manometry but updated software presents the information in a new way that may increase its clinical utility, especially when used to produce a three-dimensional picture of the anal canal. High-definition manometry uses closely spaced solid-state sensors simultaneously to measure circumferential pressures in the rectum and throughout the anal canal, so there is no need to perform a station pull-through manoeuvre.[8]

Three-dimensional anal canal manometry (vector volume manometry) utilises a radially arranged catheter setting (commonly eight-channel) that is automatically withdrawn from the anal canal during rest and squeeze, and computer software that produces a three-dimensional reconstruction of the anal canal (**Fig. 1.3**).[9] Three-dimensional manometry is also possible with high definition anal canal manometry. These systems can assess radial asymmetry or vector symmetry index (i.e. how far the radial symmetry of the anal canal differs from a perfect circle, which has a radial asymmetry of 0% or vector symmetry index of 1). Sphincter defects are associated with symmetry indices of 0.6 or less.

Three-dimensional anal canal manometry may differentiate between idiopathic and traumatic faecal incontinence by showing global external sphincter weakness rather than a localised area of scarred sphincter indicated by an asymmetrical vectogram.[9,10] Anal vector manometry has been extensively used to assess obstetric anal sphincter injury. Following caesarean section, no change in anal pressures is seen; however, after vaginal delivery a fall in rest and squeeze pressures occurs.[11] The reduction in pressures has been shown to be greatest after a third- or fourth-degree tear confirmed on AES. Functional anal sphincter length and vector volumes have been shown to decrease both at rest and during contraction after obstetric anal sphincter injury.[12] Vector volumes are decreased further in women with persistent flatus incontinence.

Pressure changes in the anal canal can be measured in a number of ways and each method has been validated for its repeatability and reproducibility, although individual methods are not interchangeable.[13] Although the correlation between measurements made using different systems and catheters is good, the absolute values are different, so that when comparing the results of different studies, it is essential to consider the method used to obtain the pressure measurements.

Significant variation exists in the results of anorectal manometry in normal asymptomatic subjects. Men have higher mean resting and squeeze pressures.[14] Pressures decline after the age of 60 years, changes most marked in women.[15] These facts must be considered when selecting appropriate control subjects for clinical studies. Normal mean anal canal resting tone in healthy adults is 50–100 mmHg. Resting tone increases in a cranial to caudal direction along the canal such that the maximal resting pressure is found 5–20 mm from the anal verge.[3,16] The high-pressure zone (the part of the anal canal where the resting pressure is >50% of the maximum resting or squeeze pressure) is similar at rest between men and women (20 mm in length) but longer in men than women when squeezing (31 mm vs 23 mm).[16] In a normal individual the rise in pressure on maximal squeezing should be at least 50–100% of the resting pressure (usually 100–180 mmHg).[17] Reflex contraction of the external sphincter should occur when the rectum is distended, on coughing, or with any rise in intra-abdominal pressure.

> ✔✔ In the assessment of patients with faecal incontinence, both resting and maximal squeeze pressures are significantly lower in patients with incontinence than in matched controls,[18] but there is considerable overlap between the pressures recorded in patients and controls.[19]

Ambulatory manometry

The use of continuous ambulatory manometry to record rectal and anal canal pressures[20] has provided

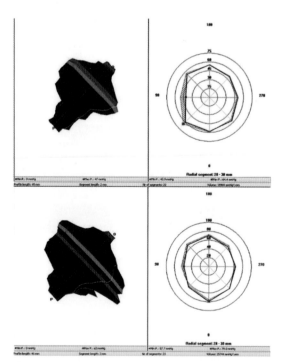

Figure 1.3 • Normal vector volume at squeeze and at rest. Note that asymmetry of the sphincter contour can be normal.

information on the functioning of the sphincter mechanism in a more physiological situation. The generation of giant waves of pressure in the rectum or neorectum may relate to episodes of incontinence in patients after restorative proctocolectomy. Ambulatory manometry has also identified patients in whom episodes of internal sphincter relaxation are not accompanied by reflex external sphincter contraction,[21] a finding that may prove useful in selecting patients likely to benefit from biofeedback treatment.

Anal and rectal sensation

The anal canal is rich in sensory receptors,[22] including those for pain, temperature and movement, with the somatic sensation of the anal transitional mucosa being more sensitive than that of the perianal skin. In contrast, the rectum is relatively insensitive to pain, although crude sensation may be transmitted by the nervi erigentes of the parasympathetic nervous system.[23]

A variety of methods have been used to measure anal sensation. Initial assessment of anal sensation used a stiff bristle to detect light touch in the anal canal, and hot and cold metal rods to detect temperature sensation.[22] Thermal sensation has been assessed with water-perfused thermodes; normal subjects can detect a change in temperature of 0.92°C.[24] The ability of the mucosa to detect a small electrical current can be assessed by the use of a double platinum electrode and a signal generator providing a square wave impulse at 5 Hz of 100 μs duration. The lowest recorded current of three readings at the point at which the subject feels a tingling or pricking sensation in the anal canal is noted as the sensation threshold. Normal electrical sensation for the most sensitive area of the anal canal (the transition zone) is 4 mA (2–7 mA). Rectal mucosal electrical sensation may also be measured using the same technique as that used for anal mucosal electrical sensation measurement, with slight modification of the stimulus (500 μs duration at a frequency of 10 Hz).[23]

The sensation of rectal filling is measured by progressively inflating a balloon placed within the rectum or by intrarectal saline infusion.[23] Normal perception of rectal filling occurs after inflation of 10–20 mL, the sensation of the urge to defecate occurs after 60 mL, and normally up to 230 mL is tolerated in total before discomfort occurs.[23]

✔ The clinical use of these measurements may be limited due to the large inter- and intra-subject variation in values and the wide normal range, reducing the discriminatory value of this technique as a clinical investigation.[25]

Temperature sensation may be vital in the discrimination of solid stool from liquid and flatus,[24] and is reduced in patients with faecal incontinence. It is thought that this sensation is important in the sampling reflex, although this is brought into question by the fact that the sensitivity of the anal mucosa to temperature change is not great enough to detect the very slight temperature gradient between the rectum and anal canal.

Anal mucosal electrical sensation threshold increases with age and thickness of the subepithelial layer of the anal canal. Anal canal electrical sensation is reduced in idiopathic faecal incontinence, diabetic neuropathy, descending perineum syndrome and haemorrhoids.[26] There are differing reports on whether there is any correlation between electrical sensation and measurement of motor function of the sphincters (pudendal terminal motor latency and single-fibre electromyography).

The sampling mechanism and maintenance of faecal continence are complex multifactorial processes, as seen by the fact that the application of local anaesthetic to the sensitive anal mucosa does not lead to incontinence and in some individuals actually improves continence.

Rectal compliance

The relation between changes in rectal volume and the associated pressure changes is termed compliance, which is calculated by dividing the change in volume by the change in pressure. Compliance is measured by inflating a rectal balloon with saline or air or by directly infusing saline at physiological temperature into the rectum. In the former method, the filling of the rectal balloon can be either incremental or continuous. When continuous inflation of the rectal balloon is used, the rate of inflation should be 70–240 mL/min.[25] Mean rectal compliance is about 4–14 mL/cmH$_2$O, with pressures of 18–90 cmH$_2$O at the maximum tolerated volume.[27] Reports on the reproducibility of the measurement of rectal compliance are varied and many have found great variation within the same subject;[25,27] the most reproducible measurement is usually the maximum tolerated volume. The use of the barostat to measure rectal compliance has been shown to be reproducible at pressures of between 36 and 48 mmHg. The compliance of the rectum does not differ between men and women up to the age of 60 years, but after this age women have more compliant rectums. Compliance is reduced in Behçet's disease and Crohn's disease and after radiotherapy in a dose-related fashion. It is also reduced in irritable bowel syndrome.

✔ The association between changes in rectal compliance and faecal incontinence is less clear. Some state that compliance is normal in incontinence whereas others have found a reduction in compliance associated with faecal incontinence,[18] although changes in compliance may be secondary to the incontinence and not causative. Altered compliance may play a role in soiling and constipation associated with megarectum.

Pelvic floor descent

Parks et al. first described the association between excessive descent of the perineum and anorectal dysfunction, and subsequently it has been described in several conditions: faecal incontinence, severe constipation, solitary rectal ulcer syndrome, and anterior mucosal and full-thickness rectal prolapse. The presumption in all these conditions is that abnormal perineal descent, especially during straining, causes traction and damage to the pudendal and pelvic floor nerves, leading to progressive neuropathy and muscular atrophy. Irreversible pudendal nerve damage occurs after a stretch of 12% of its length, and often the descent of the perineum in these patients is of the order of 2 cm, which is estimated to cause pudendal nerve stretching of 20%.

Descent of the perineum was initially measured using the St Mark's perineometer. The perineometer is placed on the ischial tuberosities and a movable Perspex cylinder is positioned on the perineal skin. The distance between the level of the perineum and the ischial tuberosities is measured at rest and during straining.[28] Negative readings indicate that the plane of the perineum is above the tuberosities and a positive value indicates descent below this level. In normal asymptomatic adults, the plane of the perineum at rest should be -2.5 ± 0.6 cm, descending to $+0.9 \pm 1.0$ cm on straining. When measured using dynamic proctography, similar measurements of pelvic floor descent are obtained. The anorectal angle normally lies on a line drawn between the coccyx and the most anterior part of the pubis, and descends by 2 ± 0.3 cm on straining.

Excessive perineal descent is found in 75% of subjects who chronically strain during defecation. The degree of descent correlates with age and is greater in women. Although increased perineal descent on straining has been shown to be associated with features of neuropathy, namely decreased anal mucosal electrical sensitivity and increased pudendal nerve terminal motor latency, not all patients with abnormal descent have abnormal neurology.[29] Perineal descent is also associated with faecal incontinence, although the degree of incontinence and the results of anorectal manometry do not correlate with the extent of pelvic floor laxity.[30]

Electrophysiology

Neurophysiological assessment of the anorectum includes assessment of the conduction of the pudendal and spinal nerves, and electromyography (EMG) of the sphincter.

Electromyography

Electromyographic traces can be recorded from the separate components of the sphincter complex, both at rest and during active contraction of the striated components. Initially, EMG was used to map sphincter defects before surgery, but AES is now so superior in its ability to map defects and is so much better tolerated by patients[31] that EMG has largely become a research tool. Broadly, two techniques of EMG are used: concentric needle studies and single-fibre studies.

Concentric needle EMG records the activity of up to 30 muscle fibres from around the area of the needle both at rest and during voluntary squeeze. The amplitude of the signal recorded correlates with the maximal squeeze pressure,[32] polyphasic long-duration action potentials indicating reinnervation subsequent to denervation injury. The main use of this technique has been in the confirmation and mapping of sphincter defects. Examination of puborectalis EMG may be more sensitive than cinedefecography in the detection of paradoxical puborectalis contraction in obstructed defecation,[33] although paradoxical puborectalis contraction is also present in normal subjects.

The use of an anal plug or sponge can record global electrical activity from the anal sphincters,[32] EMG amplitudes recorded in this way correlating with voluntary squeeze pressure. EMG performed using a needle has a smaller recording area (25 μm diameter) and the action potential from individual motor units is recorded. Denervated muscle fibres can regain innervation from branching of adjacent axons, leading to an increase in the number of muscle fibres supplied by a single axon. With multiple readings (an average of 20) using this small-diameter needle, the mean fibre density (MFD) for an area of sphincter can be calculated (i.e. the mean number of muscle action potentials per unit area or axon). Denervation and subsequent reinnervation are also indicated by neuromuscular 'jitter', which is caused by variation in the timing of triggering and non-triggering potentials.[34] An increase in sphincter MFD is often found in cases of idiopathic incontinence and is associated with recognised histological changes in sphincter structure. Atrophic sphincter muscle shows a loss of the characteristic mosaic pattern of distribution of type 1 and type 2 muscle fibres. There is also selective muscle fibre hypertrophy together with fibro-fatty fibre degeneration. These changes predominantly affect the external anal sphincter but the puborectalis and levators are also affected to a lesser extent.

MFD correlates inversely with squeeze pressure and is increased in patients with excessive perineal descent.[35] The correlation with direct assessment of the integrity of sphincter innervation (pudendal nerve terminal motor latency) is less clear.

Pudendal nerve terminal motor latency

Pudendal nerve conduction can be assessed by stimulating the nerve as it enters the ischio-rectal fossa at the ischial spine. This investigation only examines the fastest conducting fibres of the pudendal nerve and so can still be normal even in the presence of abnormal sphincter innervation. The normal value for pudendal nerve terminal motor latency (PNTML) is 2.0 ± 0.5 ms.[36]

Prolongation of PNTML is associated with idiopathic faecal incontinence, rectal prolapse, solitary rectal ulcer syndrome, severe constipation and sphincter defects. Nerve latency is delayed with increasing age and is prolonged in 24% of all faecally incontinent patients and 31% of those presenting with constipation.[36]

✔ PNTML is operator-dependent and has a poor correlation with clinical symptoms and histological findings. The American Gastroenterology Association does not recommend the use of this test for the evaluation of patients with faecal incontinence.[37]

Spinal motor latency

Transcutaneous stimulation of the sacral motor nerve roots provides further information on the innervation of the pelvic floor. The motor response from stimulation at the level of the first and fourth lumbar vertebrae can be recorded using standard EMG needles inserted into the puborectalis and external sphincter. By comparing the latency times between the two levels, the latency of the motor component of the cauda equina can be assessed. Up to 23% of patients with idiopathic faecal incontinence have cauda equina delay.[38]

Defecography/evacuation proctography

Defecography or evacuation proctography involves video fluoroscopy of the patient evacuating barium paste of stool consistency. Barium-soaked gauze may

also be inserted into the vagina and barium paste may be applied to the perineum to aid in assessing the anorectal angle and perineal descent.[39] Opacification of the small bowel with an orally ingested contrast medium or injection of contrast into the peritoneum (peritoneography) will reveal enteroceles in 18% of patients with pelvic floor weakness,[40] with only half containing bowel.[41] Defecography is a dynamic examination; it not only provides information on anorectal structural changes during defecation, but it also assesses function. While anatomical changes during evacuation (namely rectocele, enterocele, rectoanal intussusception, rectal prolapse and changes in anorectal angle) may be evident, the extent and duration of emptying is of more clinical significance.[42]

✔ Anatomical abnormalities demonstrated on proctography are of poor discriminatory value in determining patients from controls. The only measurements that can discriminate between normal subjects and those with severe constipation are the time taken to evacuate and the completeness of evacuation.[43]

During normal evacuation the anorectal angle increases because of relaxation of the puborectalis. Normal evacuation should be 90% complete (and 60% complete with a pouch). Rectoceles are significant if they are greater than 3 cm or require perianal/vaginal digitation to empty.

Dynamic pelvic MRI

Using a modified T2-weighted single-shot fast spin-echo imaging sequence or a T2-weighted fast imaging with steady-state free precession MRI sequence, anorectal and pelvic floor motion can be imaged at 1.2- to 2-second intervals. During dynamic MRI, proctography provides pelvic images at rest and when the subject strains. This gives an overview of pelvic floor movement and organ prolapse, and rectal dynamics are assessed during evacuation after adding 150 mL of ultrasound gel to the rectum[44] (**Fig. 1.4**). There are few differences in the detection of clinically relevant findings between supine MRI and seated MRI, except for detecting rectal intussusceptions, for which seated MRI is superior.[45]

✔ MRI defecography has been shown to alter the surgical approach in 67% of patients undergoing surgery for faecal incontinence.[46] It has also been shown that inter-observer agreement for assessing anorectal motion by MRI proctography is better than with barium defecography.

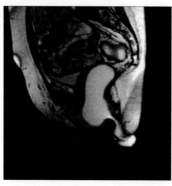

Figure 1.4 • A mid-sagittal image of the anal canal and rectum using MRI proctography, showing an anterior rectocele.

Dynamic transperineal and three-dimensional pelvic floor ultrasound

Continued developments in diagnostic ultrasound imaging can contribute to the diagnostic work-up of female patients with obstructed defecation, rectal intussusception, rectal prolapse and rectocele. Pelvic floor ultrasound scanning has the advantage of being better tolerated and cheaper than the other imaging modalities, as well as correlating well with defecating proctography and MRI.[47] Further studies are required to fully understand and validate pelvic floor ultrasound.

Scintigraphy

Scintigraphy using technetium-labelled sulphur colloid mixed with dilute veegum powder may also be used for defecography.[48] The advantages of this technique are that a quantitative result is obtained and a lower dose of radiation is used. The study is not dynamic and does not correlate with patient symptoms or manometric assessment. Radioisotope testing may also be used to assess colonic transit time to diagnose idiopathic slow transit constipation. Colonic transit time is measured more easily by tracking the progress of ingested sets of radio-opaque markers with plain abdominal radiography. A standard protocol uses a single plain abdominal radiograph 5 days after commencing ingestion of the markers (usually different-shaped markers are taken daily over the first 3 days).

Imaging the rectum and anal sphincters

The indications for anorectal imaging may be divided into three broad clinical areas: sepsis and fistula disease, malignancy and faecal incontinence.

The available techniques include surface scanning techniques, namely computed tomography (CT) and body coil MRI, and endoanal imaging, namely anal endosonography (AES), with or without subsequent multiplanar (three-dimensional) reconstruction, and endocoil MRI (largely unavailable now).

Anal endosonography/endorectal ultrasound

Three-dimensional endoluminal ultrasound uses a double-crystal design with 6–16 MHz frequency range encased in a cylindrical transducer shaft. The transducer is then used with a specially designed rectosigmoidoscope and water-filled balloon covering the transducer. This allows rectal scanning without moving or replacing the probe. The ultrasonic anatomy has been described in detail by scanning dissected specimens and comprises alternating bands of reflection created by the interfaces between the different anatomical structures present.[49] An alternating bright and dark pattern of rings is seen corresponding to the layers of the rectal wall.

To enable examination of the anal sphincters, the water-filled balloon is removed (**Fig. 1.5a**). The anal canal mucosa is generally not seen on AES; the subepithelial tissue is highly reflective and surrounded by the low reflection from the internal anal sphincter. The thickness of the internal sphincter increases with age: the normal width for a patient aged 55 years or younger is 2.4–2.7 mm, whereas in an older patient the normal range is 2.8–3.4 mm. As the width of the sphincter increases it becomes progressively more reflective and more indistinct; this may be due to a relative increase in the fibroelastic content of this muscle as a consequence of ageing. Both the external anal sphincter and the longitudinal muscle are of moderate reflectivity. The intersphincteric space often returns a bright reflection (**Fig. 1.5b**).[50]

The development of high-resolution three-dimensional AES constructed from a synthesis of standard two-dimensional cross-sectional images produces a digital volume that may be reviewed and can be used to perform measurements in any plane, yielding more information on the anal sphincter complex. This provides more reliable measurements, and volume measurements can also be performed.[51] Another development is the use of volume rendering in three-dimensional AES, allowing the analysis of information inside a three-dimensional volume by digitally enhancing individual voxels. The volume-rendered image provides better visualisation performance when there are not large differences in the signal levels of pathological structures compared with surrounding tissues.

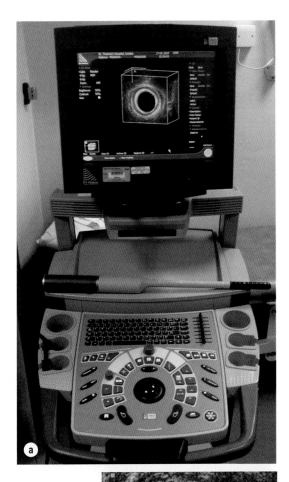

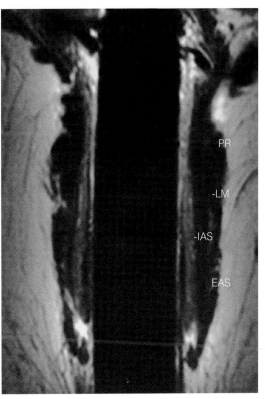

is vastly improved locally around the coil (within about 4 cm), enabling the acquisition of images of the anal sphincters with both excellent tissue differentiation and spatial resolution. Endocoils have either rectangular or saddle geometry and measure 6–10 cm in length and 7–12 mm in diameter. This increases to 17–19 mm after encasement in an acetal homopolymer (Delrin) former. The coil is inserted in the left lateral position and then secured with sandbags or with a purpose-built holder to avoid movement artefact.[50,52,53]

On T2-weighted images, the external sphincter and longitudinal muscle return a relatively low signal. The internal sphincter returns a relatively high signal and enhances with gadolinium (an intravenous contrast agent used in MRI). The subepithelial tissue has a signal intensity value between that of the internal and external sphincters (**Fig. 1.6**).

Imaging in rectal cancer

CT has an accuracy of 89% in assessing rectal tumours with extensive spread beyond the serosal layer; however, when only cases of moderate tumour spread are assessed, the accuracy is much

Figure 1.6 • A mid-coronal image of the anal canal using endocoil MRI. EAS, external anal sphincter; IAS, internal anal sphincter; LM, longitudinal muscle; PR, puborectalis.

Subepithelium
Internal sphincter
Longitudinal muscle
External sphincter

Figure 1.5 • **(a)** BK Medical three-dimensional endoanal ultrasound machine and 2050 probe. **(b)** The layers of the sphincter are depicted by the three-dimensional endoanal ultrasound probe.

Endocoil receiver MRI

MRI provides images with excellent tissue differentiation, although spatial resolution of the anal sphincters using a body coil receiver is poor. When an endoanal receiver coil is used, spatial resolution lower (55%).[54] The accuracy of CT has been improved by the advent of multislice technique CT and further improvement is expected from modern scanners with up to 64 detector rows. CT is also used to assess metastatic disease involving the liver and lungs. The development of positron emission tomography (PET) combined with CT has improved the detection of recurrent rectal carcinoma.[55] PET/CT can also yield additional pretreatment staging information in patients with low rectal cancer.[56] EUS, by comparison, can correctly T-stage rectal cancers in 75–87% of cases, with a trend to over-stage in 22%.[57] EUS is superior to CT and has a positive predictive value for tumour invasion beyond the muscularis propria of 98%. If a lymph node measures greater than 5 mm in diameter on EUS, there is a 45–70% chance that it is involved with tumour.[58]

Body coil MRI has been used to assess the stage of rectal tumours and it would appear to give comparable results to EUS,[59] with an accuracy of 88% at detecting transmural spread, 87% anal sphincter infiltration,[56] and an accuracy of T-staging of 75% and a 94% accuracy in detecting circumferential resection margin involvement.[60] A meta-analysis of 84 studies showed EUS to be slightly superior to MRI in assessing nodal status.[61]

Body coil MRI has the advantage over EUS in that it can be performed even in the presence of stenotic tumours. Furthermore, after radiotherapy EUS tends to over-stage tumours, leading to a marked reduction in its diagnostic accuracy, especially in the differentiation between T2 and T3 tumours. The other area where MRI is superior to EUS is in the assessment of recurrent tumours. The only advantage of EUS over MRI is the possibility of assessing T1 tumours that could be treated by transanal endoscopic microsurgery. The appearances of fibrosis after surgery and recurrent tumour in the pelvis are very similar using either EUS or CT, which makes assessment for recurrent disease very difficult. On MRI the signals from these two tissue types (especially on T2-weighted images) are quite different, allowing greater tissue differentiation. High resolution MRI has become the preferred imaging for the local staging of rectal cancer and helps guide surgery and identify the need for neoadjuvant treatment.[62] PET/MRI is the newest clinical hybrid imaging modality and has the potential to provide comprehensive colorectal cancer staging in one examination.

✔✔ EUS appears better at estimating the stage of T0, T1, T2 rectal tumours[63] and nodal staging.[62] However, the main determinant of local recurrence is circumferential resection margin and EUS is poor at assessing this, whereas MRI has been shown to be much more accurate.[61]

Imaging in anal sepsis and anal fistulas

Both surface imaging and endoanal imaging have been employed in the assessment of perianal sepsis. CT is unsatisfactory for the assessment of fistulas because of the poor definition of tracks, which is largely due to volume averaging. AES may be used to assess anal fistulas and has been shown to be accurate for the definition of the anatomy of anal sepsis, especially horseshoe collections and the anatomy of complex fistulas.[64] Endosonography is also able to detect and assess sphincter damage caused by chronic sepsis.

Endosonography is less accurate in the assessment of suprasphincteric sepsis and it is often difficult to differentiate between supralevator and infralevator collections, leading to inaccuracy in up to 20% of cases.[65] The internal opening on AES is identified by penetration of the internal anal sphincter by the track because of the lack of definition of the mucosa and is of limited value close to the anal margin. The diagnostic accuracy of AES is increased with the use of hydrogen peroxide injected into fistulous tracks to act as a contrast medium.[66] The use of three-dimensional AES and volume rendering improves the accuracy of AES further. MRI has the most to offer in the assessment of perianal sepsis. Anal sepsis appears on MRI as areas of very high signal, which enhance with the administration of the intravenous contrast agent gadolinium. Definition is further increased with the use of STIR (short tau inversion recovery) sequences to suppress the signal returned by fat (**Fig. 1.7**).

The Association of Coloproctology of Great Britain and Ireland position statement states that imaging is mandatory with either MRI or AES for complex fistulas. For complex or recurrent fistulas or those with horseshoe extensions, then an MRI should be obtained to guide surgery.[67]

✔✔ The use of dynamic contrast-enhanced MRI has been reported to provide better delineation of fistulas than AES, which is better than examination under anaesthetic (EUA). Correct classification with clinical examination has been achieved in 61% of cases using EUA, 81% using AES and 90% using MRI. AES predicts accurately the site of the internal opening in 91% of cases compared with 97% for MRI.[68]

✔✔ MRI and AES demonstrate comparable sensitivities at detecting perianal fistulas. However, the specificity was diagnostically poor. There was a high degree of data heterogeneity and the shortage of studies means conclusions for clinical practice are not possible.[69]

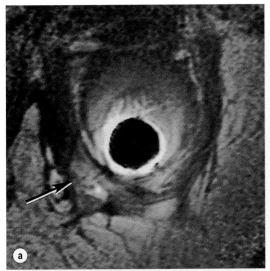

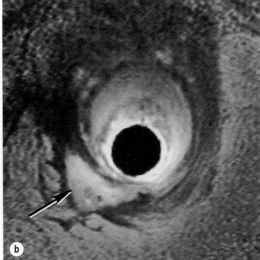

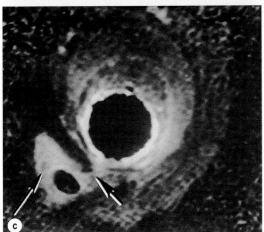

Figure 1.7 • Examples of complex perirectal sepsis as shown by the endoanal magnetic resonance probe. **(a,b)** T1-weighted images of an intersphincteric collection prior to and following gadolinium–DTPA contrast (*arrow*). **(c)** Short tau inversion recovery (STIR) image of the abscess cavity showing a central gas-containing cavity (*long arrow*) and a fistula at the 7 o'clock position (*short arrow*).

Imaging in faecal incontinence

AES has revealed that many patients who were thought to have idiopathic faecal incontinence in fact have a surgically remediable sphincter defect. It has also been shown that a much higher proportion of women sustain sphincter damage during childbirth than is suspected by clinical assessment alone. While the true incidence of sphincter tears may be lower than initially thought,[70] many women sustain important morphological changes to the sphincter following delivery.[71] The ability of AES to diagnose and correctly assess the extent of external sphincter damage has been validated by comparison with EMG studies and findings at surgery.[72] AES is superior in the differentiation between those patients with idiopathic faecal incontinence and those with a sphincter defect when compared with either simple manometric assessment or vector volume studies.

MRI is also used to assess patients with faecal incontinence and the diagnosis of sphincter defects using endocoil MRI has been validated with surgical confirmation of defect presence and extent. Endocoil MRI may be superior to AES in the detection and assessment of external sphincter defects because of better sphincter definition using MRI, although it is more important that the clinician is familiar with the imaging technique used.[73]

MRI has multiplanar capability (i.e. axial, sagittal and coronal images can be acquired), whereas standard AES provides only axially oriented images. The acquisition of volume ultrasound data has overcome this problem, and using three-dimensional AES has led to a better understanding of sphincter injury. A direct correlation exists between the length of a defect and the arc of displacement of the two ends of the sphincter.[74]

The use of endocoil MRI has shown that incontinence in the absence of a sphincter defect may be due to atrophy, where the sphincter has been replaced by fat and fibrous tissue.[53,75] The presence of external anal sphincter atrophy on endocoil MRI has been associated with poor results from anterior sphincteroplasty.

Summary

A wide variety of physiological and morphological tests is available for the assessment of the anus and rectum. Although there is no clear correlation between manometric/neurophysiological testing and clinical symptomatology in patients with idiopathic faecal incontinence, there is considerable value in performing these tests before surgery to predict long-term outcome. Anorectal investigation has revealed a large group of parous women who have occult sphincter trauma that may have a clinical impact as the women get older.

Anorectal physiological assessment is essential as an objective measure in patients with faecal incontinence and for the diagnosis of Hirschsprung's disease, and may help select those patients who will have acceptable function after coloanal anastomosis or an ileoanal pouch.

Endoanal imaging is becoming the gold standard in the preoperative determination of sphincter integrity and defines those patients most likely to benefit from surgical intervention. Endorectal imaging of early rectal tumours correlates well with histological assessment of tumour depth. MRI is the imaging modality of choice to assess the circumferential resection margin and is accurate for the diagnosis of recurrent tumour after previous resection.

In patients with primary evacuatory disorders, neurophysiological testing and defecography assist in the demonstration of unsuspected rectoanal intussusception or rectocele in patients who may benefit from surgery and those who may be suitable candidates for biofeedback therapy.

Anorectal investigation continues to have a major role in clinical research and has helped outline the anatomy of the component parts of the sphincter complex as well as to define the physiology of both defecation and anal continence. The understanding of these processes is vital to the correct management of patients with anorectal disorders.

Key points

- Normal pelvic floor function relies on a complex interplay between various mechanisms.
- Sphincter function may be assessed using anal manometry and electrophysiology.
- Sphincter anatomy may be assessed using AES and MRI, the former being the standard for the diagnosis of sphincter trauma.
- Dynamic MRI evacuation proctography and dynamic pelvic floor scans are useful in the assessment of patients with evacuatory disorders.
- Pelvic MRI or three-dimensional AES may be used to assess anorectal sepsis and can predict recurrence of anal fistulas after surgery.
- MRI is the preferred modality for the staging of rectal cancer with more accurate circumferential resection margin prediction. Preoperative staging of early T1 rectal cancer is superior with EUS.

🌐 Full references available at **http://expertconsult. inkling.com**

Key references

18. Bharucha AE, Fletcher JG, Harper CM, et al. Relationship between symptoms and disordered continence mechanisms in women with idiopathic faecal incontinence. Gut 2005;54(4): 546–55. PMID: 15753542.

    In this study 35% of patients with faecal incontinence had reduced resting pressure and 73% had reduced squeeze pressures, higher percentages than the control group. This study also found that volume and pressure thresholds for defecatory desire were lower in faecal incontinence patients.

19. McHugh SM, Diamant NE. Effect of age, gender, and parity on anal canal pressures. Contribution of impaired anal sphincter function to fecal incontinence. Dig Dis Sci 1987;32(7):726–36. PMID: 3595385.

    McHugh and Diamant found that in faecally incontinent patients, 39% of women and 44% of men had normal resting and squeeze pressures, and 9% of asymptomatic normal individuals were unable to generate an appreciable pressure on maximal squeeze.

61. Lahaye MJ, Engelen SM, Nelemans PJ, et al. Imaging for predicting the risk factors – the circumferential resection margin and nodal disease – of local recurrence

in rectal cancer: a meta-analysis. Semin Ultrasound CT MR 2005;26(4):259–68. PMID: 16152740.

This meta-analysis of the accuracy of preoperative imaging included studies between 1985 and 2004. It showed that MRI was the only investigation accurate at predicting circumferential resection margin. EUS was slightly but not significantly superior at predicting nodal status.

63. Bipat S, Glas AS, Slors FJ, et al. Rectal cancer: local staging and assessment of lymph node involvement with endoluminal US, CT, and MR imaging – a meta-analysis. Radiology 2004;232(3): 773–83. PMID: 15273331.

A meta-analysis of 90 articles showed that for muscularis propria invasion, EUS and MRI had similar sensitivities but the specificity of EUS (86%) was significantly higher than that of MRI (69%). For perirectal tissue invasion, sensitivity of EUS (90%) was significantly higher than that of CT (79%) and MRI (82%). EUS was more accurate than CT and MRI at diagnosing perirectal tissue invasion and there was no difference in diagnosis of lymph node involvement.

68. Buchanan GN, Halligan S, Bartram CI, et al. Clinical examination, endosonography, and MR imaging in preoperative assessment of fistula in ano: comparison with outcome-based reference standard. Radiology 2004;233(3):674–81. PMID: 15498901.

This prospective trial of 104 patients with anal fistulas showed that AES with a high-frequency transducer is superior to digital examination but MRI is superior to AES.

69. Siddiqui MR, Ashrafian H, Tozer P, et al. A diagnostic accuracy meta-analysis of endoanal ultrasound and MRI for perianal fistula assessment. Dis Colon Rectum 2012;55(5):576–85. PMID: 22513437.

This meta-analysis reviewed published papers for EAS and MRI between 1970 and 2010. The sensitivity of both techniques was good but the specificity was poor. Due to the significant variations between the studies, the authors suggested further work is required to advise on clinical use.

2

Colonoscopy and flexible sigmoidoscopy

Siwan Thomas-Gibson
Adam Haycock

Introduction

Since flexible endoscopy of the colon was introduced in 1963 it has become the gold-standard diagnostic test for evaluation of colonic disease. Improvements in technique and technology have also led to advances in therapeutic procedures, and the boundary between endoscopic, laparoscopic and open procedures is becoming increasingly blurred. A good understanding of both the technique and technology is essential for an endoscopist to perform high-quality, safe endoscopy. This chapter gives an insight into how colonoscopy is influencing the practice of colorectal surgery.

Indications and contraindications

Flexible sigmoidoscopy vs colonoscopy

Indications for colonoscopy or flexible sigmoidoscopy must be weighed against the risk/benefit profile. Diagnostic colonoscopy has a significantly higher risk of complications relating to sedation and bowel preparation than flexible sigmoidoscopy. Flexible sigmoidoscopy is also quicker, cheaper and easier to perform, and detection of distal pathology is now considered a marker for possible proximal pathology; for example in the English Bowel Scope Screening Programme, finding two or more tubular adenomas, a large adenoma, or a tubulovillous adenoma prompts full colonoscopy.

Contraindications

The only absolute contraindications to endoscopic examination of the colon are a competent patient who is unwilling to give consent or a known free colonic perforation. Relative contraindications include: acute diverticulitis, immediately postoperative patients, patients with a recent myocardial infarction (within 30 days), pulmonary embolism, severe coagulopathy (particularly for therapeutic procedures) or haemodynamic instability. In fulminant colitis, a limited examination with flexible sigmoidoscopy to ascertain extent of disease and acquire confirmatory biopsies is often helpful. In general, colonoscopy or flexible sigmoidoscopy is considered to be safe in pregnancy, but should only be performed for strong indications and after careful consent and liaison with an obstetrician.[1]

Sedation

Sedation during colonoscopy continues to be the subject of much debate and research. A recent large multicentre European audit of current practice[2] showed that most colonoscopies were done using moderate (conscious) sedation and that although deep sedation was associated with shorter procedure times and fewer technical difficulties, it was also more resource-intensive and required more hospitalisations for complications. American Society of Gastrointestinal Endoscopy recommendations are that routine use of deep sedation in average-risk patients cannot be endorsed. Flexible sigmoidoscopy is most often performed unsedated as the use of intravenous sedation would negate many of the potential benefits of the procedure. Unsedated colonoscopy is certainly possible and practical in a subset of patients with few complications and good acceptability.[3]

> ✅ As the practice and evidence varies widely, current recommendations are to use the minimum amount of drugs within the manufacturers' guidelines to ensure patient comfort and the success of the endoscopy.[4]

Insertion technique

Insertion technique varies greatly even amongst expert colonoscopists. Technique will depend on the local circumstances, sedation practice, endoscopist preference and equipment available. However, there are some basic principles that are recognised to contribute to safe, efficient colonoscopy.

Handling and scope control

Most skilled colonoscopists now adopt the one-person, single-handed approach where the right hand is used to manipulate the shaft and the left hand operates the angulation controls. Tip control is gained by a combination of up/down angulation with the large wheel and clockwise/anticlockwise torque applied with the right hand. The left/right angulation using the small wheel is used for maintaining the luminal view while torque is being applied with the right hand.

Insertion and steering

A digital rectal examination should be performed to lubricate the anal canal and detect any anal and distal rectal pathology prior to insertion. The initial view is often a 'red-out' due to the lens pressing against the rectal mucosa. Gentle insufflation, slow withdrawal and small amounts of tip angulation are used to gain a view of the lumen.

Tips for insertion and steering

- **Pull back more, push in less.** The first rule of expert colonoscopy is to keep the shaft straight. This allows for accurate tip control, prevents stretching of the mesentery, minimises discomfort and shortens the colon by a 'concertina' effect of telescoping the bowel wall over the shaft. Pulling back often reduces acute angles of bends, disimpacts the tip of the scope

and improves the view. In contrast, excessive pushing of the scope often results in formation of large loops, excessive pain, loss of one-to-one tip control and increases the risk of iatrogenic perforation.[5]

- **Insufflate little and suction frequently.** Pain or discomfort during colonoscopy can often be due to stretching of the bowel wall by excessive gas insufflation. Pneumatic perforation of the right colon from over-insufflation has been reported.[6] Frequent suctioning of gas prevents this and may often allow progression of the tip through the colon by the concertina effect. The use of carbon dioxide rather than air has been shown to cause less discomfort and is widely recommended.[7] The use of water-aided (either water-immersion [WI] or water-exchange [WE]) colonoscopy is also now advocated to improve comfort scores and may improve adenoma detection rate.[8]

- **Use torque frequently.** Twisting clockwise or counter-clockwise with the right hand applies torque to the shaft of the scope. With a straight shaft and bent tip, use of torque will provide lateral movement at the tip and help to stiffen the scope to prevent looping during advancement. Application of torque is also essential for loop resolution. Without the use of an image guidance device, the application of torque will be determined both by frequency of loop type and 'feel' of the instrument. The majority of sigmoid loops (N-loops, 80%; alpha loops, 10%) require clockwise torque and pull-back to resolve; atypical loops (reverse sigmoid N-spiral, 1%; reverse-alpha, 5%) require anticlockwise torque.

Patient position change

Moving the patient's position from the left lateral position during both insertion and withdrawal can shift both fluid away from and air into the uppermost segment of bowel, preventing unnecessary suctioning of fluid and insufflation of gas. It can provide mechanical advantage by opening up acute bends, especially at the rectosigmoid junction, splenic and hepatic flexures. The effective use of gravity to assist the passage of the endoscope is a simple, cost-neutral, effective technique that is easily learnt. It has been shown to be effective in promoting endoscope tip advancement in two-thirds of cases[9] but it does require cooperation from the patient and can be difficult if heavy sedation or general anaesthesia is used (**Fig. 2.1**).

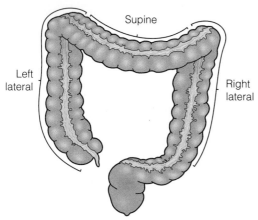

Supine

Left
lateral

Right
lateral

Figure 2.1 • Schema for optimal patient position change.

Abdominal hand pressure

The use of abdominal hand pressure aims to prevent the shaft of the endoscope looping by opposing pressure close to the anterior abdominal wall. Pressure is best used to prevent a loop from forming rather than applying it to an already formed loop, which is unlikely to be successful and may increase the discomfort felt by the patient. Specific pressure on anterior-protruding loops is more likely to be helpful as intubation progresses than non-specific pressure.[10] Magnetic imaging devices can help with guided pressure, although efficacy in promoting tip advancement is less than for patient position change,[9] as many loops do not protrude anteriorly. The use of deep inspiration can also be used to splint the diaphragm and provide pressure on the splenic and hepatic flexures if external pressure is unsuccessful.

Three-dimensional imager

Magnetic imaging systems (ScopeGuide, Olympus Optical Company; ScopePilot, Pentax Medical) use low-voltage magnetic fields to produce a real-time, three-dimensional image of the entire colonoscope shaft in both anteroposterior and lateral views, allowing the colonoscopist to visualise the configuration of the scope within the patient (see **Fig. 2.2**). This can help determine if there is an anterior component to the loop and so assist with loop resolution, as well as aiding accurate tip location. A sensor can assist with accurate hand-pressure placement.

> ✅ Meta-analysis of eight randomised controlled trials has shown real-time magnetic imaging to be of benefit in training and educating inexperienced endoscopists and improves the caecal intubation rate for experienced and inexperienced endoscopists.[11]

Withdrawal technique

It should be remembered that the aim of colonoscopy is to visualise the whole of the colonic mucosa in order to identify pathology. A systematic review of back-to-back studies[12] has shown a polyp miss rate at colonoscopy of 22% even in expert hands, although most missed polyps were small (<1 cm). All studies investigating miss rates have shown a variation in performance between endoscopists, but this can be wide even with expert examiners (>10 000 procedures), with sensitivities ranging from 17% to 48% in one large study.[13] This implies that there is a link between individual technical skill and outcome measures.

Withdrawal time

Recent publications have stressed the importance of spending sufficient time inspecting the colonic mucosa on withdrawal as a key marker for the adequacy of the examination.

> ✅✅ The current recommendation is that colonoscopists should spend more than 6 minutes during withdrawal inspecting the colonic mucosa in colonoscopies with normal results.[14] A landmark study[15] looking specifically at withdrawal time found that endoscopists who spent longer than 6 minutes on withdrawal in a negative colonoscopy had significantly higher adenoma detection rates (ADR) than their quicker colleagues.

Optimal examination technique

It seems logical that those colonoscopists who take longer to withdraw also use techniques that increase visualisation of abnormalities. In one study looking at differences in technique between two colonoscopists with different polyp miss rates,[16] a lower miss rate was judged by independent experts to be associated with superior withdrawal technique for each of the following examination criteria: (1) examining the proximal sides of flexures, folds and valves; (2) cleaning and suctioning; (3) adequacy of distension; and (4) adequacy of time spent viewing. A study looking at the quality of inspection at flexible sigmoidoscopy[17] has included similar criteria: (1) time spent viewing the mucosa; (2) re-examination of poorly viewed areas; (3) suctioning of fluid pools; (4) distension of the lumen; and (5) lower rectal examination.

The following continuous quality improvement targets regarding withdrawal (adapted from Rex

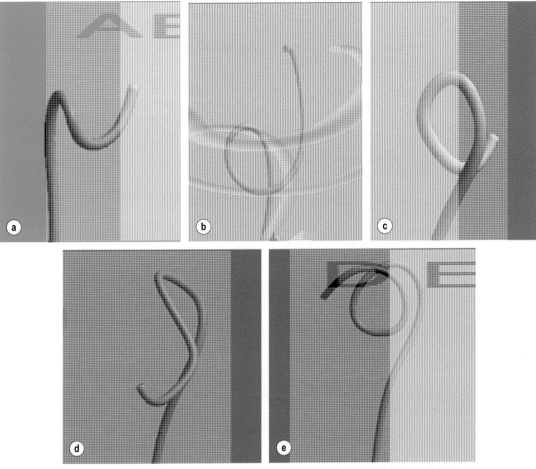

Figure 2.2 • ScopeGuide images of: **(a)** sigmoid N-loop; **(b)** alpha loop; **(c)** reverse alpha loop; **(d)** deep transverse loop; **(e)** gamma loop.

et al.[16]) aim to standardise withdrawal technique to maximise detection rates:

1. Mean examination times during withdrawal should average at least 6–10 minutes.
2. Adenoma prevalence rates detected during colonoscopy in persons over 50 years of age undergoing first-time examination should be ≥25% in men and ≥15% in women.
3. Documentation of quality of bowel preparation in all cases.

A recent publication has suggested that the implementation of systematic monitoring of withdrawal time and other quality indicators may, in itself, increase the performance of endoscopists.[18]

Bowel preparation

It is self-evident that pools of fluid or faeces will obscure good visualisation of the mucosa, and many studies have looked at the effectiveness of various bowel preparations for clearing the colon prior to colonoscopy.

✔✔ Evidence-based recommendations on bowel preparation for colonoscopy are available from many national societies.[19,20]

It has been shown that better quality preparation at flexible sigmoidoscopy results in a higher ADR,[21] but crucially important, endoscopists with a higher ADR are more likely to be critical of the quality of bowel preparation.

Position change

The use of position change has been shown in a randomised controlled trial to improve luminal distension between the hepatic flexure and sigmoid-descending junction during colonoscope withdrawal.[22] The same schema can be used for each segment as previously illustrated for insertion (see Fig. 2.1). Although four cross-over trials have shown that the improved visualisation that results can also improve polyp and adenoma detection rates, three parallel trials did not, and a meta-analysis concluded that the effectiveness is uncertain.[23]

Antispasmodics

Premedication with an antispasmodic such as hyoscine N-butyl bromide (Buscopan) has been used for colonoscopy to decrease the amount of muscular spasm caused by peristalsis. Small randomised studies have shown that this can shorten the total procedure time for flexible sigmoidoscopy as compared with placebo, and that it may be beneficial in terms of ease of insertion and the time required for caecal intubation, total procedure time, adequacy of sedation and scales of patient comfort during colonoscopy. However, a meta-analysis of the current studies concluded that the improvements may be marginal.[24] Caution must be exercised in patients with known cardiac history as there is a risk of sinus tachycardia. Other antispasmodics such as glucagon and the use of warm water irrigation may be used in patients in whom anticholinergics are contraindicated, although currently there are no data showing any significant benefit.[25]

Rectal and caecal retroflexion

Colorectal cancer is most common distally, and most experts routinely perform retroflexion in the rectum. Although the evidence that this significantly improves detection rates is still being debated,[26,27] it probably allows clearer views of the proximal sides of rectal valves and the top of the anal canal. There is a risk of iatrogenic perforation if the rectal lumen is narrow, in which case a paediatric colonoscope or thin upper gastrointestinal (GI) endoscope can be used. Recent publications have looked at the value of retroflexion in the proximal colon, but currently the data do not support this in routine practice.[28,29]

A quality improvement study has shown that a training bundle consisting of routine use of hyoscine, rectal retroflexion and minimum withdrawal time can improve global ADR, driven by improvements among the poorest performing colonoscopists.[30]

Quality assurance

There are now detailed guidelines for quality standards in colonoscopy, which include key performance indicators, measurable outcomes and minimum standards.[14,31,32] These aim to ensure a high-quality, effective and patient-centred service by setting benchmarks for both individual endoscopists and unit performance. Development of these guidelines has in a large measure been driven by the implementation of bowel cancer screening programmes, which involve asymptomatic individuals choosing to undergo invasive investigations. It is imperative to minimise risk for this group by provision of a safe, high-quality service. This has had the benefit of improving quality assurance standards for the whole of endoscopy.[33]

Endoscopy training

Guidelines on training have been published both in the UK and USA to improve access to and quality of endoscopy training.[34,35] Accredited national courses in endoscopy have been developed to provide more readily available and structured training, and have now become essential components of gastroenterology training. Focus has also been placed on ensuring that those endoscopists responsible for training or performing screening procedures on healthy populations are themselves competent to do so. 'Training the Trainers' courses teach experienced endoscopists adult education theory and its application to skills training in endoscopy. Accreditation for colonoscopists wishing to undertake colorectal cancer screening is now mandatory in England and Wales. Both initiatives are aimed at maximising the provision of high-quality endoscopy and training on a national basis and not just in teaching centres. A national audit in 2011 of all colonoscopies done in England has demonstrated improvements in virtually all aspects of colonoscopy,[33] including training, validating the rigorous quality assurance process undertaken in recent years.

The use of both computer and animal endoscopic simulation has now been shown to be of value in the early phase of colonoscopy training,[36] with transfer of skills to live patients. The importance of non-technical skills and teamwork is now considered to be vital to the performance of high-quality endoscopy. Training can improve safety-related knowledge and attitudes,[37] and observation of behavioural markers relating to these non-technical skills now forms part of the UK assessment and credentialing process.[38]

> ✅ Current European recommendations are that endoscopy simulators, where available, should be used to allow training to occur in a safe, controlled environment.[39]

New techniques in endoscopic mucosal visualisation

There are many new developments in colonoscopic technique and technology that may improve polyp detection and identification of pathology.

Assisted-viewing devices

Cuffs, caps and rings have been developed that attach to the distal tip of a colonoscope and aim to improve the view by flattening the folds of the colon during withdrawal, allowing for improved visibility behind folds. They have all been shown to increase the polyp and adenoma detection rates, particularly for small proximal polyps, and there may also be additional benefit of rings and cuffs in improved caecal intubation rates and decreased pain scores.[40] Retrograde (Third-Eye RetroScope) and 360-degree viewing endoscopes (Third-Eye Panoramic, Fuse FullSpectrum Endoscopy, Ewave) have shown some efficacy in improving adenoma detection rates,[41] but research is still ongoing and none has yet shown benefit when incorporated into routine practice.[42]

Chromoendoscopy

Chromoendoscopy is a technique that uses a surface dye such as indigo carmine to make irregularities in the colonic mucosa more readily apparent to the endoscopist (**Fig. 2.3**).

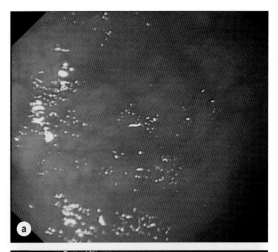
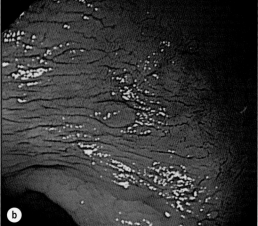

Figure 2.3 • (a) Polyp in white light. **(b)** With indigo carmine dye-spray.

> ✓✓ The use of chromoendoscopy has been shown to significantly improve adenoma detection during surveillance of high-risk groups such as ulcerative colitis[43–45] and familial colorectal cancer syndromes.[46]

It has also been shown to aid identification of flat or depressed adenomas, which are much more prevalent than was previously thought and have a high risk of malignant transformation. It can, however, be time-consuming and currently there is no substantive evidence for its use during routine colonoscopy.

Optical enhancement (electronic chromoendoscopy or electronic chromoendoscopy) uses optical filters to narrow the bandwidth of white light (narrow-band imaging, NBI), or spectral emission processing of white light (I-scan, Flexible Spectrum Imaging Colour Enhancement, FICE) to enhance the visualisation of the capillary network or microsurface pattern of colonic adenomas[47] (**Fig. 2.4**). These technologies are activated by the push of a button on enabled scopes, which has clear advantages over the use of dye-spray. They are recommended for use in high-risk groups such as Lynch syndrome patients where spotting even diminutive adenomas is crucial, but randomised trials have not shown significant benefit in routine endoscopy.[48,49] Confocal laser endomicroscopy combines a standard video endoscope with a miniaturised laser microscope. Using intravenous sodium fluorescein as a contrast agent, 'virtual histology' can be created, allowing visualisation of both the surface epithelium and some of the lamina propria, including the microvasculature. This can potentially provide accurate identification of colonic intra-epithelial neoplasia and carcinoma, although many barriers have so far prevented uptake in routine use.[50]

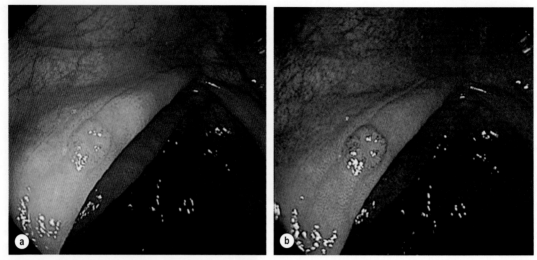

Figure 2.4 • **(a)** Polyp in white light. **(b)** With narrow band imaging.

High-magnification endoscopy

High-magnification endoscopes can magnify the image up to 100 times, and newer high-definition scopes have a much greater pixel density and ability to improve detail discrimination. In conjunction with dye-spray or electronic chromoendoscopy, their use permits identification of a polyp's surface 'pit pattern' to assist in distinguishing between cancerous, adenomatous and non-adenomatous polyps. A classification system devised by Kudo et al. in 1994[51] has been shown to have a reasonable diagnostic accuracy (overall 86.1%, sensitivity 90.8%, specificity 72.7%) when compared to histological findings[52] (**Fig. 2.5**). There is a learning curve in identification of the patterns, however, so for inexperienced endoscopists it does not significantly reduce the number of histological samples taken. Further work has resulted in a simple classification system, the Narrow-band Imaging International Colorectal Endoscopic (NICE) Classification,[53] but studies have yet to confirm its real-world utility, and current evidence does not support a 'resect-and-discard' approach.[54]

Endoscopic therapy

One of the exciting benefits of improving endoscopic skills and technology is the increasingly successful application of novel therapeutic techniques. Therapy that previously required open surgical procedures can now be performed in a minimally invasive way.

Basic therapy

Polypectomy

The ability to remove abnormal tissue endoscopically forms the basis of all cancer prevention and surveillance programmes. The resectability of a polyp depends on its size, characteristics and accessibility. Polyps that are unlikely to be removable endoscopically are those with submucosal invasion,

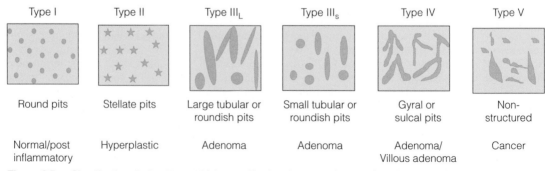

Type I	Type II	Type III$_L$	Type III$_s$	Type IV	Type V
Round pits	Stellate pits	Large tubular or roundish pits	Small tubular or roundish pits	Gyral or sulcal pits	Non-structured
Normal/post inflammatory	Hyperplastic	Adenoma	Adenoma	Adenoma/ Villous adenoma	Cancer

Figure 2.5 • Classification of pit pattern at high-magnification chromoendoscopy (after Kudo et al.).

large sessile polyps extending beyond 50% of the bowel wall circumference, low rectal polyps extending beyond the dentate line, or lesions encircling the appendix orifice.[55]

It is recognized that serrated lesions are also more difficult to resect as they have indistinct edges.[56]

Small polyps less than 4 mm in size can be removed by cold forceps or cold snare. Hot biopsy is now no longer recommended by either the American or European endoscopy societies. Larger-stalked polyps are best removed using a conventional large or mini-snare. The stalk should be transected approximately halfway between the polyp and the bowel wall. This ensures a clear resection margin whilst leaving sufficient stalk in place to facilitate endoscopic treatment should post-polypectomy bleeding occur. Diathermy unit settings should be chosen to ensure enough coagulating current is applied to allow adequate haemostasis of the blood vessels within the polyp stalk. A validated Direct Observation of Polypectomy Skills (DOPyS) assessment tool has been developed to assist with the training and evaluation of polypectomy technique,[57] and is now in clinical use for competency assessment of trainees and in the Bowel Cancer Screening accreditation processes in England.

Retrieval of the polyp is important to determine the histology and grade of dysplasia. Small polyps can be sucked through the scope into a polyp trap, while larger polyps can be grasped or snared and withdrawn with the scope. Retrieval baskets or nets are particularly useful for retrieving more than one piece of tissue or multiple polyps.

Endoscopic mucosal resection (EMR)

EMR involves injection of fluid into the submucosal space to lift the mucosa (and the polyp) away from the muscle layer of the bowel wall (**Fig. 2.6**). This facilitates removal of sessile or flat lesions, reducing the risk of thermal injury to the bowel wall.[58] The authors find the addition of adrenaline (1:200 000) to improve haemostasis and a few drops of methylene blue to differentiate the submucosal plane helpful. Large lesions (>2 cm) can be removed in a piecemeal fashion safely using a submucosal lift.

✓✓ Polyp recurrence may be reduced following piecemeal resection by the judicious use of argon plasma coagulation (APC) to destroy small areas of residual polyp around the resected margin.[59]

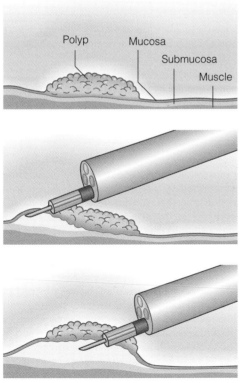
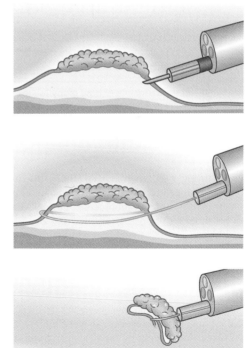

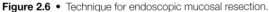
Figure 2.6 • Technique for endoscopic mucosal resection.

Revised St Mark's Colonoscopic Tattooing Protocol 2011

Indications	Equipment	Procedure
• Prior to surgery to localise pathology • To mark lesions for endoscopic surveillance • **Do not tattoo rectal lesions** as they disrupt surgical planes • There is no need to tattoo lesions in the caecum; however, **if in doubt, then place a tattoo**	• Primed variceal injection needle with 10mL syringe filled with normal saline • 5mL syringe filled with Spot® (or 0.9mL sterilised Black (Indian) Ink made up to 5mL with normal saline)	• Direct needle at an angle to mucosa • Raise a bleb using 1-2mL of saline • Swap to syringe filled with Spot® or Indian Ink • Inject 1mL into the bleb to create tattoo • Swap to syringe filled with saline and flush ink out with 1mL saline before removing needle • Repeat process for 3 tattoos

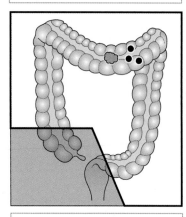

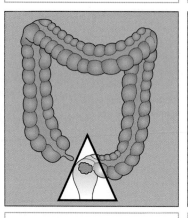

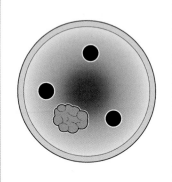

Place 3 tattoos **distal** to lesion	**Do not** place tattoo below 20cm but clearly record distance of LESION from anal verge	Place tattoos 120° apart **as close to lesion as possible** but separate from it

Remember: To document **how many** tattoos were placed and **the position relative to the lesion**

Figure 2.7 • St Mark's colonoscopic tattooing protocol.

The 'non-lifting' sign, when a polyp fails to lift with a submucosal injection, should raise a suspicion of malignant invasion of the submucosa. Lesions that do not lift should be biopsied, tattooed (**Fig 2.7**) and referred for expert assessment and consideration of surgical resection.

Investigation of acute lower gastrointestinal (GI) bleeding

The lower GI tract accounts for a quarter to a third of all hospitalised cases of GI bleeding,[60] with diverticular disease being by far the most common cause. Colitis, cancer, polyps and angiodysplasia account for the majority of the rest. Most lower GI bleeding stops spontaneously and in those cases an elective colonoscopy with standard bowel preparation is appropriate. In the uncommon case of continued bleeding, a rapid purge to allow endoscopic therapy can be considered to decrease both the recurrence of bleeding and the need for surgical intervention.[61] Surgery is reserved for cases of recurrent, uncontrolled or massive bleeding.

Colonic decompression

The three main causes of bowel obstruction are cancer, diverticular disease and sigmoid volvulus. Flexible sigmoidoscopy with placement of a decompression tube is the initial treatment of choice for a volvulus. It has a high initial success rate (78%) but is only a temporising measure as recurrence is common and elective surgery is therefore still considered the definitive treatment. Emergency surgery is reserved for a volvulus unresponsive to endoscopic therapy or for patients with bowel ischaemia or peritonitis.

Acute colonic pseudo-obstruction (Ogilvie's syndrome) may mimic the signs and symptoms of bowel obstruction. It may be initially treated conservatively with removal of any triggering factors, mobilisation and the use of a parasympathomimetic agent such as neostigmine (if not contraindicated). If this approach fails, then endoscopic placement of a decompression tube is generally accepted as the first invasive therapeutic manoeuvre. Emergency surgery is again only indicated in resistant or complicated cases, such as those with perforation or ischaemia.

Advanced therapy

Endoscopic submucosal dissection (ESD)
ESD is a technique that has been developed for 'en bloc' resection of large lesions in the gastrointestinal tract. A deep, submucosal lift is created using a viscous solution such as sodium hyaluronate or 10% glycerine. Mucosal and submucosal incisions are made using a modified needle knife to dissect the mucosa from the submucosa. A transparent hood is attached to the endoscope tip to help retract tissue and maintain the submucosal field of view. The benefit of this technique is that it produces excellent specimens for histological analysis, but the technique itself is difficult, and success depends on excellent endoscopic and haemostatic skills. It is also quite time-consuming, usually taking between 2 and 3 hours in expert hands, and should be performed only when surgical backup is available. It does achieve a higher rate of en bloc and R0 resection compared to EMR, at the cost of a higher risk of complications.[62]

Stricture dilatation and stenting
The dilatation of colonic strictures is generally reserved for benign disease, whereas the use of self-expandable metal stents (SEMS) is usually indicated for malignant disease.[63]

Through-the-scope (TTS) balloon dilators have been used in the management of strictures associated with inflammatory bowel disease, non-steroidal anti-inflammatory drug (NSAID)-induced colonic strictures and anastomotic strictures. Success rates vary, with recent studies suggesting short-term relief in 70–100%, but with frequent recurrence. Complication rates are significant, with a risk of perforation of 2% and bleeding between 4% and 11%.

SEMS are usually inserted through the scope and can be deployed as far as the proximal ascending colon. Preoperative stenting of malignant strictures can, in carefully selected cases, allow for one-stage surgical procedures, but are mostly used for palliation, with patency established up to a year. SEMS can also be considered as a potential therapy for selected benign strictures and has been reported with anastomotic strictures unresponsive to dilatation, Crohn's disease, diverticular disease and radiation-induced strictures.

Novel therapies

As technology and endoscopic skill evolve, the lines between what is possible endoscopically, laparoscopically and traditionally have become increasingly blurred. Although initial interest in Natural Orifice Transluminal Endoscopic Surgery (NOTES) was high, most studies have concluded that the standard laparoscopic techniques are quicker and safer. However, enthusiasts continue to innovate. A novel trans-anal endo-surgical approach to large, complex rectal polyps (TASER) may allow for minimally invasive management of polyps that were previously destined for surgery.[64] Endoscopic full-thickness resection (EFTR) techniques are being developed that may allow for wider oncological resection, although new platforms and prospective clinical trials are required before they are taken up in routine clinical practice.[65] Balloon-assisted colonoscopy can be used to provide a stable platform for advanced endoscopic therapy and may enable access in cases that were previously incomplete due to technical difficulties.

Competing technologies

Currently, optical colonoscopy remains the gold-standard test for examination of the colon due to its relatively high pathology detection rate and the ability to perform therapy. However, newer techniques are emerging that may be considered as 'disruptive technologies' that will undoubtedly change the current position.

Computed tomography colonography (or virtual colonoscopy)

Computed tomography colonography (CTC), also known as virtual colonoscopy (VC; or 'CT pneumocolon'), is now an established technique for detecting colon cancer and colonic polyps. It comprises two low-dose CT scans of the abdomen and pelvis, and is less invasive than optical colonoscopy, requires no conscious sedation and is better tolerated by patients. The diagnostic performance characteristics are potentially comparable to expert optical colonoscopy with sensitivity for detecting large polyps (>10 mm in maximal diameter) exceeding 90% and 96% for cancer,[66] but it lacks the facility for mucosal biopsy or polyp removal. It has, however, now superseded barium enema as the radiological test of choice for the colon.

Self-propelling colonoscopes

One disadvantage of traditional optical colonoscopy is the prolonged training required for expertise. There would be significant advantages to providing the same examination and potential for therapy without the need for an experienced operator. A number of self-propelling or self-navigating colonoscopes have been developed, but these have not been widely adopted despite initial tests showing them to be safe and effective. The current trend is clearly towards greater quality and accuracy of traditional colonoscopy performance, rather than widespread adoption of new technology.

Colon capsule

Wireless capsule endoscopy (WCE) is a safe, minimally invasive, non-sedation requiring, patient-friendly modality to visualise the bowel, and is now considered first line for investigation of small bowel disease. The development of the PillCam colon capsule (Given Imaging Ltd, Yoqneam, Israel) aims to widen the application to investigation of colonic disease. It is attractive for similar reasons and, unlike optical colonoscopy, only requires expertise in image interpretation. The second-generation PillCam Colon Capsule 2 has a wider field of view and adaptive frame rate than the first-generation, and a meta-analysis has demonstrated high specificity for polyps over 10 mm in a screening setting.[67]

Conclusions

This chapter has given an overview of the role of flexible sigmoidoscopy and colonoscopy in the diagnosis, treatment and prevention of colorectal disease. Traditional optical endoscopy is becoming more refined and new technologies are emerging that will impact on the need for open or laparoscopic surgery. The current focus is on quality assurance and improvements in training with continual skill development essential for all those endoscopists wishing to perform high-quality, safe endoscopy.

Key points

- Good technique is vital for high-quality safe endoscopy.
- Sedation practice should be standardised and use the minimum amount of drug required for patient comfort.
- Withdrawal times should be in excess of 6 minutes in normal colonoscopies.
- Advanced imaging techniques are now becoming more widely available and may impact on current practice.
- All endoscopists should be familiar with basic therapeutic techniques (polypectomy, diathermy, decompression) and indications for referral for advanced therapy (EMR, ESD, stenting).
- Competing technologies are evolving and need to be evaluated for their utility in clinical practice.
- Performance in technical skills should be considered in conjunction with non-technical skills and team working.

▶ Video resources:

- http://www.stmarksacademicinstitute.org.uk/resources/colonoscopy-insertion-steering-and-examination/
- http://www.stmarksacademicinstitute.org.uk/resources/colonoscopy-experts-in-action-part-1/
- http://www.stmarksacademicinstitute.org.uk/resources/colonoscopy-experts-in-action-part-2/
- http://www.stmarksacademicinstitute.org.uk/resources/colonoscopy-equipment-and-accessories/
- http://www.stmarksacademicinstitute.org.uk/resources/olympus-scopeguide-3d-imager/
- http://www.stmarksacademicinstitute.org.uk/resources/polypectomy-training-polypectomy-in-detail/

🌐 Full references available at **http://expertconsult.inkling.com**

Key references

14. Rizk MK, Sawhney MS, Cohen J, et al. Quality indicators common to all GI endoscopic procedures. Gastrointest Endosc 2015;81(1):3–16. PMID: 25480102.

15. Barclay RL, Vicari JJ, Doughty AS, et al. Colonoscopic withdrawal times and adenoma detection during screening colonoscopy. N Engl J Med 2006;355(24):2533–41. PMID: 17167136.

Observational study of 12 experienced colonoscopists over 7882 colonoscopies showing a 10-fold difference in ADR between endoscopists and a significant difference in those who spent more or less than 6 minutes during withdrawal in normal colonoscopies.

19. ASGE Standards of Practice Committee. Bowel preparation before colonoscopy. Gastrointest Endosc 2015;81(4):781–94. PMID: 25595062.

20. Connor A, Tolan D, Hughes S, et al. Consensus guidelines for the safe prescription and administration of oral bowel-cleansing agents. Gut 2012;61(11): 1525–32. PMID: 22842619.

43. Hurlstone DP, Sanders DS, McAlindon ME, et al. High-magnification chromoscopic colonoscopy in ulcerative colitis: a valid tool for in vivo optical biopsy and assessment of disease extent. Endoscopy 2006;38(12): 1213–7. PMID: 17163321.
Biphasic examination with 1800 images from 300 patients obtained via conventional or magnification imaging. Magnification imaging was significantly better than conventional colonoscopy for predicting disease extent in vivo ($P < 0.0001$).

44. Kiesslich R, Fritsch J, Holtmann M, et al. Methylene blue-aided chromoendoscopy for the detection of intraepithelial neoplasia and colon cancer in ulcerative colitis. Gastroenterology 2003;124(4):880–8. PMID: 12671882.
Randomised controlled trial of 165 patients showing a significantly better correlation between the endoscopic assessment of degree ($P=0.0002$) and extent (89% vs 52%; $P <0.0001$) of colonic inflammation and the histopathological findings in the chromoendoscopy group compared with the conventional colonoscopy group. More targeted biopsies were possible and significantly more neoplasias were detected (32 vs 10; $P=0.003$).

45. Rutter MD, Saunders BP, Schofield G, et al. Pancolonic indigo carmine dye spraying for the detection of dysplasia in ulcerative colitis. Gut 2004;53(2):256–60. PMID: 14724160.
Back-to-back colonoscopies in 100 patients showing significantly more dysplasia detection with chromoendoscopy and targeted biopsies ($P=0.02$). Chromoendoscopy required fewer biopsies (157 vs 2904) yet detected nine dysplastic lesions, seven of which were only visible after indigo carmine application.

46. Hurlstone DP, Karajeh M, Cross SS, et al. The role of high-magnification-chromoscopic colonoscopy in hereditary nonpolyposis colorectal cancer screening: a prospective 'back-to-back' endoscopic study. Am J Gastroenterol 2005;100(10):2167–73. PMID: 16181364.
Back-to-back colonoscopies in 25 asymptomatic HNPCC patients. Pan-chromoscopy identified significantly more adenomas than conventional colonoscopy ($P=0.001$) and a significantly higher number of flat adenomas ($P=0.004$).

59. Brooker JC, Saunders BP, Shah SG, et al. Treatment with argon plasma coagulation reduces recurrence after piecemeal resection of large sessile colonic polyps: a randomized trial and recommendations. Gastrointest Endosc 2002;55(3):371–5. PMID: 11868011.
Patients with apparent complete excision of adenomatous polyps were randomised to application of APC to the margins or not. Postpolypectomy application of APC reduced recurrence at 3 months (1/10 APC, 7/11 no APC; $P=0.02$).

3

Colorectal cancer

Robert J.C. Steele

Introduction

Colorectal cancer is a major health problem. In the UK, it is the second most common cause of cancer death, accounting for some 16 000 deaths in 2014. In 2013 there were approximately 41 000 new cases, of which about 15 000 were rectal and 26 000 colonic.[1] The overall numbers in men are higher than in women, and this is more pronounced in the rectum than in the colon. The 5-year relative survival rate is currently in the region of 57% and has improved over the last 30 years from a figure of around 20% in 1971–75.[1]

Surprisingly, there is no precise definition of the colon and the rectum. Although the colon comprises the large bowel proximal to the rectum, the definition of the rectum is unclear. Anatomical texts describe the top of the rectum as the point where the sigmoid mesocolon ends or that part of the large bowel level with the third sacral vertebra.[2] Surgeons, on the other hand, prefer to think of the rectum as the segment of large bowel lying within the true pelvis. As far as rectal cancer is concerned, the UK definition is a tumour within 15 cm of the anal verge on rigid sigmoidoscopy,[3] whereas authorities from the USA have preferred 11 or 12 cm.[4] Perhaps the simplest definition is the intraoperative identification of the fusion of the two antemesenteric taenia into an amorphous area where the true rectum begins.

These distinctions are important for two reasons. First, radiotherapy is not appropriate for colonic tumours and, secondly, comparisons between outcomes for colorectal cancer surgery are impossible unless uniform definitions are adopted. This problem has yet to be addressed by international consensus.

Natural history

Within the large bowel, about 50% of cancers arise in the rectum and left colon and 25% in the right (**Fig. 3.1**); in 4–5% of cases there are synchronous lesions. It is now widely accepted that the majority of colorectal cancers arise from pre-existing adenomatous polyps, the supporting evidence being as follows:[5]

1. The prevalence of adenomas correlates well with that of carcinomas, the average age of adenoma patients being around 5 years younger than patients with carcinomas.
2. Adenomatous tissue often accompanies cancer, and it is unusual to find small cancers with no contiguous adenomatous tissue.
3. Most sporadic adenomas are identical histologically to the adenomas of familial adenomatous polyposis (FAP), and this condition is unequivocally premalignant.
4. Large adenomas are more likely to display cellular atypia and genetic abnormalities than small lesions.
5. The distribution of adenomas throughout the large bowel is similar to that of carcinomas.
6. Adenomas are found in up to one-third of all surgical specimens resected for colorectal cancer.
7. The incidence of colorectal cancer has been shown to fall with a long-term screening programme involving colonoscopy and polypectomy.

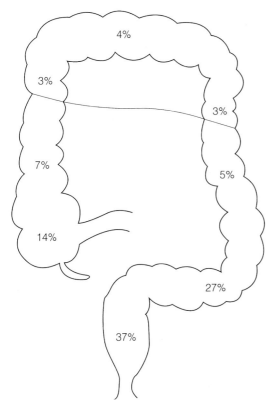

Figure 3.1 • Frequency of anatomical locations of colorectal cancer.
Based on data from The Wales-Trent Bowel Cancer Audit, 1993

Although the majority of adenomas diagnosed in the West are polypoid or exophytic, the flat adenoma, defined as an adenoma where the depth of the dysplastic tissue is no more than twice that of the mucosa, is now a recognised entity. These are difficult to find, but may account for up to 40% of all adenomas. In addition, the serrated lesion, which is histologically distinct from the adenoma and related to the hyperplastic polyp, is now recognised as a premalignant condition, particularly on the right side of the colon.[6] Reliable diagnosis of these subtle lesions requires a skilful, experienced colonoscopist and the use of dye sprayed on to the colonic mucosa to highlight the contours of the abnormal tissue.

When invasion has taken place, colonic cancer can spread directly and via the lymphatic, blood and transcoelomic routes.

Direct spread

Direct spread occurs longitudinally, transversely and radially, but as adequate proximal and distal clearance is technically feasible in the majority of colorectal cancers, it is radial spread that is of most importance.

In a retroperitoneal colonic cancer, radial spread may involve the ureter, duodenum and muscles of the posterior abdominal wall; the intraperitoneal tumour may involve small intestine, stomach, pelvic organs or the anterior abdominal wall. Rectal tumours may involve the pelvic organs or side walls.

Lymphatic spread

In general, the lymphatic spread of colonic cancer progresses from the paracolic nodes along the main colonic vessels to the nodes associated with either cephalad or caudal vessels, eventually reaching the para-aortic glands in advanced disease. This orderly process does not always occur, however, and in about 30% of cases nodal involvement can skip a tier of glands.[7] In contrast to rectal disease, it is rare for a colonic cancer that has not breached the muscle wall to exhibit lymph node metastases[7] (overall, about 15% of cases confined to the bowel wall will be found to have lymph node metastases). In the rectum, drainage is via the mesorectal nodes.

Blood-borne spread

The most common site for blood-borne spread of colorectal cancer is the liver, presumably arriving by the portal venous system. Up to 37% of patients may have occult liver metastases at the time of operation, and around 50% of patients may be expected to develop overt disease at some time. The lung is the next most common site, with around 10% of patients developing lung metastases at some stage; other reported sites include ovary, adrenal, bone, brain and kidney.

Transcoelomic spread

Colonic cancer may spread throughout the peritoneum, either via the subperitoneal lymphatics or by virtue of viable cells being shed from the serosal surface of a tumour, giving rise to malignant ascites, which is relatively rare.

Aetiology

Knowledge of molecular genetics in sporadic colorectal cancer has increased rapidly in recent years, but the stimuli that lead to these carcinogenic changes are still obscure.

Genetic factors

The predisposing genetic factors and molecular changes underlying colorectal cancer have been widely studied, and are dealt with in detail in Chapter 4. In summary, the most commonly inherited forms of colorectal cancer are Lynch syndrome, caused by mutations to the DNA mismatch repair genes, and familial adenomatous polyposis (FAP), caused by germline mutations in the *APC* gene. However, any family history can confer a degree of risk, which is presumably accounted for by a combination of shared environmental factors and inherited genetic polymorphisms. In all colorectal cancers, there appear to be two main pathways to carcinogenesis – chromosomal and microsatellite instability – but more refined methods of classifying the molecular pathways have recently been developed that are consistent with this concept.[8]

Diet and lifestyle

In 2007, the World Cancer Research Fund (WCRF) published its report on Food, Nutrition, Physical Activity and the Prevention of Cancer based on a systematic review of the world literature.[9]

✔✔ With respect to colorectal cancer,[9] evidence for decreased risk was found for physical exercise, dietary fibre, calcium, garlic, non-starchy vegetables and pulses. Evidence for increased risk was uncovered for obesity, red meat, processed meat, alcohol, animal fat and sugar. It is clear that being overweight and underactive stand out as major risk factors, and governments worldwide have recognised this as an area for action. Smoking is also important and long-term smoking is associated with relative risks of between 1.5 and 3.0.[10]

Predisposing conditions

Long-standing inflammatory bowel disease, both ulcerative colitis and Crohn's disease, increases the risk of colorectal cancer. Previous gastric surgery has also been implicated, and although the association is controversial, the risk may be about twofold. Altered bile acid metabolism may play a role in this process, both after gastrectomy and after vagotomy. The risk after ureterosigmoidostomy is well established, although this operation has now been largely superseded by the use of an isolated ileal conduit for urinary diversion.

Presentation

Colorectal cancer can present as an emergency or with chronic symptoms that are well recognised. Right-sided cancer typically presents with anaemia, as the liquid nature of the faeces and the wider diameter of the colon make obstructive symptoms unusual. When the tumour is situated in the descending or sigmoid colon, change of bowel habit, colicky abdominal pain and blood in the stool are the commonest symptoms. In the rectum, bleeding is predominant, and with a large tumour, tenesmus is common. Occasionally, the patient may notice the primary tumour as a mass and even more rarely a sigmoid cancer may cause pneumaturia and urinary infection by fistulation into the bladder, or a gastrocolic fistula may cause faecal vomiting or severe diarrhoea.

Unfortunately, many of the symptoms of colorectal cancer are common and non-specific, and although there have been sustained public awareness campaigns in the UK to increase the number of patients consulting their GPs for these symptoms, this has had the unfortunate effect of greatly increasing the number of patients being investigated with no effect on the stage at diagnosis. Guidelines have been developed to classify those at high risk warranting urgent investigation based on change in bowel habit, rectal bleeding in the absence of anal symptoms, palpable abdominal or rectal masses and anaemia (Box 3.1).[11] These guidelines are not

Box 3.1 • UK Department of Health criteria for high and low risk of colorectal cancer

Higher risk
- Rectal bleeding with a change in bowel habit to looser stools or increased frequency of defecation persisting for 6 weeks (all ages)
- Change in bowel habit as above without rectal bleeding and persisting for 6 weeks (>60 years)
- Persistent rectal bleeding without anal symptoms* (>60 years)
- Palpable right-sided abdominal mass (all ages)
- Palpable rectal mass (not pelvic) (all ages)
- Unexplained iron deficiency anaemia (all ages)

Low risk
- Patients with no iron deficiency anaemia, no palpable rectal or abdominal mass
- Rectal bleeding with anal symptoms and no persistent change in bowel habit (all ages)
- Rectal bleeding with an obvious external cause, e.g. anal fissure (all ages)
- Change in bowel habit without rectal bleeding (<60 years)
- Transient changes in bowel habit, particularly to harder or decreased frequency of defecation
- Abdominal pain as a single symptom without signs and symptoms of intestinal obstruction (all ages)

* Soreness, discomfort, itching, lumps, prolapse or pain.
Reproduced from Thompson MR, Heath I, Ellis BG, et al. Identifying and managing patients at low risk of bowel cancer in general practice. Br Med J 2003; 327:263–5. With permission from BMJ Publishing Group Ltd.

particularly discriminatory, however, and there is currently great interest in developing the role of sensitive faecal immunochemical testing (FIT) for haemoglobin to assist in determining which symptomatic patients warrant colonoscopy.

Investigation

Currently, the main investigative techniques include sigmoidoscopy, colonoscopy and computed tomography (CT) colonography. Barium enema, formerly the mainstay of investigation, has fallen out of favour owing to false-positive and false-negative results occurring in up to 1% and 7% of cases, respectively, with errors usually occurring in the sigmoid colon and caecum.[12]

Although rigid sigmoidoscopy may provide satisfactory rectal visualisation, it has been largely superseded by flexible sigmoidoscopy for examination of the rectum and distal colon. The extent to which the colon can be examined by this means is highly variable, however, and it can be argued that colonoscopy should be the investigation of choice. However, it does carry a risk of perforation, and even in good hands failure to achieve caecal intubation can be expected in around 5% of cases. In addition, precise localisation of a tumour seen at colonoscopy is difficult as the only reliable landmarks are the anus and the terminal ileum, although the use of magnetic scope guides allows more accurate estimation of the site of a lesion.

> ✅ CT as a primary investigative modality is now coming to the fore with the widespread introduction of CT colonography or 'virtual colonoscopy', which is effective in detecting polypoid lesions down to 6 mm in diameter and superior to barium enema for the detection of cancers and significant polyps.[13]

This is fast becoming a standard investigation and has replaced the barium enema as the radiological investigation of choice in the majority of centres. Capsule endoscopy, until recently used only to visualise the small bowel, has now been modified to allow examination of the large bowel, and may become a very important tool in the investigation of colorectal symptoms and in screening and surveillance.

When the diagnosis has been made, staging of the primary tumour, liver and lungs is now considered mandatory in the majority of cases. A fit patient with metastatic disease may be suitable for active treatment, whereas an elderly patient with a relatively asymptomatic primary and evidence of widespread dissemination may escape resection.

> ✅ CT of the chest and abdomen is now regarded as the staging modality of choice, supplanting chest X-ray and ultrasound. In a patient with a rectal cancer, MRI of the rectum is now considered mandatory to allow accurate preoperative staging and treatment planning. Endorectal ultrasound is used in some centres to assist with the assessment of early rectal cancer as it is reasonably accurate in distinguishing T1 from T2 tumours, but it is highly operator-dependent and not universally employed. PET-CT scanning has a limited role, but is recommended when surgical resection of metastases is being considered in order to exclude occult disease.[14]

Screening

Colorectal cancer is a suitable candidate for screening. Prognosis after treatment is much better in early stage disease and the polyp–carcinoma sequence offers an opportunity to prevent cancer by treating premalignant disease. The ideal screening test should detect the majority of tumours without a large number of false positives, i.e. it should have high sensitivity and specificity. In addition, it must be safe and acceptable to the population offered screening. In colorectal cancer, the most widely studied test is Haemoccult, a guaiac-based test that detects the peroxidase-like activity of haematin in faeces. Because this activity is diminished as haemoglobin travels through the gastrointestinal tract,[15] upper gastrointestinal bleeding is less likely to be detected than colonic bleeding. On the other hand, false-positive results may be produced by ingestion of animal haemoglobin or vegetables containing peroxidase, and because of the intermittent nature of bleeding from tumours, the sensitivity of Haemoccult is only about 50–70%.[16]

Screen-detected tumours are much more likely to be at an early stage than symptomatic disease, but this does not prove that screening is beneficial. Even improved survival in patients whose tumours are detected by screening is not conclusive because of the biases inherent in screening. These biases are threefold, and comprise selection bias, length bias and lead-time bias.

Selection bias arises from the tendency of people who accept screening to be particularly health conscious and therefore atypical of the population as a whole. Length bias indicates the tendency for screening to detect a disproportionate number of cancers that are slow growing, and thereby have a good prognosis. Lead-time bias results from the time between the date of detection of a cancer by screening and the date when it would have been diagnosed had the subject not been screened. As survival is measured from the time of diagnosis, screening advances the date at which diagnosis is made, thus lengthening the survival time without necessarily altering the date of death.

✓✓ Because of these biases, effectiveness can be assessed only by comparing disease-specific mortality in a population offered screening with that in an identical population not offered screening. This has to be done in the context of a well-designed randomised controlled trial, and for colorectal cancer three trials using faecal occult blood (FOB) have reported mortality data.[17–19] The first of these was carried out in Minnesota,[17] and showed a significant 33% reduction in colorectal cancer-specific mortality with annual FOB testing and a significant 21% reduction in a group offered biennial screening. In Nottingham, a trial of biennial FOB testing demonstrated a 15% reduction in cumulative mortality[18] and an almost identical study carried out in Funen, Denmark, showed an 18% reduction in mortality.[19]

There seems little doubt that FOB screening can reduce mortality from colorectal cancer, when applied to unselected populations, and the challenges for the future are to increase uptake and to improve the sensitivity and specificity of the screening test. Worldwide there is increasing interest in using faecal immunological testing (FIT) for blood, which is not affected by dietary peroxidase or animal haemoglobin and is therefore more accurate than the indirect guaiac test.[20] It is also associated with higher uptake, as, unlike the guaiac test, only one sample is required, and the collection device is more hygienic. Of particular interest is the use of quantitative FIT, which is automated (**Fig. 3.2**),

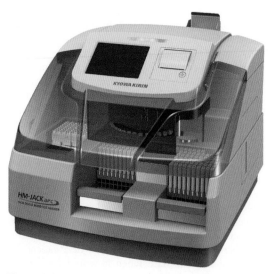

Figure 3.2 • A quantitative faecal immunochemical test (FIT) analyser.

and therefore not subject to human observational error, and provides the user with the facility to set the performance characteristics to suit the screening programme.

Another approach is to use endoscopy as a primary screening test. As 70% of cancers and large adenomas are found in the distal 60 cm of the large bowel, flexible sigmoidoscopy has been proposed as a screening test, and there is good evidence that it is more sensitive than FOB testing.

✓✓ Once-only flexible sigmoidoscopy between the ages of 55 and 64 has been investigated as a screening modality in a multicentre randomised study,[21] and has been shown to reduce colorectal cancer mortality *and* incidence, particularly in the rectum and left colon; the incidence reduction is undoubtedly due to adenoma removal at the time of flexible sigmoidoscopy. In the UK, flexible sigmoidoscopy is being introduced as part of the national bowel screening programme, and the guaiac test is being replaced by FIT.

Surveillance after adenoma detection

Surveillance of patients diagnosed as having adenomatous polyps poses a significant challenge in terms of the use of colonoscopy resources, particularly with the introduction of population screening. For this reason, guidelines have been developed that classify patients as being at low, intermediate or high risk for adenoma recurrence.[22] The low-risk category includes those with one or two adenomas less than 1 cm in diameter, and either no follow-up or a repeat colonoscopy at 5 years is recommended. For those at intermediate risk, defined as three to four adenomas or at least one adenoma greater than 1 cm in diameter, colonoscopy at 3 years is recommended. High-risk patients, those with five or more small adenomas or three or more where at least one is greater than 1 cm in diameter, should have another colonoscopy at 1 year. While the evidence upon which these guidelines is based is not very strong, they represent a sensible approach, and one that has been adopted widely in the UK.

The malignant polyp

After colonoscopic polypectomy, subsequent histological examination of the specimen may reveal a focus of invasive cancer (**Fig. 3.3**). A relatively rare situation in the past, this has rapidly become a common occurrence with the introduction of colorectal population screening and it poses the problem of what to do next. Clearly, if there is a risk of residual tumour, either

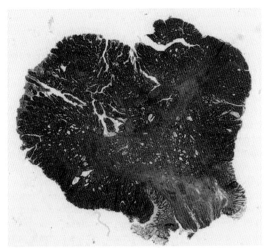

Figure 3.3 • Polyp cancer. The resection margin is clear of tumour, but the stroma of the centre of the polyp is occupied by invasive adenocarcinoma.

in the bowel wall or in the regional lymph nodes, then formal resection is advisable, but quantifying this risk is by no means simple.

When a completion colectomy is required, one difficulty that can be encountered by the surgeon is identifying the section of colon that is to be removed. Colonoscopic localisation of a lesion is notoriously unreliable, and polypectomy scars heal very quickly. For these reasons, if an endoscopist has any reason to suspect that a polyp may be harbouring invasive

malignancy, then the polypectomy site should be marked with injection of submucosal ink (tatoo – see Chapter 2 for protocol) in order to guide the surgeon in the event of further intervention.

The second issue to consider is whether the polyp cancer has been cured. After endoscopic resection of a malignant polyp, assuming staging CT scans do not reveal either residual disease or distant spread, the pathologist's assessment of the resected cancer becomes crucial. Haggitt and colleagues reported that if a tumour infiltrates the head, neck or stalk of a peduculated polyp the risk of residual disease is less than 1%.[23] In contrast, if it involves submucosa at the base of the stalk – known as Haggitt level 4 – the risk is far greater (**Fig. 3.4**). Sessile adenomas have similar risks to Haggitt level 4 lesions.

Risk prediction was also categorized by Kikuchi in full-thickness rectal biopsies taken at transanal surgery and involved subdividing the depth of invasion into thirds of the submucosa. The most superficial invasion is termed sm1, and the deepest sm3: risks of nodal mestastasis have been quoted to be as high as 2, 8 and 23% for the respective levels.[24]

Clearance of the tumour on histology is another way of assessing the risk of recurrent disease and a clearance of less than 1 mm has the same clinical significance as a positive margin. In this situation the risk of residual disease is quoted as 21–33%,[25] variation depending on other adverse histological features. However, when the margin of excision was over 1 mm and there were no adverse histological features the risk of residual disease was reported

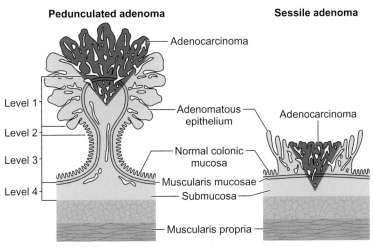

Figure 3.4 • Haggitt classification[23] describing invasion depth of pedunculated and sessile malignant polyps. The focus of invasive cancer is represented by dark shading as having penetrated through the muscularis mucosae to level 1 (carcinoma limited to the head of the polyp). Level 2 is where carcinoma invades to the level of the neck (the junction of the head and stalk) of the adenoma. Level 3 is carcinoma invading any part of the stalk. Level 4 is where carcinoma invades into the submucosa of the bowel wall below the level of the stalk. In the sessile adenoma a stalk is absent and so, by definition, the lesion is defined as being level 4.
Adapted from Williams JG, Pullan RD, Hill J, et al. Management of the malignant colorectal polyp: ACPGBI position statement. Colorectal Dis 2013;15(Suppl.2):1–38.

Table 3.1 • The risk of residual disease in the bowel wall or lymph nodes based on histological features identified after endoscopic resection of a malignant polyp[23]

Histological feature	Grade of risk	Estimated risk of residual disease
Resection margin <1 mm	Very high	20%
Pedunculated Haggitt level 4	Very high	20%
Kikuchi sm3	Very high	20%
Poor differentiation	High	8–15%
Kikuchi sm2	Medium	5–10%
Lymphovascular invasion	Medium	5–10%
Resection margin 1–2 mm	Low	5%
Tumour budding	Low	5%

Reproduced with permission from Williams JG, Pullan RD, Hill J, et al. Management of the malignant colorectal polyp: ACPGBI position statement. Colorectal Dis 2013;15(Suppl.2):1–38.

as zero in 46 patients. When the depth of invasion from the muscularis mucosae in sessile lesions was less than 1 mm in 122 patients without other adverse features,[26] there was similarly no residual disease.

'Adverse' features that worsen prognosis are poor differentiation, lymphovascular invasion and tumour budding, Varying figures have been published for the histological predictors of risk described above but this is not an exact science as much of the data come from small studies. When weighing up the risk of residual disease it is important to recognize the limitations associated with piecemeal EMR specimens as, unless all the submucosa is included, predictions are unreliable. When there is a margin of excision of 1 mm or more, a depth of invasion below muscularis mucosae of 1 mm or less, and there are no adverse features, there is little evidence to recommend resection.[27]

In discussing these issues with the patient, it is important to present the predicted risk of residual disease as well as the risks of intervention to enable an informed choice (Table 3.1). Even when dealing with malignant polyps that have the highest risk of residual disease, 70–90% of patients will not have cancer within the specimen and the patient should be aware of that when considering surgery.

Surgery

Surgical excision remains the mainstay of treatment for colorectal cancer (see Chapters 5 and 6). For colon cancer, the commonest operations are right hemicolectomy, extended right hemicolectomy, left hemicolectomy, sigmoid colectomy and (sub) total colectomy depending on the site and number of cancers. Increasingly, these procedures are being performed laparoscopically with attendant improvements in short-term outcomes, but there is still a definite role for open surgery in the more challenging cases. For rectal cancer the choice is usually between anterior resection where intestinal continuity is preserved and abdomino-perineal excision (APER), which results in a permanent colostomy. In both operations, the principle of mesorectal excision to ensure a clear circumferential margin whenever possible is established, and in APER, there is increasing emphasis on pelvic floor excision (often referred to as extralevator abdomino-perineal or ELAP excision) to ensure adequate clearance of very low cancers.

Quality of surgery is paramount, both in terms of avoiding postoperative morbidity and obtaining good long-term outcomes. There is now unequivocal evidence that both volume and specialisation are associated with better short-term outcomes in a range of cancer operations,[28,29] and in the UK it is recognised that colorectal cancer surgery should only be performed by appropriately trained surgeons whose work is audited.[14]

Adjuvant therapy

Because of the high risk of radiation enteritis affecting adjacent small bowel, adjuvant radiotherapy is not recommended for primary colon cancer. Thus, adjuvant therapy for colon cancer is restricted to systemic treatment, and continues to be based on fluoropyrimidines (5-fluorouracil and the orally available derivative, capcitabine). More recently, combinations with oxaliplatin have proved to be more effective, but these are only appropriate for fitter patients. The more targeted agents bevacizumab (anti-VEGF) and cetuximab (anti-EGF) have not been found to be effective in the adjuvant setting in randomised trials. Until recently, the only indication for adjuvant chemotherapy has been stage III disease, but there is now a move to a more personalised approach; the presence of microsatellite instability is now recognised as an indication for surgery alone in stage II, and the presence of *BRAF* and *KRAS* mutations can be used as predictors of risk that can be used to guide the use of chemotherapy. Traditionally, adjuvant chemotherapy is given after surgery, guided by the pathological findings in the resection specimen, but the FOxTROT trial, designed to test the efficacy of preoperative chemotherapy in patients with colon cancer staged radiologically as T3/4 will report soon.[30]

The same principles for postoperative adjuvant therapy apply to rectal cancer, but preoperative or neoadjuvant treatment has become standard for a proportion of cases of rectal cancer. However, despite a considerable amount of research over the years, there is still no precise consensus as to an optimal neoadjuvant strategy. In broad terms, however, it can be stated that in patients considered to be at moderate risk of local recurrence with mesorectal excision, but in whom the circumferential margin is not seen to be involved on MRI, preoperative radiotherapy (25 Gy in five fractions over 1 week) followed by immediate surgery may be appropriate. Those where MRI does indicate margin involvement, on the other hand, should be considered for combination chemotherapy and radiotherapy followed by a period of up to 3 months to allow for cytoreduction before surgery.[14] It is now firmly established that preoperative radiotherapy produces better disease control and less morbidity than postoperative treatment, and with adequate perioperative staging of the primary tumour with MRI, the latter should no longer be necessary.

In some cases, particularly with earlier tumours, preoperative treatment of this sort can result in a complete clinical response, and there is currently debate as to how to manage such patients, with a strategy of watchful waiting gaining traction.[31] In patients staged as having early cancer (T1 and sometimes T2), particularly when the patient has comorbidities, there is increasing interest in organ preservation, but it is far from clear how this is best achieved. Until recently, local excision was the preferred option, but the strategy of preoperative radiotherapy followed by local excision of any residual disease after a period of around 6 weeks is being tested by the STAR TREC trial. However, there is emerging evidence that those who do not respond completely to radiotherapy have a very high risk of recurrence after local excision, and this is a rapidly moving field which is assuming increasing importance as the proportion of rectal cancers diagnosed at an early stage is rising with the advent of national screening programmes.

Management of advanced disease

The surgical management of the advanced primary tumour is covered in Chapter 8. In colonic cancer, local recurrence usually occurs at the suture line and, in the absence of disseminated disease, re-resection should be attempted, although palliative bypass may be all that can be achieved. The patient with distant metastases poses different challenges.

Operable metastases

Hepatic resection for colorectal cancer metastases is now widely practised, but it has never been tested by a randomised trial, and all comparative studies have used retrospective data from historical controls.[32] With careful patient selection, hepatectomy for colorectal metastases can be associated with a 5-year survival of around 33%,[33] and although the most widely accepted criterion for resection is one to three resectable metastases in one lobe of the liver, many surgeons are now extending their indications.

The role of preoperative chemotherapy in these patients is currently unclear, and the results of a phase III multicentre international trial are awaited. There is, however, some non-randomised evidence that preoperative treatment with 5-fluorouracil plus folinic acid (FUFA) and oxaliplatin may improve both resectability and long-term survival. In a proportion of patients with liver disease that is not amenable to resection, ablation using radiofrequency energy may be employed.[33] This may prolong survival, but as yet must be regarded as palliative.

Pulmonary metastases may also be amenable to resection, but as only 10% of patients develop such metastases and only 10% of these have disease confined to the lung, very few patients will be suitable. Although segmental resection of the lung may be associated with 5-year survival rates of 20–40%, there is sufficient uncertainty to support a randomised trial of resection versus best supportive care (PULMICC), and the results are eagerly awaited.[34]

Advanced local disease

In patients with advanced local disease, be it primary or recurrent, careful thought must be given to appropriate palliation, and, where possible, potential cure. In advanced colon cancer, bypass surgery may be appropriate, but multi-organ en bloc resection may be curative, and suitable patients should be given this option, even when it means referring them on to a tertiary centre. Likewise, in rectal cancer, although palliative radiotherapy with or without a defunctioning stoma may produce a degree of symptom control, consideration should always be given to pelvic exenteration, particularly in younger, fitter patients.

In patients with peritoneal spread alone, or with easily operable liver metastases, peritonectomy combined with heated intraperitoneal chemotherapy (HIPEC) may result in long-term survival.[35] However, this has never been subjected to a randomised trial, and the small number of suitable patients make it very unlikely that this will ever happen.

Inoperable disseminated disease

In the patient with widespread disease, chemotherapy containing fluoropyrimidines is the only established therapeutic option, but this can only be regarded as palliative. Recently, the oral 5FU prodrugs UFT and capecitabine have come into use, and as they have been found to offer equivalent survival with the advantage of increased ease of delivery they are now regarded as suitable single agents for first-line use. Even more recently, combination chemotherapy with intravenous 5FU and either irinotecan or oxaliplatin has been demonstrated to enhance survival as both first- and second-line therapy. If oxaliplatin has been used as first-line treatment, then irinotecan should be considered for second-line therapy and vice versa.

Monoclonal antibody treatment, either in the form of bevacizumab (an antibody against vascular endothelial growth factor (VEGF)) or cetuximab (an antibody against epidermal growth factor (EGF) receptor), has been shown to confer survival advantages in combination with conventional chemotherapy. Cetuximab is now recommended for use along with 5-fluorouracil/leucovorin/oxaliplatin or fluorouracil/irinotecan as first-line treatment for patients with metastatic *KRAS* wild-type disease, as a functioning KRAS pathway is necessary for EGF-receptor signal transduction. Bevacizumab has not been recommended in the UK by NICE (National Institute for Health and Care Excellence) on the grounds that it is not cost-effective.

Pathological staging

Accurate, detailed and consistent pathology reporting for colorectal cancer is important for estimating prognosis and planning further treatment in terms of adjuvant therapy. Both macroscopic and histological appearances must be described in some detail, and the following information should be available.

Microscopic description

1. Size of the tumour (greatest dimension).
2. Site of the tumour in relation to the resection margins.
3. Any abnormalities of the background bowel.

Macroscopic description

1. Histological type.
2. Differentiation of the tumour, based on the predominant grade within the tumour.[36]
3. Maximum extent of invasion into/through the bowel wall (submucosa, muscularis propria, extramural).
4. Serosal involvement by tumour, if present.[37]

5. A statement on the completeness of excision at the cut ends (including the 'doughnuts' from stapling devices) and at any radial margin.
6. The number of lymph nodes examined, the number containing metastases, and whether or not the apical node is involved.
7. Extramural vascular invasion if present.[38]
8. Pathological staging of the tumour according to Dukes' classification.[39]

Dukes' staging is simple, reproducible and widely recognised, but TNM staging is becoming increasingly recognised as the international standard;[40] the two systems are described in Table 3.2. Some pathologists use the Jass classification,[41] although its usefulness may be limited by observer variation in the degree of lymphocytic infiltration at the advancing margin of the tumour (one of the four parameters that contribute to the classification) and the fact that its prognostic value appears to be confined to rectal tumours.

After curative resection, cancer registry data indicate that age-adjusted 5-year survival for Dukes' stage A colonic cancer is 82%, 69% for stage B, 53% for stage C and 6% for those with distant metastases (stage 'D').[42] These results can be improved on, as evidenced by individual series, although the 'Will Rogers' effect (stage migration owing to variable quality of pathology reporting) may play a role in this respect.

Summary recommendations for best practice

Investigation

1. Patients with suspicious symptoms or proven colorectal cancer should be investigated with either endoscopic visualisation of the whole of the large colon by total colonoscopy or CT colonography.
2. Unless it cannot alter management, all patients should have screening (preoperative where possible) for lung and liver metastases by CT scanning, and patients with rectal cancer should have MRI of the rectum.

Elective surgical treatment

1. Any tumour with a distal margin at 15 cm or less from the anal verge using a rigid sigmoidoscope should be classified as rectal and treated as such.
2. Surgery for colorectal cancer should be performed only by appropriately trained surgeons whose workload volume permits meaningful audit.

Table 3.2 • Clinicopathological staging of colorectal cancer

Dukes' staging* (based on histological examination of the resection specimen)	
A	Invasive carcinoma not breaching the muscularis propria
B	Invasive carcinoma breaching the muscularis propria, but not involving regional lymph nodes
C1	Invasive carcinoma involving the regional lymph nodes (apical node negative)
C2	Invasive carcinoma involving the regional lymph nodes (apical node positive)
TNM staging[†]	
T	Primary tumour
TX	Primary tumour cannot be assessed
T0	No evidence of primary tumour
Tis	Carcinoma in situ
T1	Tumour invades submucosa
T2	Tumour invades muscularis propria
T3	Tumour invades through muscularis propria into subserosa or into non-peritonealised pericolic or perirectal tissues
T4	Tumour perforates the visceral peritoneum or directly invades other organs or structures[‡]
N	Regional lymph nodes
NX	Regional lymph nodes cannot be assessed
N0	No regional lymph node metastasis
N1	Metastasis in 1–3 pericolic or perirectal lymph nodes
N2	Metastasis in 4 or more pericolic or perirectal lymph nodes
M	Distant metastasis
M0	No distant metastases
M1	Distant metastases

* Dukes' stage D has come to mean the presence of distant metastases.
[†] UT, ultrasound depth; yT, following neoadjuvant therapy.
[‡] Direct invasion in T4 includes invasion of other segments of the colorectum by way of the serosa, e.g. invasion of the sigmoid colon by a carcinoma of the caecum.

Emergency treatment

1. Emergency surgery should be carried out during daytime hours as far as possible by experienced surgeons and anaesthetists.
2. In patients presenting with obstruction, steps should be taken to exclude pseudo-obstruction before operation.
3. Stoma formation should be carried out in the patient's interests only, and not as a result of lack of experienced surgical staff or appropriate stenting facilities.
4. The overall mortality for emergency/urgent surgery should be 20% or less.

Treatment of advanced disease

1. It is recommended that effective palliation with optimal quality of remaining life should be the main aim of therapy in advanced disease.

2. Consideration should be given to palliative chemotherapy in patients with local advanced and metastatic disease. Thus, patients with advanced disease who remain in good general condition should have the opportunity to discuss the possible benefits of palliative therapy with an oncologist.
3. Consideration should be given to surgical treatment in selected patients with locally advanced and metastatic disease. In particular, the patient with limited hepatic involvement should be considered for partial hepatectomy by an experienced liver surgeon.

Outcomes

Surgeons should carefully audit the outcome of their colorectal cancer surgery:

1. They should expect to achieve an operative mortality of less than 20% for emergency surgery and 5% for elective surgery for colorectal cancer.

2. Wound infection rates after surgery for colorectal cancer should be less than 10%.

3. Surgeons should expect to achieve an overall anastomotic leak rate below 4% for colonic resection.

4. Surgeons should examine carefully their practice with a view to meeting or improving on targets set by national long-term mortality statistics.

Pathology

All resected colorectal tumours should be submitted for histological examination. The report should reach an acceptable standard, providing information that will be useful in assessing prognosis, planning treatment and carrying out audit.

Key points

- It is now accepted that most if not all colon cancers arise from pre-existing adenomas and serrated polyps. Flat adenomas, which are difficult to detect without special endoscopic techniques, may be a significant precursor lesion.
- The main lifestyle factors that predispose to colorectal cancer are currently recognised as obesity, lack of exercise, red and processed meat, a low-fibre diet, alcohol and smoking.
- Colonoscopy is the gold standard investigative technique, but CT colonography is an adequate alternative. CT scanning is the optimal method of preoperative staging.
- Faecal occult blood (FOB) and flexible sigmoidoscopy screening can reduce colon cancer mortality, and both are currently available in the UK and in many other countries.
- The range of agents available for treating advanced disease is rapidly expanding and, although many will not be suitable, all patients with metastases should be considered for surgical treatment.

🌐 Full references available at **http://expertconsult. inkling.com**

Key references

9. World Cancer Research Fund. Food, nutrition, physical activity and the prevention of cancer; a global perspective. Washington, DC: AICR; 2007.
   This report lays out all the life-style-associated risk factors for all common cancers.

10. Giovannucci E. An updated review of the epidemiological evidence that cigarette smoking increases risk of colorectal cancer. Cancer Epidemiol Biomarkers Prev 2001;10:725–31. PMID: 11440957.

14. Scottish Intercollegiate Guidelines Network. SIGN 126 Diagnosis and management of colorectal cancer: a national clinical guideline. Health Improvement Scotland; 2015 Revised.
   Up-to-date evidence-based guideline on the management of colorectal cancer.

17. Mandel JS, Church TR, Ederer F, et al. Colorectal cancer mortality: effectiveness of biennial screening for fecal occult blood. J Natl Cancer Inst 1999;91:434–7. PMID: 10070942.
   These three randomised trials (references 17–19) provide evidence that disease-specific mortality can be reduced by faecal occult blood screening for colorectal cancer, and form the basis for current debates regarding the introduction of national screening programmes in several countries.

18. Hardcastle JD, Robinson MHE, Moss SM, et al. Randomised controlled trial of faecal occult blood screening for colorectal cancer. Lancet 1996;348: 1472–7. PMID: 8942775.
   These three randomised trials (references 17–19) provide evidence that disease-specific mortality can be reduced by faecal occult blood screening for colorectal cancer, and form the basis for current debates regarding the introduction of national screening programmes in several countries.

19. Kronborg O, Fenger C, Olsen J, et al. A randomized study of screening for colorectal cancer with fecal occult blood test at Funen in Denmark. Lancet 1996;348:1467–71. PMID: 8942774.
   These three randomised trials (references 17–19) provide evidence that disease-specific mortality can be reduced by faecal occult blood screening for colorectal cancer, and form the basis for current debates regarding the introduction of national screening programmes in several countries.

21. Atkin WS, Edwards R, Kralj-Hans I, et al. Once-only flexible sigmoidoscopy screening in prevention of colorectal cancer: a multicentre randomised controlled trial. Lancet 2010;375:1624–33. PMID: 20430429.
   Main evidence base for flexible sigmoidoscopy screening and first definitive evidence that polypectomy prevents colorectal cancer.

4

Colorectal cancer and genetics

Sue Clark
Andrew Latchford

Introduction

Individuals develop colorectal cancer as a result of interaction between their genotype and the environment to which they are exposed. The lifetime risk of colorectal cancer in the UK population is about 5%. As it is common, many people by chance alone have at least one affected relative;[1] as the number of affected relatives increases, so does the risk of developing the disease.[2] As far as genetic factors are concerned, there is a spectrum of risk: at one end are those with no particular genetic predisposition, and at the other those very rare individuals who will inevitably develop bowel cancer. Between the extremes lie those whose genetic constitution plays some role. While open to error, it is possible to divide the population into three broad categories of risk for colorectal cancer: low, moderate and high risk.

In the high-risk group, the contribution of inheritance (genotype) is overwhelming, though environmental influences may modify disease severity (phenotype). It is this minority (accounting for less than 5% of large-bowel cancer) that is traditionally described as being at risk of 'inherited bowel cancer'.

In the low- and moderate-risk groups, genotype may still contribute to risk but less markedly, and is thought to account for about 30% of colorectal cancer risk.[3] This may be due to low penetrance genes that influence dietary carcinogen metabolism, DNA repair and a variety of other functions.

This chapter deals predominantly with those in the high-risk group. Although these individuals comprise a minority of those at risk overall, there is sufficient knowledge about the specific syndromes that fall within this category to provide important opportunities for cancer prevention.

Assessment of risk

The crucial step in allocating individuals to one of these risk categories is the documentation of an accurate family history allowing an empirical assessment of risk.[2] It should focus on site and age at diagnosis of all cancers in family members, as well as the presence of related features such as colorectal adenomas. This can be time-consuming, especially when the information needs to be verified. Few surgeons are able to devote the necessary time or skill to do this, and it is here that family cancer clinics or registries for inherited bowel cancer have an important role.[4]

A full personal history should also be taken, focused on:

- symptoms (e.g. rectal bleeding, change in bowel habit), which should be investigated as usual;
- previous large-bowel polyps;
- previous large-bowel cancers;
- cancers at other sites;
- other risk factors for colorectal cancer (inflammatory bowel disease, ureterosigmoidostomy, acromegaly); these conditions are not discussed further in this chapter, but may warrant surveillance of the large bowel.

The family history has many limitations, particularly in small families. Other difficulties arise because of incorrect information or early death of individuals before they develop cancers. A vast range of complex pedigrees arise, and rather than try to devise guidelines to cover all of them, common sense is needed. If a family seems to fall between risk groups it is safest to manage the family as if in the higher-risk group. Despite this, some families will appear to be at high risk simply because of chance clustering of sporadic cancer while some, particularly small families with Lynch syndrome, will be assigned to the low- or moderate-risk groups. Even in families affected with an autosomal dominant condition, 50% of family members will not have inherited the causative mutation and will therefore not be at any increased risk of developing cancer.

Family histories evolve, so that the allocation of an individual to a particular risk group may change if further family members develop tumours. It is important that patients are informed of this, particularly if they are in the low- or moderate-risk groups and therefore not undergoing regular surveillance.

Low-risk group

Individuals in this group have:

1. no personal history of bowel cancer; and
2. no first-degree relative (i.e. parent, sibling or child) with bowel cancer; or
3. one first-degree relative with bowel cancer diagnosed at age 50 years or older.

Moderate-risk group

This has been divided into high- and lower-risk subgroups.

Low-moderate risk
This group comprises:

1. those with one affected first-degree relative diagnosed under 50 years; or
2. two affected first-degree relatives diagnosed at age 60 years or older.

High-moderate risk
This group comprises those with:

1. three or more affected relatives in a first-degree kinship (none under 50 years); or
2. two affected relatives diagnosed under 60 years (or with a mean age at diagnosis under 60 years) in a first-degree kinship.

High-risk group

This category encompasses Lynch syndrome and the various polyposis syndromes. Criteria for inclusion include:

1. member of a family with known familial adenomatous polyposis (FAP) or other polyposis syndrome; or
2. member of a family with known Lynch syndrome; or
3. pedigree suggestive of autosomal dominantly inherited colorectal (or other Lynch syndrome-associated) cancer; or
4. pedigree indicative of autosomal recessive inheritance, suggestive of MYH-associated polyposis (MAP).

Diagnosis of the polyposis syndromes is comparatively straightforward as there is a recognisable phenotype in each. Lynch syndrome is much more difficult as there is no such characteristic phenotype, other than the occurrence of cancers.

Management

Low-risk group

The risk of bowel cancer even in these individuals may be up to twice the average risk,[2] although this tends to be expressed after the sixth decade of life.

✔ There is no evidence to support invasive surveillance in this group.[5]

It is important to explain to these individuals that they are at only marginally increased risk of developing colorectal cancer, and that this risk is not sufficient to outweigh the disadvantages of colonoscopy. They should be aware of the symptoms of colorectal cancer, the importance of reporting if further members of the family develop tumours, and be encouraged to take part in population colorectal cancer screening.

Moderate-risk group

✔ There is a three- to sixfold relative risk for individuals in this category,[2] but probably only a marginal benefit from surveillance.[5]

Part of the reason for this is that the incidence of colorectal cancer is very low in the young and rises markedly in the elderly. Even those aged 50 who have a sixfold relative risk by virtue of their family history are less likely to develop colorectal cancer in the following 10 years than are 60-year-olds at average risk.[6]

✅ Current recommendations[5] are that individuals at high-moderate risk should be offered colonoscopy 5-yearly starting at 50 years of age; those in the low-moderate risk group should be offered a one-off colonoscopy age 55 years.

Again, these individuals should be informed of the symptoms of colorectal cancer, the importance of reporting changes in family history and that they should take part in population screening when they reach the appropriate age.

High-risk group

There is up to a 1 in 2 chance of inheriting a lifetime risk in excess of 50% of developing bowel cancer in this group, and referral to a clinical genetics service is essential. The polyposis syndromes are usually diagnosed from the phenotype, supplemented by genetic testing. Diagnostic confusion can arise, particularly in cases where there are adenomatous polyps insufficient to be diagnostic of FAP. This may occur in MAP, FAP with an attenuated phenotype, or Lynch syndrome. A careful search for extracolonic features, mismatch repair immunohistochemistry and microsatellite instability assessment of tumour tissue, and germline mutation detection can sometimes help. Despite this, the diagnosis in some families remains in doubt. In these circumstances the family members should be offered thorough surveillance.

Lynch syndrome

Lynch syndrome is inherited in an autosomal dominant fashion, is responsible for about 3% of colorectal cancers and is the commonest of the inherited bowel cancer syndromes, with current estimates that it occurs in up to 1:400 of the population. The terminology in this area is extremely confusing and has recently been revised.[7] Labelled first as the 'cancer family syndrome', the name was changed to hereditary non-polyposis colorectal cancer (HNPCC) to distinguish it from the polyposis syndromes and to highlight the absence of the large numbers of colorectal adenomas found in FAP. However, scanty adenomatous polyps are a feature of Lynch syndrome.

Various different diagnostic criteria have been used, including different definitions based on family history. Mutations in mismatch repair (MMR) genes were identified in some, but not all, families with an apparent dominantly inherited cancer syndrome. The term Lynch syndrome should be used where there is evidence of mismatch repair mutation. For those families where there is a strong family history fulfilling the Amsterdam criteria (see below), but MMR mutation has been excluded, the term 'familial colorectal cancer type X' should be used. HNPCC has been used to cover both of these groups but is largely obsolete.

Clinical features

Lynch syndrome is characterised by early onset of colorectal cancer, the average age at diagnosis being 45 years. These tumours have certain distinguishing pathological features. There is a predilection for the proximal colon, and tumours are frequently multiple (synchronous and metachronous). They tend to be mucinous, poorly differentiated and of 'signet-ring' appearance, with marked infiltration by lymphocytes and lymphoid aggregation at their margins. The associated cancers and their frequencies are detailed in Table 4.1.[8] The prognosis of these cancers tends to be better than in the same tumours arising sporadically.

Genetics

Lynch syndrome is due to germline mutations in MMR genes, whose role is to correct errors in basepair matching during replication of DNA or to initiate apoptosis when DNA damage is beyond repair. The vast majority of cases are due to mutations in the MMR genes *hMLH1*, *hMSH2*, *hMSH6*, *hPMS2*. Recently, transmissible epimutations in the non-MMR gene *EPCAM* have been identified as a cause of Lynch syndrome. Other MMR gene mutations (*hMLH3*, *hMSH3*, *hPMS1*) have been reported in some families with Lynch syndrome but their clinical significance is not established.

The MMR genes are tumour-suppressor genes: patients with Lynch syndrome inherit a defective copy from one parent and tumourigenesis is

Table 4.1 • Cancers associated with Lynch syndrome

Site	Frequency (%)
Large bowel	30–75
Endometrium	30–70 (of women)
Stomach	5–10
Ovary	5–10 (of women)
Urothelium (renal pelvis, ureter, bladder)	5
Other (small bowel, pancreas, brain)	<5

triggered when the solitary normal gene in a cell becomes mutated or lost, so that DNA mismatches are no longer repaired in that cell. Defective MMR results in the accumulation of mutations in a host of other genes, leading to tumour formation.

A hallmark of tumours with defective MMR is microsatellite instability (MSI). Microsatellites are regions where a short DNA sequence (up to five nucleotides) is repeated. There are large numbers of such sequences in the human genome, the majority in non-coding DNA. Base-pair mismatches occurring during DNA replication are normally repaired by the MMR proteins. In tumours with a deficiency of these proteins, this mechanism fails and microsatellites become mutated, resulting in a change in the number of sequence repeats and hence the length of the microsatellite (microsatellite instability). Typically in such a tumour over half of all microsatellites will exhibit this phenomenon.

About 15% of sporadic colorectal cancers show MSI. Most occur in older patients and are due to inactivation of the MMR gene *hMLH1* by promoter methylation, which is not, as far as we know, related to any inherited factor.

Diagnosis

Pedigree

Over the years a confusing range of 'criteria' have emerged. The International Collaborative Group on HNPCC (ICG-HNPCC) proposed the Amsterdam criteria in 1990. These were not intended as a diagnostic definition but rather to target genetic research by identifying families very likely to have a dominantly inherited cancer predisposition. The Amsterdam criteria were modified by the ICG-HNPCC in 1999 (Box 4.1) to include Lynch syndrome-associated cancers other than colorectal cancer (Amsterdam II criteria).[9] Subsequent studies have shown that approximately half the families that meet these criteria have Lynch syndrome (i.e. an MMR mutation is identified), and a similar proportion of individuals with Lynch syndrome come from families not meeting

these criteria (i.e. 50% of Lynch syndrome families do not meet the Amsterdam criteria).

Therefore although family history alone may be used to highlight high-risk families, it is insufficient to make a diagnosis of Lynch syndrome and a combination of tumour analysis and/or genetic testing is used in addition to family history to make the diagnosis.

Analysis of tumour tissue

A reference panel of five microsatellite markers is used to detect MSI; if two of the markers show instability, the tumour is designated 'MSI-high'. The value of MSI testing is that Lynch syndrome is due to MMR mutation and therefore virtually all colorectal cancers arising as a result of Lynch syndrome will be MSI-high. The Bethesda guidelines[10] (Box 4.2) were proposed to determine whether tumour tissue from an individual should be tested for MSI. The aim was to provide a sensitive set of guidelines that would encompass nearly all Lynch syndrome-associated colorectal cancers but also many 'sporadic cancers', and to use MSI testing to exclude those individuals lacking MSI-high, whose cancers are extremely unlikely to be caused by Lynch syndrome. Those designated MSI-high can then be further investigated using immunohistochemistry and genetic testing.

MSI testing is expensive and requires DNA extraction. A simpler approach is to use standard immunohistochemical techniques to identify MMR proteins.[11] This technique has the benefit of identifying the gene that is likely to be mutated and therefore can be used to direct further genetic testing. However, it is not 100% sensitive, particularly in benign adenomatous colonic polyps and endometrial cancer, and so care is needed in interpreting the results.

> ✅✅ NICE has recently recommended universal testing of new cases of colorectal cancer to screen for evidence of Lynch syndrome (https://www.nice.org.uk/guidance/DG27). This may be done by either MSI or MMR immunohistochemistry and their analysis shows this to be cost-effective.

Genetic testing

The decision whether to perform germline genetic testing on a blood sample from an at-risk or affected person takes the features of the patient, family and tumour into account. This cautious approach is currently justified on the grounds of cost, since genetic testing for MMR genes in the first member of the family (mutation detection) costs around £600. Once a mutation has been detected in a family, testing other at-risk family members to determine whether they too carry

Box 4.1 • Amsterdam criteria II

- At least three relatives with a Lynch syndrome-associated cancer (colorectal, endometrial, small bowel, ureter, renal pelvis), one of whom should be a first-degree relative of the other two
- At least two successive generations should be affected
- At least one cancer should be diagnosed before age 50 years
- FAP should be excluded
- Tumours should be verified by pathological examination

- Colorectal cancer diagnosed at age <50 years
- Multiple colorectal or other Lynch syndrome-associated tumours, either at the same time (synchronous) or occurring over a period of time (metachronous)
- Individuals diagnosed with colorectal cancer at <60 years, in whom the tumour has microscopic characteristics indicative of microsatellite instability;
- Individuals with colorectal cancer who have one or more first-degree relatives diagnosed with a Lynch syndrome-related tumour at age 50 years or younger
- Individuals with colorectal cancer who have two or more first- or second-degree relatives diagnosed with a Lynch syndrome-related tumour at any age

the abnormal gene (predictive testing) is much more straightforward, and allows those without the mutation to be discharged from further surveillance.

As with the other syndromes described in this chapter, testing should be undertaken only after the patient has been counselled appropriately and given informed consent. The consent process should include an offer to provide written information, including a frank discussion of the benefits and risks (e.g. to employment, insurance) of genetic testing. A multidisciplinary clinic where counselling is available is ideal.[12] However, not every individual will accept an offer of genetic testing. Significant predictors of test uptake by individuals include an increased perception of risk, greater confidence in the ability to cope with unfavourable genetic news, more frequent thoughts of cancer and having had at least one colonoscopy.[13]

Germline gene testing may have several outcomes (Box 4.3) and the results should be relayed via the multidisciplinary clinic, where counselling is available.[14] There are also complexities of interpretation of results that mandate this (missense mutations, genetic heterogeneity).[15] Unregulated genetic testing for cancer risk has led to errors and adverse outcomes for individuals. Failure to detect a mutation may be due to a variety of factors:

Box 4.3 • Outcomes of genetic testing

Mutation detected

Test at-risk family members (predictive testing): if positive, surveillance and/or other management (e.g. surgery); if negative, no surveillance required

Mutation not detected

Keep all at-risk members under surveillance

some cases may be due to mutation in regulatory genes rather than the MMR genes themselves; there may be other genes involved that have not yet been identified; there may be a technical failure to identify a mutation which is present; or the family history may be a cluster of sporadic tumours. When this happens, the at-risk family members should continue to be screened.

✅ Familial colorectal cancer type X, i.e. families meeting the Amsterdam criteria but with MSI-negative tumours, are at lower risk, so that 3- to 5-yearly colonoscopy is sufficient.[16]

Surveillance

✅✅ Colonoscopic surveillance reduces the risk of colorectal cancer in Lynch syndrome patients by 63%.[17]

Colonoscopy must be meticulous, because tiny cancers may be present[18] and interval cancers are common. Chromoendoscopy increases the pick up of neoplastic lesions in Lynch syndrome and is recommended.

✅ Colonoscopy every 1–2 years from age 25 years (or 5 years younger than the youngest affected relative, whichever is the earlier)[11] is recommended for Lynch syndrome. Surveillance should continue until about 75 years or until the causative mutation in that family has been excluded.[11]

Screening for extracolonic cancers is available, but there is currently little evidence of benefit. Recommendations vary from centre to centre, but surveillance is generally advised where there is a family history of cancers at a particular site. Box 4.4 shows the options for extracolonic surveillance.[11]

Box 4.4 • Extracolonic surveillance in Lynch syndrome

- Annual transvaginal ultrasound ± colour flow Doppler imaging ± endometrial sampling
- Annual CA125 level and clinical examination (pelvic and abdominal)
- Upper gastrointestinal endoscopy every 2 years
- Annual urinalysis/cytology
- Annual abdominal ultrasound of renal tracts, pelvis, pancreas
- Annual liver function tests, CA19–9, CEA

Intervention

Surgery

Prophylactic

The option of prophylactic colectomy rather than colonoscopic surveillance should be discussed with mutation carriers, because of the high risk of colorectal cancer. A similar situation pertains to prophylactic hysterectomy and bilateral salpingo-oophorectomy in women who have completed their families.

Colectomy might be subtotal, with an ileorectal anastomosis, or might take the form of a restorative proctocolectomy. The risk of metachronous cancer in the retained rectum after ileorectal anastomosis has been estimated to be about 12% at 12 years.[19] Regular endoscopy of residual large bowel should be carried out postoperatively, at intervals no greater than 12 months.

✔ Use of a decision analysis model indicates large gains in life expectancy for carriers of MMR mutation when offered some intervention. Benefits were quantified as 13.5 years from surveillance, 15.6 years from proctocolectomy and 15.3 years from subtotal colectomy compared with no intervention.[20] However, recognition that short (1- to 2-year) intervals between high-quality colonoscopies are needed for surveillance in Lynch syndrome, and that aspirin reduces cancer risk, means that there may be no advantages of prophylactic surgery over good-quality surveillance.

Adjusting for quality of life showed that surveillance led to the greatest quality-adjusted life expectancy benefit. This study provides a mathematically based indication of benefit only: individual circumstances need to be incorporated into the decision-making process when making recommendations.

Treatment

For those with colonic tumours, the main choice lies between segmental colectomy and colectomy with ileorectal anastomosis (IRA). Segmental resection leads to better function but an increased risk of metachronous cancers and need for full colonoscopic surveillance. Colectomy and IRA has a prophylactic element in that the entire colon is removed, but without the additional morbidity of proctectomy, reducing metachronous cancer risk; furthermore, ongoing surveillance is much easier and more acceptable. Proctocolectomy (with or without ileoanal pouch reconstruction) can be considered in patients who present with rectal cancer.

✔ There is a risk of metachronous bowel tumour of 16% after 10 years of follow-up.[21]

Medical

Studies of colorectal cancer cell lines deficient in MMR genes have shown that MSI is reduced in cells exposed to non-steroidal anti-inflammatory drugs (NSAIDs).[22]

✔✔ The CAPP2 (Colorectal Adenoma/Carcinoma Prevention Programme 2) study[23] was an RCT of aspirin and resistant starch as chemopreventive agents in Lynch syndrome. This study reported a significant reduction in colorectal cancer rates in those treated with 600 mg aspirin daily, and certainly draws into question the benefits of prophylactic or extended therapeutic large-bowel excision. CAPP3 is currently recruiting to help determine optimum dose and duration of treatment. Individuals with Lynch syndrome should be offered aspirin to reduce their cancer risk.

The benefit of adjuvant cytotoxic chemotherapy (notably 5-fluorouracil) for cancers in the setting of Lynch syndrome has been questioned.[11] This may be because some agents act by damaging DNA, which results in apoptosis. MMR proteins are thought to play a part in signalling the presence of irreversible DNA damage and initiating apoptosis, a pathway absent in these tumours. The current European Society for Medical Oncology guidelines suggest that the small (10%–15%) subset of patients with Dukes' B (stage II) tumours which have deficient MMR (due either to germline mutation [Lynch syndrome] or to inactivation by promoter methylation) are at a very low risk of recurrence and are unlikely to benefit from chemotherapy. They do not therefore recommend the use of adjuvant 5FU for those in this group whose tumour demonstrates poor prognostic features. There is no evidence that deficient MMR influences the benefit from oxaliplatin, therefore the Dukes' C (stage III) disease is treated using the same chemotherapy regimes as colorectal cancer with proficient MMR. Currently there is a great deal of interest in immunotherapy in the treatment of colorectal cancer with deficient MMR. Data regarding the use of checkpoint inhibitors are promising but they are not yet used in routine clinical practice.

Familial adenomatous polyposis

Less common than Lynch syndrome, the risk of colorectal cancer in patients with FAP is nearly 100%. FAP is usually characterised by:

- hundreds of colorectal adenomatous polyps at a young age (second or third decade of life) (**Fig. 4.1**);
- duodenal adenomatous polyps;

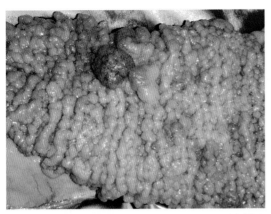

Figure 4.1 • Colectomy specimen from a patient with FAP.

Box 4.5 • Extracolonic manifestations in FAP

Ectodermal origin
- Epidermoid cysts
- Pilomatrixoma
- Tumours of central nervous system
- Congenital hypertrophy of the retinal pigment epithelium

Mesodermal origin
- Connective tissue: desmoid tumours, excessive adhesions
- Bone: osteoma, exostosis, sclerosis
- Dental: dentigerous cyst, odontoma, supernumerary teeth, unerupted teeth

Endodermal origin
- Adenomas and carcinomas of duodenum, stomach, small intestine, biliary tract, thyroid, adrenal cortex
- Fundic gland polyps
- Hepatoblastoma

- multiple extraintestinal manifestations (Box 4.5);
- mutation in the tumour-suppressor adenomatous polyposis coli (*APC*) gene on chromosome 5q;
- autosomal dominant inheritance (offspring of affected individuals have a 1 in 2 chance of inheriting FAP).

Diagnosis

FAP was originally defined by the presence of over 100 colorectal adenomas. This clinical definition is still useful, as a mutation in the *APC* gene can only be identified in up to 80% of affected individuals. The majority of new cases come from families with a known history of the disease, but confusion can arise as approximately 20% are due to a new mutation.[24] In these circumstances there will be no family history of colorectal cancers at a young age or of multiple polyps. Further potential sources of confusion are the recent discovery of MAP and the well-documented existence of attenuated FAP characterised by a relative paucity of polyps (10–100) and a later age of developing colorectal cancer.[25]

Inadequate colonoscopy may lead to a false diagnosis of attenuation, an error that can be avoided by the use of dye-spray (chromoendoscopy).[26] A further point that should be borne in mind is that some individuals with Lynch syndrome have a number of adenomatous polyps. Where the diagnosis requires confirmation, the use of dye-spray and random biopsies looking for microadenomas (a hallmark of FAP and MAP, but not seen in Lynch syndrome) are helpful, as are upper gastrointestinal (GI) endoscopy (up to 80% of FAP patients have gastric fundic gland polyps and the lifetime risk of duodenal adenomas is over 90%), and testing for MSI and immunohistochemistry of tumours.

Genetic testing

☑ The issue of genetic testing is a useful paradigm highlighting the fundamental role played by registries. Identification of at-risk family members who might be offered gene testing is critical and is usually made possible by the comprehensive collation of family pedigrees that such registries are uniquely positioned to obtain and update.

An uncontrolled approach to testing and the release of results can lead to inadequate counselling and the provision of incorrect information to patients.[27]

An affected family member should be tested first. The mutation can be located in approximately 80% of affected individuals. Once the mutation has been identified, at-risk members of the family can be offered simple blood testing. Should the known family mutation not be found in the at-risk individual, that person can be discharged from further surveillance[28] but should be informed that he or she remains at the same risk of sporadic colorectal cancer as any member of the general population. Such an approach eliminates unnecessary colonic examination and costs less than conventional clinical screening.[29]

Genotype–phenotype correlation

The site of the mutation in the *APC* gene can influence the expression of FAP.[30] Genotype–phenotype correlation is seen in the association between certain mutations and severe FAP (dense colorectal polyposis with relatively early colorectal cancer development), and between other mutations and less severe FAP ('attenuated' polyposis).[31] However, individuals with identical mutations can display differences in phenotypic expression, suggesting that other modifier genes and the environment play a role in disease expression.[32]

Some of the multiple extracolonic manifestations of FAP (see Box 4.5),[33] such as desmoid disease, also show some correlation with the mutation site; others, notably duodenal polyposis and malignancy, do not.

These genotype–phenotype correlations have led to suggestions that the findings of molecular analysis might guide both surveillance and treatment.[31,34,35] At present, however, it is important to emphasise that prophylactic colectomy or proctocolectomy (almost always with an ileoanal pouch) remain the management options of choice for the large bowel in all patients with proven FAP.

Surveillance

If the family mutation is known, at-risk family members are usually offered predictive genetic testing in their early teens. If this is not possible, then clinical surveillance is required. It is very unusual for significant colorectal polyps to develop before the teenage years and while cancers have been described in children, they are exceptionally rare. If an individual has symptoms attributable to the large bowel (anaemia, rectal bleeding or change in bowel habit), colonoscopy should be performed. Otherwise annual flexible sigmoidoscopy starting at 13–15 years of age is recommended. If no polyps are detected, 5-yearly colonoscopy should be started at the age of about 20 years, with annual flexible sigmoidoscopy in the intervening years. Decision-making regarding the age at which such surveillance can be stopped depends on the specific family history.

The large bowel

Surgery

Prophylactic

Once the diagnosis has been made, either by predictive genetic testing or by the detection of adenomatous polyposis during surveillance of an at-risk family member, the aim is to offer prophylactic surgery before a cancer develops. If the diagnosis has been made on the basis of flexible sigmoidoscopy, colonoscopy should be performed to assess the colonic polyp burden. If the individual is symptomatic or the polyps are dense or large, surgery should be undertaken as soon as is practicable. In other cases it is usual to defer surgery until a time when its social and educational impact will be minimised, usually a long summer vacation or 'gap' after leaving school.

As the surgical options have increased, so has the controversy surrounding the choice between them. Increasingly, laparoscopically assisted surgery is becoming available and has great attractions in this group, where a good cosmetic result makes surgery more acceptable. The available operations are:

- colectomy and ileorectal anastomosis (IRA);
- restorative proctocolectomy (RPC) with an ileal pouch–anal anastomosis;
- total proctocolectomy and end ileostomy (almost exclusively for those with very low rectal cancer).

Most young people facing prophylactic colectomy want to avoid a permanent ileostomy, so the choice really lies between the first two options. The biggest attraction of RPC is that the entire large bowel is removed, so that there is no risk of polyps or cancer developing in a retained rectum. However, a cuff of rectal mucosa is retained when a stapled anastomosis is performed, and cancers at this site have been reported.[36] A mucosectomy can be done to remove this area and a handsewn pouch anal anastomosis created, but this is a more technically demanding technique, which probably also results in poorer functional outcome, and does not fully protect against cancer, probably as a result of incomplete mucosectomy. Furthermore, follow-up studies have shown adenoma formation within ileoanal pouches[37] and the development of cancer has been reported.

The advantages of IRA are that it is a one-stage procedure (whereas RPC often involves a temporary defunctioning ileostomy) with lower morbidity and mortality.

✔ The functional results in terms of defaecatory frequency and leakage are generally slightly better after IRA than after RPC.[38]

Sexual and reproductive function can both be compromised by proctectomy. There is a small but definite risk of erectile and ejaculatory dysfunction in men undergoing proctectomy. In addition there is a pouch failure rate of about 10%, resulting in the need for a permanent ileostomy. These potential complications are particularly difficult to accept for essentially healthy young people undergoing surgery for prophylaxis rather than treatment.

✔ Recent studies have shown that RPC for both FAP[39] and ulcerative colitis adversely affects fertility in women.

It is known that some groups are at particular risk of developing rectal cancer after IRA. These are individuals with numerous rectal polyps and carriers of certain mutations (such as at codon 1309). Historical data show a cumulative rectal cancer risk of up to 30% by 60 years of age, but at the time many of these patients underwent IRA, RPC was not available. IRA was the only option to avoid a permanent ileostomy, and thus was done in circumstances when it would not now be recommended.

✔ In selected cases the risk of rectal cancer is low and IRA is a reasonable option.[40]

Many patients will have experience of one or both operations from other family members who have undergone them, which may affect their choice. Ultimately, they need to be informed about the advantages and disadvantages of both procedures, as well as the implications of their genotype (if identified) so that their decision can be as informed as possible.

Treatment

In the presence of a colonic cancer, the surgical decision-making is essentially the same as in prophylactic surgery. In individuals with severe rectal polyposis or in those carrying a mutation at codon 1309 of the *APC* gene, the risk of subsequent uncontrollable rectal polyposis requiring completion proctectomy, or of rectal cancer itself, are high and outweigh the disadvantages of RPC. In those with few rectal polyps, mutations at other sites and the few patients with a genuine attenuated phenotype, IRA may represent a better option. Ultimately, it remains for the informed patient to make a choice.

When rectal cancer is present, the choice is between RPC and proctocolectomy and ileostomy. As in any case of rectal cancer, a very low tumour precludes sphincter preservation. Careful local staging and multidisciplinary management are crucial in these cases.

Surveillance after surgery

Follow-up is required after all procedures. After IRA or RPC, per anal digital and flexible endoscopic examination are mandatory, at intervals of up to 12 months, depending on findings. The NSAID sulindac has been used to control rectal adenomas[41] and pouch adenomas.[42] There are, however, no robust published long-term data to support the use of NSAIDs and indeed there are reports of cancer despite NSAID 'chemoprevention' and surveillance in this setting. The selective cyclo-oxygenase (COX)-2 inhibitor celecoxib showed a moderate reduction in large-bowel polyps in treated patients[43] but no longer has a licence and can no longer be recommended in FAP. More recently the use of omega-3 fish oil supplements has been shown to have a similar beneficial effect to these NSAIDs in control of colorectal polyps[44] but again this was a short-term study and there are no long-term data on cancer prevention. Aspirin has not been shown to have a significant effect in reduction of polyp burden.[45] Following colectomy, the major causes of mortality and morbidity are duodenal cancers and desmoid tumours. This knowledge guides postoperative management.[46]

Upper gastrointestinal tract polyps

Non-adenomatous gastric polyps (fundic gland polyps) occur in up to 80% of patients with FAP. It is doubted whether these lesions have malignant potential, which at most is extremely low.[47] There are few data regarding gastric adenomas in FAP. There does appear to be an increased risk for these polyps in FAP, although this has not been well quantified. These may undergo malignant transformation but it is likely that they behave in a relatively indolent manner, as gastric cancer is not seen commonly in this patient group. There are no guidelines for the surveillance or management of gastric adenomas in FAP.

✔ Duodenal adenomas occur in nearly all patients with FAP but are severe in only 10%, with malignant change occurring in 5%.[48]

Surveillance of the upper gastrointestinal tract

Surveillance usually begins in the third decade of life (in the asymptomatic patient), with endoscopies at intervals of between 6 months and 5 years depending on the severity of duodenal polyposis.[49] A staging system for duodenal polyposis has been developed (Table 4.2) to allow surveillance to be tailored to disease severity and to identify individuals at high risk of developing malignancy.[50]

✔✔ Duodenal surveillance is beneficial. Duodenal cancer detected at surveillance endoscopy has a significantly improved overall survival compared to symptomatic cancers.[51]

The ampulla and periampullary area must be examined, being at particularly high risk, so a side-viewing as well as end-viewing scope should be used in the examination. If the ampulla is abnormal due to the development of an adenoma the frequency

Table 4.2 • Spigelman staging of severity of duodenal polyposis in FAP

	Points allocated		
	1	**2**	**3**
Number of polyps	1–4	5–20	>20
Polyp size (mm)	1–4	5–10	>10
Histological type	Tubular	Tubulovillous	Villous
Degree of dysplasia	Mild	Moderate	Severe
Total points	**Spigelman stage**	**Recommended follow-up interval**	
0	0	5 years	
1–4	I	5 years	
5–6	II	3 years	
7–8	III	1 year and consider endoscopic therapy	
9–12	IV	Consider prophylactic duodenectomy	

of endoscopic surveillance may need to be altered according to the severity of the ampullary disease.[52]

Management of duodenal polyposis

> ✔ Management of severe duodenal polyposis is difficult. No chemopreventive options are available and endoscopic therapy does not have robust data to support its use.

Open duodenotomy and polypectomy is associated with high recurrence rates and is not recommended.[53] The role of advanced endoscopic techniques, often under general anaesthesia, is not established but may be used to manage those with more severe disease and delay the need for definitive surgery.

While prophylactic pancreatico-duodenectomy or pylorus-preserving pancreatico-duodenectomy has been described with good outcomes, associated morbidity and mortality are substantial.[54] However, the poor prognosis once invasive disease is present and the high rate of progression to cancer of advanced polyposis (36% over 10 years in one series) mean that this aggressive approach can be justified in some cases with Spigelman stage IV disease. Cancer risk and hence the need for intervention is minimal in patients with stage 0–II disease.

Desmoid tumours

Desmoid tumours are fibromatous lesions consisting of clonal proliferations of myofibroblasts (**Fig. 4.2**). They occur in approximately 15% of individuals with FAP, with a mortality rate of about 10%.[55] Most exhibit cycles of growth and resolution and, while causing discomfort and being unsightly, may not cause

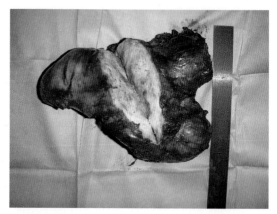

Figure 4.2 • A desmoid tumour excised from the abdominal wall.

significant problems. Most desmoids associated with FAP arise either intra-abdominally (usually within the small-bowel mesentery) or on the abdominal wall, although they can appear in the extremities and trunk. They are histologically benign, but within the abdomen can cause small-bowel and ureteric obstruction, intestinal ischaemia or perforation, all of which can be fatal. A model of desmoid tumour development, based on the appearance of a precursor plaque-like lesion, has been proposed, offering a possibility for prevention or early treatment.[56]

The aetiology of desmoid tumours is multifactorial, with contributions from trauma (e.g. operative), oestrogens, specific *APC* gene mutations and modifier genes.

Management

The challenge in the management of these bizarre tumours is to identify the minority that are rapidly and relentlessly progressive, and to avoid harming patients with unnecessarily aggressive attempts to treat the rest. Ureteric obstruction is not infrequent, and as the consequences can be obviated by ureteric stenting it is wise to perform regular renal tract imaging in patients otherwise being managed non-operatively every 6–12 months.

Computed tomography (CT) provides the best imaging with respect to size and relationship to surrounding structures, but T2-weighted magnetic resonance imaging (MRI) sequences may provide useful information about cellularity and growth potential. Ultrasound can be used to monitor the ureters.

✔ Treatment options include NSAIDs, antioestrogens, surgical excision and cytotoxic chemotherapy.[57]

Anecdotal successes with a variety of NSAIDs and antioestrogens abound (e.g. sulindac 150–200 mg twice daily alone or in combination with a high-dose antioestrogen such as raloxifene 120 mg daily), although good evidence of efficacy is lacking. Evaluation of these treatments is further hampered by the natural history of desmoids, which have been documented to regress spontaneously and exhibit relentless growth in only a small minority of patients.

✔ Evidence[55] supports the use of surgery as first-line treatment for abdominal wall and extra-abdominal desmoids, although the recurrence rate is high.

There is no evidence to support the concern that recurrence might be increased by the use of prosthetic materials to repair any resulting defect. Historical evidence of significant morbidity and mortality has led to the recommendation that surgery should usually be avoided where possible for intra-abdominal desmoids. If such surgery is required, because of progressive disease or desmoid-related complications, then careful patient selection and a referral to a specialist centre may lead to good outcomes with low morbidity and mortality, although recurrence remains a problem.[58]

MYH-associated polyposis (MAP)

Study of patients with the phenotype of FAP but no identifiable *APC* mutation has led to the discovery of this form of adenomatous polyposis, which has considerable clinical overlap with FAP, but is genetically distinct.[59]

Clinical features

The large bowel

As in FAP, the most consistent feature of MAP is the development of colorectal adenomas and carcinomas. The number of polyps is very variable,[60] with about half the patients in one series having a phenotype consistent with classical FAP (hundreds of polyps) and half having an attenuated phenotype with fewer than 100 polyps. Some cases of cancer have been reported in individuals with a definite genetic diagnosis of MAP, but very few polyps indeed, and the lifetime risk of colorectal cancer is almost 100% by the age of 60. The distribution differs from FAP in that there is a greater proportion of right-sided cancers, which also develop slightly later, at an average of 47 years.

The upper gastrointestinal tract

Duodenal adenomas are seen in MAP but they seem to be less of a clinical problem than in FAP, with a later onset and the suggestion of different disease pattern to FAP.[61] Gastric fundic gland polyps and duodenal adenomas occur in MAP, but less commonly, with 20–30% having duodenal polyps.[61]

Other manifestations

It has been suggested that there is an increased frequency of breast cancer in MAP, up to 18% in one series.[62] Osteomas and dental cysts have also been documented. To date no MAP patient with desmoid has been reported.

Genetics

This condition is due to biallelic mutation of the MutY human homologue (*MYH*) gene on chromosome 1p. Thus, for the first time, autosomal recessive inheritance has been described in the context of inherited bowel cancer. The frequency of mutation carriage (heterozygosity) in the general population may be as high as 1 in 200, but individuals who are heterozygotes appear to be at most only at minimally increased risk of colorectal cancer.

Genetic testing is available, and should be considered in individuals with a clinical diagnosis of FAP, but no detectable *APC* mutation, as well as patients presenting with fewer adenomas. The recessive inheritance means that there will often be no family history of colorectal cancer or polyps. This mode of inheritance also poses challenges in terms of genetic counselling and family testing strategies.

Management

The management of an affected individual is essentially the same as for FAP, although as a higher proportion has an attenuated phenotype, and the age of onset may be a little later, it may be that more patients can be managed, at least initially, by annual colonoscopy and polypectomy. Upper gastrointestinal tract surveillance is started at around the age of 25.

There is insufficient evidence currently to support breast screening, but female patients should be informed of the potentially increased risk. Breast self-examination and participation in population-based breast cancer screening should be encouraged.

The lifetime risk of a heterozygote carrier developing colorectal cancer has not yet been fully clarified, but studies to date indicate that any increase in risk is modest (in the range 1.5–2 times). Thus surveillance is not currently recommended.

Peutz–Jeghers syndrome

Peutz–Jeghers syndrome (PJS) is an autosomal dominant condition characterised by mucocutaneous pigmentation (**Fig. 4.3**) together with multiple gastrointestinal hamartomatous polyps. The gene responsible in some patients is *STK11* (*LKB1*) on chromosome 19p13, although there is evidence of genetic heterogeneity as mutation at this site has been excluded in some families.

A 78-year follow-up of the original family described by Peutz is instructive.[63] Survival of affected family members was found to be reduced as a result of bowel obstruction and the development of a range of cancers.

Bowel obstruction

The commonest polyp-related complication is small-bowel obstruction, often caused by intussusception

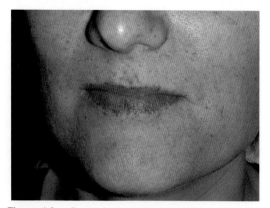

Figure 4.3 • Peutz–Jeghers pigmentation.

with a polyp at the apex. Repeated episodes result in increasingly difficult laparotomies and loss of bowel length.

> ✅ The incidence of subsequent small-bowel obstruction can be reduced by adequate intraoperative small-bowel enteroscopy, allowing identification and removal of all polyps at the time of initial laparotomy.[64]

Cancer risk

Individuals with PJS are at significantly increased risk of gastrointestinal malignancy, although the risk has not been well defined. Other areas at increased risk include the breasts (female), ovaries, cervix, pancreas and testes.[65]

Surveillance and management

Up-to-date surveillance protocols are best obtained from local registries. Most involve annual review with physical examination and measurement of haemoglobin. Upper and lower gastrointestinal endoscopies (with polypectomy) and capsule endoscopy or MRI enterography are performed every 2–3 years. Endoscopic surveillance and polypectomy may reduce the risk of cancer development but further data are required.[66] Surveillance also identifies polyps that may become symptomatic; if large polyps are seen in the small bowel or symptoms suggesting intermittent small bowel obstruction occur, or if there are small-bowel polyps with anaemia, a double-balloon enteroscopy or laparotomy with intraoperative enteroscopy and polypectomy is recommended to clear the small bowel of polyps and prevent frank obstruction.

As far as malignancy at other sites is concerned, where surveillance programmes have been shown to be useful in the general population they should be used. Breast surveillance has been recommended due to the very high risk of breast cancer and PJS has been included in the conditions for which breast cancer surveillance is recommended by NICE. Patients with PJS should be referred to their local breast screening centre.[67] There is currently no evidence to support ovarian or pancreatic surveillance in PJS.[67,68]

Juvenile polyposis

Not to be confused with the finding of an isolated juvenile polyp (which has very low, if any, malignant potential), juvenile polyposis is an autosomal dominant condition where multiple characteristic hamartomatous juvenile polyps occur, mostly in the colon but also in the upper gastrointestinal tract. Some affected individuals harbour germline mutations in the *SMAD4* gene,[67] (some of whom also have hereditary haemorrhagic telangiectasia) while others have germline mutations in the *BMPR1A* gene.

There is a risk of colorectal cancer approaching 40% and an increased risk of gastric cancer, particularly in those with an *SMAD4* germline mutation. Regular endoscopic screening,[69] by OGD and colonoscopy, with polypectomy for large polyps, is mandatory. Occasionally prophylactic colectomy or gastrectomy is required.

Serrated polyposis syndrome

Serrated polyposis syndrome (SPS) is being diagnosed increasingly commonly. It is thought that there is a genetic component to SPS, but it has not been identified. Certainly there are some families with SPS which display an autosomal dominant pattern of inheritance. In addition it is established that first-degree relatives of an individual with SPS have an increased risk of colorectal cancer.[70] Most patients can be managed endoscopically.[71] The British Society of Gastroenterology has recently produced a position statement with guidelines covering diagnosis, endoscopic management and surgery.[72] There are few data about surgery in SPS. The choice of operation will be determined by the colonic phenotype but in the prophylactic setting IRA is likely to be the operation of choice and there seems little rationale to consider RPC. In the setting of cancer, the extent of the resection will be in part determined by the density and distribution of the polyp burden as well as the

site of the cancer, whilst also taking into account the age and comorbidity of the patient and the likely functional outcome from surgery.

Other inherited colorectal cancer syndromes

There are a number of extremely rare syndromes where the phenotype and cancer risk are still being defined, but for which surveillance is recommended. The patients with these conditions are best referred to a specialist unit.

Cowden's syndrome, caused by mutations in the *PTEN* gene, consists of gastrointestinal hamartomas and cancers, together with a high risk of cancer of the breast, thyroid, endometrium and cervix, benign fibrocystic breast disease, non-toxic goitre and varied benign mucocutaneous lesions, particularly trichilemmomas. Targeted screening seems sensible, but there is little evidence to support it.

Molecular pathways of colorectal cancer development

It has long been known that colorectal cancer develops through the adenoma–carcinoma sequence, with accompanying accumulation of genetic changes, in a process of evolution. It has become clear that there are actually several alternative pathways (**Fig. 4.4**), something that was first identified by studying the cancers arising in Lynch syndrome. While the study of cancers arising in the inherited

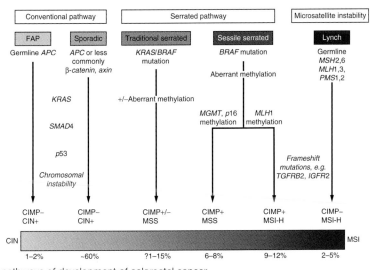

Figure 4.4 • The pathways of development of colorectal cancer.
Modified from East JE, Atkin WS, Bateman AC, et al. British Society of Gastroenterology position statement on serrated polyps in the colon and rectum. Gut 2017;66:1181–96, with permission.

syndromes has highlighted these different pathways, an appreciation and understanding of the differences between them is becoming increasingly important in managing all patients with colorectal cancer.

Summary

The emerging complexity of the relationship between genetics and bowel cancer, coupled with rapid advances in knowledge, reinforce the need for the availability of experienced, informed and up-to-date opinion in the areas of diagnosis and management. Individual surgeons will rarely be able to meet all of these needs. Patients and their families are best served by the existence of good working relationships between managing clinicians, family cancer clinics and registries based in expert centres.

Key points

- Genetic factors make a significant contribution to colorectal cancer.
- High-risk families should be referred to specialised registries, genetics units or clinical groups.
- Lynch syndrome and FAP are the commonest autosomal dominant high-risk conditions.
- In the UK, NICE has recommended that all colorectal cancers are tested for mismatch repair function using MMR immunohistochemistry or tumour DNA microsatellite instability assessment, to identify patients with Lynch syndrome.
- An understanding of these conditions is required to recognise and diagnose them.
- Individuals with these conditions are at risk of a range of extracolonic tumours, so need specialised follow-up.

Full references available at **http://expertconsult. inkling.com**

Key references

17. Jarvinen HJ, Aarnio M, Mustonen H, et al. Controlled 15-year trial on screening for colorectal cancer in families with hereditary nonpolyposis colorectal cancer. Gastroenterology 2000;118:829–34. PMID: 10784581.

A prospective controlled trial showing that colonoscopic surveillance in Lynch syndrome led to a 63% reduction in colorectal cancer and a significant decrease in mortality.

23. Burn J., Gerdes A.M., Macrae F., et al. Long-term effect of aspirin on cancer risk in carriers of hereditary colorectal cancer: an analysis from the CAPP2 randomised controlled trial. Lancet 2011;378:2081–7. PMID: 22036019.

A prospective, randomised trial whose primary endpoint was colorectal cancer development in patients with Lynch syndrome. It showed that taking 600 mg aspirin for 25 months signicantly reduced risk of both colorectal and all Lynch syndrome-associated cancers after 55 months.

51. Bulow S, Christensen IJ, Hojen H, et al. Duodenal surveillance improves the prognosis after duodenal cancer in familial adenomatous polyposis. Colorectal Dis 2012;14:947–52. PMID: 21973191.

A series of 304 patients from a previous study were followed up. This is the first study to show a survival benefit from surveillance of the duodenum in FAP. Survival after a surveillance-detected cancer was significantly better than after a symptomatic cancer (8 years vs 0.8 years; $P < 0.0001$).

5

Surgery for colon cancer

Robin Kennedy

The development of enhanced recovery after surgery (ERAS) protocols,[1] introduction of laparoscopic surgery and increased focus on careful assessment of outcomes have resulted in significant recent change in surgery for colon cancer.

Preparation of the patient for elective surgery

General issues

Prior to admission, reversible risk factors should be identified and treated to optimise fitness and improve outcomes. When there is significant likelihood of ischaemic heart disease preoperative functional testing is necessary to establish the level of risk, and it should be treated if necessary. The disease, planned treatment, risk of death and complications, should be discussed and a written summary provided to enable informed consent.

Before elective surgery in the author's practice all colonic cancers will have been biopsied endoscopically to confirm histology and their location defined by injection of India ink (a suggested tattoo protocol is shown in Chapter 2). Staging CT scanning of the thorax and abdomen with intravenous contrast will have been undertaken and synchronous cancer excluded using colonoscopy or CT colonography.

Bowel preparation

Mechanical bowel preparation (MBP) may be poorly tolerated, ineffective and has adverse consequences due to dehydration, particularly in the elderly. A Cochrane review in 2011 did not find significant benefit from it in terms of anastomotic leakage, re-operation or wound infection[2] and recommended avoidance of MBP in elective colectomy patients. Anastomotic leakage is, however, a devastating complication and construction of an upstream, defunctioning stoma will decrease it and should be considered in high-risk and emergency patients.[1,3] In view of this, MBP is generally used if a stoma is planned, in order to reduce the amount of faecal material between the stoma and anastomosis. Whether MBP is necessary to gain benefit from an upstream stoma in this situation, rather than merely diversion of gas, is debatable and needs clarification by randomised trial (RCT).

Venous thromboembolism prophylaxis

Venous thromboembolism (VTE) after colorectal surgery is a risk which increases with malignancy, prior pelvic surgery, preoperative corticosteroid use, significant comorbidity and hypercoagulability.[1] Graduated compression stockings and subcutaneous low molecular weight heparin are recommended prophylaxis. Although fatal pulmonary embolism has been reported in 0.5–1% of patients after colorectal resection, the benefits seen from laparoscopy and ERAS care now make this a rare event. It is therefore doubtful that continuing subcutaneous prophylaxis after discharge is necessary, except when there has been a prolonged stay due to complications.[1]

Blood transfusion

Transfusion is required for elective surgery only when oxygen delivery becomes compromised due to anaemia. A haemoglobin level of 70–80 g/L is considered the trigger for this, as a restrictive approach is most appropriate.[4] The three determinants of oxygen delivery are cardiac output (which in turn depends on stroke volume and heart rate), oxygen saturation and haemoglobin concentration. Thus in patients who cannot increase oxygen delivery, such as those with ischaemic heart disease, or who are symptomatic from anaemia, it is appropriate to transfuse at a higher level of haemoglobin (e.g. 80–90 g/L). Preoperative oral iron therapy should also be used to optimise functional status prior to surgery. In our practice the vast majority of elective patients do not have blood cross-matched, but have a sample saved for urgent cross-matching if necessary.

Antibiotic prophylaxis

Antibiotics should be administered routinely 30–60 minutes prior to commencing surgery as there is good evidence that this reduces the incidence of wound infection.[1] Additional doses of the drugs may be given during a particularly long procedure, but repeated postoperative administration is only necessary when there has been significant contamination.

The principles of surgery

The primary aim of cancer surgery should be to optimise oncological outcome, while providing the best possible short- and long-term recovery. On occasions, the radicality of surgery may need to be balanced against compromising recovery, but in the vast majority of patients this is not the case. Optimal outcome requires complete local removal of the tumour with its associated lymphovascular package and any contiguous organ involvement – this has become known as complete mesocolic excision (CME).

The term CME was introduced in 2009 by Hohenberger[5] and embodies three principles:

1. Dissection in the embryologically defined mesocolic plane.
2. Central ligation of the vascular pedicle (CVL).
3. Resection of an adequate length of colon on either side of the tumour.

Hohenberger reported impressive results from Ehrlangen with cancer-related 5-year survival of 89.1% after resection in stage I–III patients.[5]

Cancer-related survival (CRS) is defined as survival from postoperative death, whether from recurrence or postoperative complications, including re-operation. In the same centre, patients operated between 2003 and 2009 had an overall survival (OS) of 78% after curative resection[6] and CRS of 90.6%. The outcomes reported from this relatively wealthy area of Southern Germany are reproducible, with similar data coming from Australia.[7]

CME aims to include all the mesentery and potentially involved lymph nodes associated with the colonic cancer, thus reducing the chance of leaving disease. It is analogous to total mesorectal excision (TME), in which minimising residual local disease reduces local recurrence and improves outcome.

The evidence for CME

As there is debate regarding the utility of CME and the relative contributions to cure of the different elements, a brief review of the literature on the three principles of CME will be presented to guide surgeons.

Dissection in the mesocolic plane

Various authors have stressed the importance of specimen quality, but it was West and Quirke[8] who first presented robust evidence that dissection within the mesocolic plane is associated with improved survival. In univariate analysis of cohort data this approach improved 5-year survival by 15%. In multivariate analysis the differences were only significant in stage III patients, conferring a 27% improvement in survival.

These authors suggested the following: 'poor quality muscularis plane surgery, in which one or more large defects are seen in the mesocolon going down on to the muscle layer, might not remove the entire primary tumour and disrupts the lymphatic and vascular drainage, potentially resulting in a poor outcome'.[8] Dissection in the mesocolic plane is a key element in improving oncological outcome.

Central vascular ligation

The difficulty faced by the surgeon is in understanding what the different components of CME contribute to oncological outcome and whether CVL confers increased perioperative risk in certain situations. One might accept that dissection within the mesocolic plane should be relatively straightforward and therefore applied universally, but what is the evidence for taking vessels close to their origin? CVL is known as 'D3 resection' and removes N3 nodes – also known as main, central, or apical nodes. **Figure 5.1** demonstrates this schematically, distinguishing it from a D1 resection, which removes just pericolic nodes. In contrast, a D2

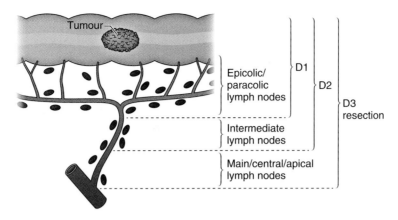

Figure 5.1 • Description of D1, D2 and D3 resection depending on the level of nodal dissection.

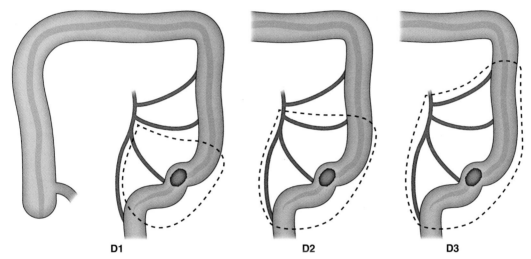

Figure 5.2 • Examples of D1, D2 and D3 resections for sigmoid cancer.

resection includes both pericolic and intermediate nodes (see **Fig. 5.2**).

There is some evidence supporting D3 resection of central nodes, versus D2 resection of intermediate and pericolic nodes. Kanemitsu[9] reported D3 right hemicolectomy in 370 consecutive patients and identified metastases in main nodes in 3% (11/370). The 5-year survival in the D3-positive patients was 36%, suggesting D3 resection would benefit only approximately 1% of all patients (⅓ of 3%).

In the publication by Kotake[10] from a multi-institutional database, the incidence of metastases in D3 nodes was also small at 4.9% and the 5-year survival of these patients was similar at 37%, excision of these nodes theoretically benefiting less than 2% (37% of 4.9%) of the total population. However, when the data from Kotake's collaborative group were examined in a multivariate analysis, in

6580 patients in whom D3 dissection was performed for T3 or T4 disease there was an 18% reduction in death by comparison with D2 resection. The data demonstrated that the survival benefit occurred in node-positive as well as node-negative patients and the authors concluded that it might have been secondary to the removal of undetected micro-metastatic disease within the mesentery, as well as resection of positive nodes. When micrometastases (tumour deposits <2 mm in diameter) and isolated tumour cells (<0.2 mm diameter) are identified in specimens that would otherwise be classified as stage I or II, the patient's prognosis worsens.[11,12] Since we know from the calculations above that resection of D3 nodes themselves improves survival by less than 2%, Kotake's reported improvement in survival of 18% after D3 resection should perhaps be interpreted as emphasising the importance of accurate mesocolic plane dissection, rather than the relatively small potential benefit from origin ligation. In contrast to the oncological benefit of D3 dissection in T3 and T4 disease, there was no benefit from D3 dissection in T2 disease when the same authors examined that with the same methodology.[13]

A difficulty confronted by the surgeon is accurate prediction of the T stage in order to undertake the most appropriate operation. One approach is to perform D3 resection as the default procedure unless there are particular circumstances making it inappropriate (e.g. the patient's comorbidity combined with a low chance of positive D3 nodes). Currently most surgeons rely on CT scanning for preoperative T staging and that has limited accuracy. This situation is likely to continue unless preoperative endoluminal ultrasound for T staging increases.

Lymphatic drainage may vary due to vascular variations and/or fusion of mesocolic and omental planes in the transverse colon. Lymph nodes are positive in the sub-pyloric area in 1.1–3.8% of patients with ascending or transverse colon cancer.[12] In addition, nodes along the gastroepiploic vessels may be involved in 4% of such tumours. Where nodes are clearly involved, resection with a view to cure should be attempted. However, in the author's practice removal of gastroepiploic nodes is undertaken only when their involvement is likely.

The concept of tumour cells missing certain nodes on their centripetal journey is known as 'skip' metastasis. This seems to occur in 1–2% of patients[12,14] and in the study by Tan[14] it was an isolated N3 node in 0.7%. 'Flush' ligation of the inferior mesenteric artery (IMA) on the aorta is often described, but unless N3 nodes dictate, ligation 1 cm from the origin of the IMA is preferred in order to avoid damage to the hypogastric plexus, thus minimising urinary and sexual dysfunction. Similarly, damage to autonomic nerves on the superior mesenteric artery (SMA) may result in severe diarrhoea. Although some authors[5] prefer to dissect the ileocolic artery to its origin on the SMA by displacing bowel and mesentery fully to the left and upwards, Japanese data[12] have suggested lymphatic drainage from the right colon is limited to the front of the SMV and resection behind the vein is not recommended.

The extent of longitudinal resection

The last element of CME is resection of an adequate length of bowel. An excellent consensus review[12] summarised this. Lymphatic flow is towards the nearest feeding or main vessel. Guidance from the Japanese Society for Cancer of the Colon and Rectum[15] is that when the lesion has a clear main vessel the resection does not need to proceed more than 5 cm past that main vessel, or 10 cm past the tumour in the opposite direction.[12] When a tumour is directly opposite a main vessel then resection 10 cm away from the tumour on either side will suffice. Should the tumour be equidistant between two vessels, resection 5 cm lateral to each vessel is necessary (**Fig. 5.3a**).

These guidelines appear simple, but surgeons should be aware that certain authors have suggested[16,17] that nodal positivity may occur in areas not being resected, despite following such guidelines. For example, in the Korean study[16] by Park, 6% of patients with caecal cancer had nodal metastases located adjacent to the right branch of the middle colic artery. Similarly, 20% of patients with hepatic flexure tumours were reported to have positive nodes along the left branch of the middle colic artery and 8% at the origin of the middle colic.

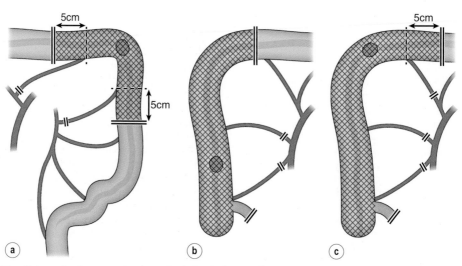

Figure 5.3 • Schematic diagrams showing extent of colonic resection recommended for different tumour sites.

The data from Park were from a population in which nodal metastases were more frequent than currently in Western literature. Nodal metastases were present in 44.2% of Park's population, as opposed to 32% in Hohenberger's most recent publication.[6] As the frequency of positive nodes reduces, as is occurring with earlier diagnosis, then the need for a more extensive D3 resection (as opposed to a standard D3 resection) decreases. There is little doubt that more detailed pathological analysis of nodal status is required in cancer of the colon in order to clarify what benefit derives from more extensive surgery.

The Japanese guidelines are specific and potentially retain more colon than is normal in Western practice. Hohenberger's recommendations are relatively radical by comparison, recommending removal of the transverse colon for tumours of either colonic flexure.[5] When nodal disease would not otherwise be resected, this radicality is appropriate and increases the chance of cure. The presence of residual disease, at the tumour margin or in nodes, should be regarded as predicting treatment failure and be avoided whenever possible. However, radical surgery has to be balanced against the potential for morbidity arising from resection of N3 nodes close to major vessels, and more extensive bowel resections requiring longer operations and resulting in more complications.

In an important study undertaken in Copenhagen, patients underwent either CME or more traditional surgery.[18] The CME group had more extended resections than in the non-CME group (17.4% vs 3.6%). Intraoperative organ injuries were more common in the CME group (9.1% vs 3.6%, P <0.001) with rates of postoperative sepsis and certain complications being significantly higher,[19] possibly reflecting a development phase. These data highlight the issues when taking on CME, but with appropriate training and experience it should be possible to perform CME without excess morbidity. It is, however, important for the surgeon to be aware what oncological value derives from different components of an intervention, in order to weigh that against the potential morbidity.

✅ Colonic cancer resection should proceed within the mesocolic plane in order to improve cancer outcomes. The specimen should include intermediate lymph nodes as this confers most of the oncological benefit from nodal resection. When a surgeon is confident to perform CVL without morbidity, inclusion of main nodes should improve results.

A randomised trial examining the extent of surgery would be welcome but may not occur due to problems with the size of such a study and surgical equipoise. However, the population study from Copenhagen mentioned above examined results following CME in one hospital, comparing them to outcomes from the other three hospitals where CME was not routinely performed.[18] Surgeons were trained to undertake CME and results were examined over a 3½-year period starting in 2008. Pathologists were also trained in the CME hospital to more accurately stage specimens. After propensity score matching, disease-free survival was significantly higher following CME, irrespective of stage, with 4-year disease-free survival of 85.8% (95% CI 81.4–90.1) after CME and 73.4% (66.2–80.6) after non-CME surgery (log rank $P=0.0014$). This finding is important as the phenomenon of stage migration will explain a within-stage improvement in survival associated with the correct categorisation of stage I–III patients. It will not, however, result in improved survival of the total group as identified in this research. Further research is necessary regarding the relative contributions of different components of CME to the oncological outcome.

Practical guidance on the extent of resection

The author's preference is to perform right hemicolectomy for any tumour involving the caecum, right colon or right transverse colon (Figs 5.3b, 5.3c) (see Recommended Videos 1 and 2). The ileocolic vein is transected at its junction with the superior mesenteric vein, or within 1 cm of that, and the accompanying artery at the same site. The right colic artery with or without the right branch of the middle colic artery is divided close to, or at its origin.

Transverse colectomy is performed when the Japanese guidelines on the extent of longitudinal resection[12,15] cannot be fulfilled by either right hemicolectomy or segmental left colectomy. In this situation the middle colic artery is transected at its origin, preserving the rest of the colon. Although extended right hemicolectomy has been advocated for transverse colon cancer by many, it is a more difficult operation that is likely to be accompanied by greater morbidity[20] than more limited resections.

When a tumour is present at the splenic flexure a 'segmental left colectomy' (see Recommended Video 3) is undertaken, dividing the origin of the left branch of the middle colic artery and that of the ascending left colic vessel (Fig. 5.3a). All nodal tissue is also dissected from the left aspect of the middle colic artery and the left side of the inferior mesenteric artery. Five centimetres of bowel away from the lesion on the other side of each vessel is included in the resection. This is satisfactory from an oncological perspective and is preferred to an extended right hemicolectomy as function is preserved.

In virtually all patients with left colon cancer distal to the ascending left colic artery, a left hemicolectomy (see Recommended Video 4) will be performed with CVL and anastomosis of the proximal descending colon to the rectum at 15 cm from the anal verge. This routinely involves mobilisation of the splenic flexure, including the left half of the transverse colon, with division of the inferior mesenteric vein at the inferior border of the pancreas to allow anastomosis to the rectum without tension. In the very rare circumstance that there is a large descending left colic artery arising from the middle colic it is preserved, as division of this vessel may result in ischaemia of the distal colon. In distal sigmoid cancer, resection is performed as described above for left hemicolectomy, but taking 5 cm distal to the cancer and performing an anastomosis to the rectum.

Radicality of surgery may be modified when there is a stage I cancer of the distal half of the sigmoid colon. In this situation the author may sometimes preserve bowel by dividing the blood supply immediately distal to the ascending left colic artery, providing there is a long enough sigmoid colon to allow anastomosis without tension between the proximal sigmoid and rectum, at 15 cm or less from the anal verge. There are clear limitations to accurate preoperative diagnosis of T stage, as described above, thus this more limited resection is performed rarely.

Laparoscopic or open surgery?

Although laparoscopic colorectal resection was reported first in 1991[21] it was used by a minority of surgeons for many years due to the challenges posed by the acquisition of technical competence and early reports of recurrence at port sites.[22] In 2004 and 2005 a number of large multicentre trials[23,24] completed recruitment and demonstrated equivalent oncological outcomes when laparoscopic resection of cancer was compared to conventional open surgery. There had been encouraging reports of improvements in postoperative recovery when laparoscopic resection was possible.[25,26]

Perioperative care was transformed in early 2000 by publications from Henrik Kehlet in Copenhagen, who pioneered the practice of enhanced recovery after surgery (ERAS). Kehlet reported cohort data on patients undergoing open colectomy for cancer with a median postoperative stay of 2½ days[27] and similar results with laparoscopic surgery.[28] This transformation in postoperative outcomes has been one of the most important surgical advances within the last 20 years, improving recovery by reducing complications.[29] In the author's practice, after introducing ERAS care and the application of laparoscopic surgery in over 90% of elective

patients, median stay since 2001 has been consistent: 4–5 days after colonic cancer resection and 5–6 days for rectal cancer.[30,31]

The debate regarding the benefits of laparoscopic versus conventional open surgery has been extensive, largely due to difficulty demonstrating differences in recovery that reflect those clearly perceived by surgeons who are adept at laparoscopic colorectal resection. Difficulty acquiring technical competence, the cost of laparoscopic instruments and entrenched views have slowed adoption.

The most appropriate evidence demonstrating a convincing argument for minimally invasive surgery in colorectal cancer derives from two multicentre RCTs comparing the two approaches within an ERAS programme.

> ✅✅ The LAFA and EnROL trials demonstrated a 2-day reduction in total hospital stay after laparoscopic surgery when compared to conventional open surgery.[32,33] The earlier of these two studies reported that the only factor in multivariate analysis associated with a reduction in complications was laparoscopy.

A recent multinational study from the ERAS Compliance Group[34] confirmed the conclusions from these two RCTs. In 2350 patients with colorectal cancer treated within an ERAS programme, the only factors reducing both complications and hospital stay were the use of laparoscopy and the extent of compliance within the ERAS programme – improvements in recovery being proportional to the number of pre- and intraoperative ERAS interventions. Late outcome analysis within the LAFA trial[35] has also demonstrated a significant reduction in incisional hernias [10.1% vs 16.8% ($P = 0.05$)] and adhesion obstruction [2.4% vs 7.3% ($P = 0.02$)], for laparoscopic versus open surgery, respectively.

Whether there is also an oncological benefit from laparoscopic cancer resection compared to open surgery is unclear, but some data from rectal cancer trials suggest this may be the case. Within the COREAN RCT,[36] rectal cancer resected laparoscopically had a 3-year disease-free survival that was greater than following open surgery: 79.2% (95% CI 72.3–84.6) versus 72.5% (65.0–78.6) respectively, the difference being lower than the prespecified non-inferiority margin (–6.7%, 95% CI –15.5 to 2.4; $P < 0.0001$). In the COLOR II multicentre European RCT,[37] stage III rectal cancer 3-year disease-free survival was 64.9% after laparoscopy versus 52.0% after open resection (difference 12.9%; 95% CI 2.2–23.6): this difference was not described as significant as the analysis was not a prespecified endpoint. Perioperative immunosuppression is greater after conventional open surgery than laparoscopy[38] and thus open surgery might adversely impact cancer outcome. Further research is, however, necessary to clarify this.

✅ In the author's view there is clear evidence that laparoscopic surgery decreases complications after surgery, and shortens recovery. It needs to be undertaken by surgeons who are competent in the technique and, in conjunction with an ERAS programme, should be considered our gold standard of practice. Open surgery within an ERAS programme is, however, appropriate in the treatment of some complex and re-operative problems, or when laparoscopy is contraindicated or unavailable.

Vascular variations of the colon

Vascular variations are particularly common in the arteries and veins to and from the transverse and right colon (see Recommended Video 5). They are described in **Figs 5.4** and **5.5** and it is important that the surgeon is familiar with them when performing laparoscopic CME, particularly in the obese. The author's preference in right hemicolectomy is to perform the operation from a position standing between the patient's legs. This facilitates dissection of the middle colic vascular branches and precise, safe, origin ligation of appropriate vessels as described above. The vessels are also used as reference points to guide dissection as their origins are relatively consistent.

During recent years preoperative mapping of the vascular anatomy on staging CT scans has simplified this. Currently vascular mapping employs portal venous phase 1 mm scans. It is hoped that bolus-tracked arterial, as well as portal venous phase images, will become available soon and that, with appropriate software, 3-D reconstructions of vascular anatomy will be provided routinely for surgeons.

Variations in vascular anatomy affecting the IMA are less important than those of the SMA if the IMA is being divided near its origin for D3 resection. If, however, the ascending left colic artery is being preserved or being divided selectively – for D2 high anterior resection (Fig. 5.2) or segmental left colectomy (Fig. 5.3a), respectively – it is important to recognise that it usually arises at around 3.5 cm from the aorta. It may, however, arise between 1 cm and 7 cm from the parent vessel.[39,40] For this reason, training is directed to enabling surgeons to precisely skeletonise and transect all named vessels without blood loss.

Obesity and difficulties in laparoscopic surgery

Obesity poses problems for surgeons and in laparoscopic surgery it may be appropriate to compromise on the site of transection of the right branch of the middle colic artery or the right colic branch by dividing the vessel at the base of the mesentery, just to the right of the midline, as it runs towards the hepatic flexure. Although this is not at the origin of the vessel it will not be more than 1–2 cm from it and reduces the potential morbidity of a precise D3 resection at this site in the obese patient. In such patients, and those with other significant comorbidities, it is important to bear in mind that there seems little disadvantage in oncological outcome (less than 2% reduction in 5-year survival – see above), by comparison with an origin ligation, provided the surgeon can perform resection in the mesocolic plane and remove all intermediate nodes.

It is important during laparoscopic surgery in the obese (and also in patients of height less than 1.55 m) for surgeons to employ extra strategies. The following are essential: use of an operating table that can simultaneously tilt patients 30 degrees head down and 20 degrees to the right, and a method of securing the patient to the table so they cannot move during tilting. The surgeon should also not hesitate to increase intra-abdominal pressure from 12 to 15 mmHg and use extra 5-mm ports and an expanding foam retractor intra-abdominally to position small bowel. While some report benefit from using a 'handport', that has not been the author's experience.

Due to difficulties in becoming proficient in laparoscopic colorectal surgery, a national programme for training specialists was established successfully in England.[42] This demonstrated that preceptorship in over 20 cancer resections significantly improved clinical outcomes for patients,[43] over and above the volume of unsupervised operations performed. Avoiding the disadvantage of a learning curve for patients is essential. The English programme also emphasised the need for a consistent theatre team and the avoidance of adverse outcomes resulting from non-technical aspects of surgery (e.g. distractions and interruptions, limited time allocation, dysfunctional teamwork, equipment problems). The programme employed proven educational strategies in order to shorten learning curves (e.g. mental rehearsal, structured and regular appraisal, repetition, use of training videos).

Anastomotic leakage

With use of laparoscopic surgery in up to 98%[31] of elective colorectal resections and routine use of ERAS pathways, the speed of postoperative recovery has been transformed. A median postoperative stay of 4 days after colectomy is now routine. These advances bring anastomotic leakage into clear focus as the most worrying postoperative problem. It is associated with a 4–15% postoperative mortality,[44]

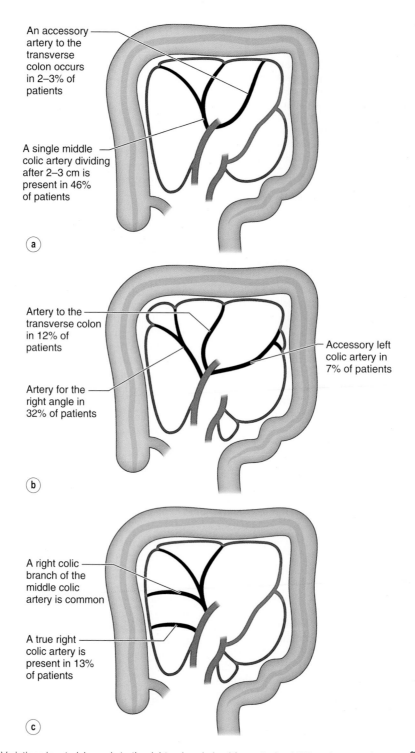

An accessory artery to the transverse colon occurs in 2–3% of patients

A single middle colic artery dividing after 2–3 cm is present in 46% of patients

(a)

Artery to the transverse colon in 12% of patients

Artery for the right angle in 32% of patients

Accessory left colic artery in 7% of patients

(b)

A right colic branch of the middle colic artery is common

A true right colic artery is present in 13% of patients

(c)

Figure 5.4 • Variations in arterial supply to the right colon derived from study of 156 cadaver angiograms.[39,40]

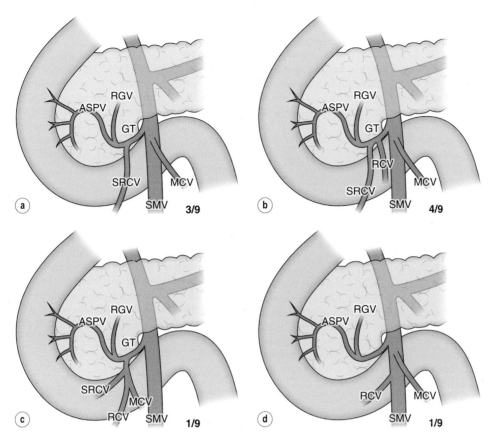

Figure 5.5 • Variations in venous anatomy of the superior mesenteric vein at the inferior border of the pancreas. Numbers indicate number of subjects. SRCV, superior right colic vein; ASPV, anterior superior pancreatico-duodenal vein; MCV, middle colic vein; RCV, right colic vein; RGV, right gastroepiploic vein; SMV, superior mesenteric vein; GT, gastrocolic trunk.
Adapted from Jin et al.[41]

increased hospital stay and reduced long-term survival.[45]

The pathogenesis of anastomotic leakage has traditionally been considered to be either due to technical problems or ischaemia – the former said to occur within a day or two of surgery and the latter after approximately 5 days. This supposition seems very unlikely to be correct when tachycardia can be observed within 24 hours of surgery in fit patients who have undergone technically satisfactory surgery and in whom leakage becomes apparent some days later.

Diagnosis

In the era of surgery that is optimised using laparoscopy and ERAS care, it is very clear when patients are not achieving their milestones. One would expect the vast majority of patients to have had all tubes, catheters and physical intervention removed and be walking, eating and drinking satisfactorily on day 1 or at the latest day 2 after surgery, and to have opened their bowel by day 2 or 3.

Thus, if tachycardia persists or other complications occur such as pyrexia, arrhythmia, respiratory problems, abdominal pain or abdominal distension, one should consider early investigation to exclude anastomotic leakage. To do this we examine C-reactive protein (CRP) daily, looking specifically for a rise in CRP >200.[46] Subtle clinical signs such as slight tachycardia or high CRP may well alert the clinician to leakage when a patient is still eating and walking around the ward on day 2 or 3. In that situation a contrast-enhanced CT scan of chest, abdomen and pelvis (without rectal contrast, which complicates subsequent water-soluble contrast examination) should be requested in order to exclude subtle signs such as gas bubbles adjacent to the anastomosis, or other areas of free intraperitoneal air. If CT scanning is negative for anastomotic dehiscence,[44] and other complications are excluded, a water-soluble contrast enema is performed on the same day by a radiologist with a specialist interest in this area. Although it may be dubious whether to intervene when patients are well, if there is subsequent deterioration clinically or of laboratory results, the identification of leakage clarifies management and expedites re-operation. All surgeons who perform colorectal surgery will encounter such complications and it is the expeditious diagnosis of them and urgent re-intervention when necessary that distinguishes the quality of postoperative care.

Management

The options to treat leakage from an intraperitoneal anastomosis include the use of antibiotics when there is minimal physical upset and the patient is stable – unfortunately this rarely seems to be the case. If at surgical intervention there is minimal soiling around the anastomosis it may be reasonable to preserve it, perform an upstream defunctioning loop stoma and wash the bowel through from the stoma, with a proctoscope placed transanally to evacuate the effluent, leaving drain(s) adjacent to the anastomosis. This can sometimes be performed laparoscopically but requires considerable laparoscopic colorectal surgical expertise. When soiling is evident either around the anastomosis or generally, it is not possible to preserve the anastomosis and a Hartmann's procedure should be performed as the safest approach.

Defunctioning stoma

Reducing anastomotic leakage and its consequences is achieved in low rectal surgery by defunctioning the bowel,[3] and although the evidence for improvement after colonic resection is not as clear, a parallel is likely. Thus when there is a high risk of leakage, defunctioning should be considered. McDermott and colleagues[44] reported a number of factors that increase the chance of leakage and can be used to guide decision-making: male sex, American Society of Anesthesiologists fitness grade above II, renal disease, comorbidity, historic radiotherapy, size of tumour over 3 cm, advanced tumour stage, emergency surgery, metastatic disease, smoking, obesity, poor nutrition, alcohol excess, immunosuppressants, bevacizumab, blood loss/transfusion and duration of surgery in excess of 4 hours.

Emergency management

Emergency presentation of colonic cancer increases postoperative complications and worsens cancer outcomes. This is clearly demonstrated by the UK national audit of practice for 2014–15,[47] which reported a 90-day mortality after emergency or urgent surgery of 12.3%, compared with 2.1% for planned surgery.

In the UK, about 20% of patients with colonic cancer present as an emergency and 16% present with obstruction. Bleeding and perforation are less common modes of emergency presentation; when perforation occurs, it is often in the caecum as a result of distal obstruction in the face of a competent ileocaecal valve. Obstruction is thus the most likely reason for emergency or urgent operation.

Obstruction

At presentation with obstruction a CT scan to clarify diagnosis is preferred to plain abdominal X-rays and if doubt exists regarding whether there is pseudo-obstruction, either a water-soluble contrast enema or endoscopy is necessary. Management should be expedited when there are signs of sepsis, when there is localised tenderness over the caecum suggesting imminent perforation, or when the caecal diameter is 12 cm or more.

Management of obstruction

The options to treat obstructing colonic cancer are either emergency surgery or stenting.

Emergency surgery requires preoperative resuscitation of the patient.

Surgery should be performed by experienced surgical and anaesthetic staff, preferably during daylight hours. Initially it is usually necessary to decompress the bowel using either a 19-gauge needle connected to suction, or a 28-gauge Foley catheter inserted via the caecum. Once decompressed, the bowel can be safely handled and if the obstruction is right-sided a standard right hemicolectomy performed.

If the tumour is more distal, the options are an extended resection or segmental left colectomy. The SCOTIA study[48] randomised between these treatments, reporting that patients treated by left hemicolectomy had more acceptable bowel function. In the case of obstruction with a competent ileocaecal valve, extended resection may be mandated by perforation of the caecum or doubt about caecal viability. When a more distal colonic obstruction is present decompression intraoperatively is usually necessary to allow resection. This has been described using intraoperative prograde lavage through a large-bore caecal catheter, with effluent evacuated via anaesthetic scavenger tubing inserted into the left colon[49] (**Fig. 5.6**). The author's personal preference is, however, to progradely aspirate the colon via a 28-gauge Foley catheter placed through

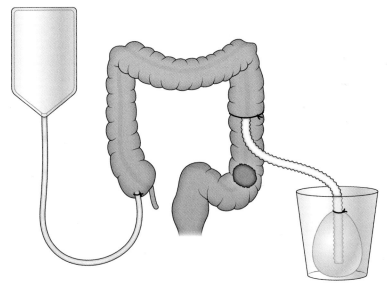

Figure 5.6 • On-table colonic irrigation.

an appendicostomy, provided the contents of the colon are predominantly gas as is normally the case. Retrograde aspiration using the same catheter, threaded up the small bowel, can also usually be achieved, allowing a more satisfactory procedure.

As outcomes in the emergency setting are inferior to elective surgery and many patients are physiologically compromised, it is advisable to defunction an anastomosis. When treating the severely ill or those with gross intra-abdominal sepsis it is safer not to anastomose at all, but to perform a Hartmann's procedure, and in the most physiologically compromised obstructed patients, only to defunction without resection.

Stenting of left colonic obstructions is an attractive option as it allows relief of obstruction and elective resection of the tumour approximately 2 weeks later (**Fig. 5.7**). In the largest RCT to date stenting followed by elective surgery reduced stoma rates from 69% for emergency surgery to 45% in the stented patients ($P < 0.001$).[50] Stenting also has the advantage that in the palliative setting it may be the definitive treatment. It is not without problems, such as failure to relieve obstruction and perforation, and it is important to recognise that technical expertise is crucial.

Perforation

Perforation, apart from in the obstructed caecum, may be at the tumour or may be in a segment of diverticulitis proximal to a tumour; in this situation

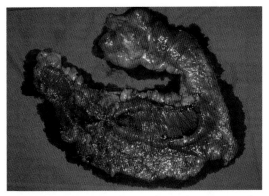

Figure 5.7 • Stent crossing an obstructing cancer at the splenic flexure that was subsequently treated by elective subtotal colectomy.

the primary is easily missed. Treatment of perforated patients is preferably by resection, but the degree of contamination and fitness of the patient will dictate whether reconstruction is advisable, as described above.

Future developments

Preoperative chemotherapy for locally advanced colon cancer patients has shown promise within the FOxTROT trial;[51] in the first 150 patients there was significant downstaging after neoadjuvant chemotherapy. Long-term outcomes are awaited from the full trial to evaluate oncological outcomes, but it looks very promising.

> **Key points**
>
> - Optimal outcomes are achieved by performing surgery for colon cancer laparoscopically, within an enhanced recovery programme.
> - High-quality training in laparoscopic surgery is required.
> - Complete mesocolic excision is associated with improved oncological outcomes.
> - Colorectal surgeons must be aware of the variable vascular anatomy of the colon. Improved imaging will allow planning of surgery for individual patients.
> - Anastomotic leak should be suspected and diagnosed early.
> - Stenting provides an attractive alternative to emergency surgery for obstruction when appropriate expertise is available. Useful data on complications and case selection are emerging from clinical trials.

Acknowledgements

The author and editor are indebted to Professor Fumio Konishi, Honorary Consultant, Department of Surgery, Nerima Hikarigaoka Hospital, Tokyo, Japan; Professor Emeritus, Visiting Professor, Jichi Medical University, Tochigi and Saitama, Japan for his assistance with this chapter.

▶ Recommended videos:

1. Right hemicolectomy (Thorn, Jenkins, Kennedy) – https://tinyurl.com/y8e23usa
2. Right hemicolectomy using Thunderbeat (Thorn, Jenkins, Kennedy – no sound track) – https://tinyurl.com/y6vncknc
3. Segmental left colectomy for splenic flexure tumours (Uraiqat, Jenkins, Kennedy) – https://tinyurl.com/y8xdrvc4
4. Left hemicolectomy (Ouro, Jenkins, Kennedy) – https://tinyurl.com/yat674ta
5. Vascular variations in the right colon (Thorn, Jenkins, Kennedy) – https://tinyurl.com/y6wodwjy

Key references

8. West NP, Morris EJA, Rotimi O, et al. Pathology grading of colon cancer surgical resection and its association with survival: a retrospective observational study. Lancet Oncol 2008;9:857–65. PMID: 18667357.
12. Søndenaa K, Quirke P, Hohenberger W, et al. The rationale behind complete mesocolic excision (CME) and a central vascular ligation for colon cancer in open and laparoscopic surgery. Int J Colorectal Dis 2014;29:419–28. PMID: 24477788.

27. Basse L, Hjort Jakobsen D, Billesbolle P, et al. A clinical pathway to accelerate recovery after colonic resection. Ann Surg 2000;232:51–7. PMID: 10862195.
32. Vlug MS, Wind J, Hollmann MW, et al. Laparoscopy in combination with fast track multimodal management is the best perioperative strategy in patients undergoing colonic surgery: a randomized clinical trial (LAFA study). Ann Surg 2011; 254:868–75. PMID: 21597360.
   The first multicentre RCT demonstrating laparoscopic colon cancer resection improves outcome even when open surgery is optimised within an ERAS programme. Laparoscopy was the only factor to reduce both complications and hospital stay.
33. Kennedy RH, Francis EA, Wharton R, et al. Multicenter randomized controlled trial of conventional versus laparoscopic surgery for colorectal cancer within an enhanced recovery program: EnROL. J Clin Oncol 2014;32: 1804–11. PMID: 24799480.
   Showed very similar results to LAFA trial: that laparoscopic surgery within an ERAS programme significantly improves outcome. Results also showed laparoscopy improved rectal cancer outcomes and that independent pathological assessment of specimen quality was equivalent between the two approaches.

6

Surgery for rectal cancer

John Bunni
Brendan J. Moran

Introduction

Cancer of the rectum, defined as an adenocarcinoma within 15 cm from the anal verge, accounts for approximately 30% of all colorectal malignancies. There were 14 440 new cases of rectal cancer registered in the UK in 2008.[1] This incidence is likely to increase in the short term due to the Bowel Cancer Screening Programme implemented in the UK in 2009.

Treatment is predominantly surgical excision with the addition of neoadjuvant therapy (radiotherapy or chemoradiotherapy administered preoperatively) in selected cases. Total mesorectal excision (TME) is now considered the gold standard, with fewer local recurrences and better overall survival.[2–6] Major resectional surgery is technically challenging due to relative inaccessibility within the confines of the bony pelvis, difficulty in reconstruction, risk of anastomotic leakage and local recurrence.

Major surgery is associated with significant morbidity and mortality, and may be inappropriate in some cases. Availability of a range of treatments, both surgical and non-surgical, for management of rectal cancer makes it critical that patient assessment, cancer staging (Box 6.1), perioperative optimisation (Box 6.2) and selection of appropriate therapy are carried out in a multidisciplinary team (MDT) setting.

Objectives of surgery

The aims of rectal cancer surgery are to cure the patient and if possible preserve normal bowel, bladder and sexual function. Mechanisms to achieve these aims encompass two key treatment modalities,
namely surgical technique[2,3] and neoadjuvant therapy, both of which have been shown to reduce local recurrence.[4,6] Optimal surgery, in the form of TME, reduces local recurrence and improves survival.[2–8] Evidence from randomized trials has reported reduction in local recurrence with neoadjuvant radiotherapy,[2,6,9] though to date only one trial has reported improved survival.[10] Preoperative radiotherapy can 'downstage' the primary tumour, but caution is warranted. The original histology provides an estimate of the likelihood of occult hepatic and other systemic metastases already present at the time of resection. Neoadjuvant radiotherapy has no effect on this original estimate: even if the primary tumour shrinks or disappears completely (pathologically complete response, pCR) in a subset (approximately 10–20% after chemoradiotherapy). A tumour that is truly locally confined will be cured by adequate locoregional therapy and inadequate locoregional therapy will result in local recurrence. In the presence of occult metastases, the outcome will be determined by the metastases.

The rectal cancer surgeon can impact on:

1. in-hospital mortality;
2. local recurrence;
3. quality of life.

In-hospital mortality

Postoperative deaths in hospital involve patient, tumour and surgeon-related factors. Clearly, in an elderly patient with comorbidity who presents in an emergency with an obstructing tumour, the risks of death are much higher than in a younger patient undergoing elective surgery. Elective surgery under the age of 80 years has an overall in-hospital mortality of 1–8% compared with 6–16% mortality in those over 80.[7,11] A patient over 80 with malignant large bowel obstruction has a 1 in 3 chance of in-hospital mortality.[12] Similarly, the in-hospital mortality in the presence of an anastomotic leak is much higher.[13] Anastomotic leak rates vary between surgeons. Whilst a low anastomosis, preoperative radiotherapy and other factors increase the risk of leakage, the one major consistent mechanism to reduce the rate and consequences of leakage is a defunctioning stoma. This surgical decision to defunction, or not, is crucial and increasingly most authorities agree that defunctioning should be considered in all patients who have had a TME for rectal cancer. From time to time the decision to adopt a local treatment approach avoiding major surgery, particularly for early tumours, may be optimal for a patient. Thus, a decision for local excision, transanal endoscopic microsurgery (TEMS) or even local radiotherapy will be influenced by weighing up the likely benefit of the alternative, and fitness of the patient for a major resection.

Local recurrence

Local recurrence after rectal surgery is defined as disease in the pelvis, including recurrence at the site of anastomosis and in the perineum.[14] Local recurrence is for the most part incurable and results in major morbidity with debilitating symptoms of pelvic pain, ureteric obstruction, intestinal and urinary tract fistulation, and poor bowel and urinary function. Increasingly, local recurrence is recognized as failure of complete tumour excision at primary surgery. Thus, local 'recurrence' may, in many cases, represent persistent and progressive disease, rather than true recurrence. There are a number of predictors of risk of local recurrence (Box 6.3). Practically all are associated with both locally advanced tumours and frequently metastatic disease at presentation. Additionally, they predict for a high risk of subsequent postoperative systemic recurrence. Fortunately, some of these factors can be identified preoperatively, which helps in planning the appropriate management in an MDT setting, employing appropriate neoadjuvant treatments in selective cases.

Reported local recurrence rates vary from 2.6% to 32% and are probably most influenced by surgical technique.[15,16] The lowest recurrence rates and best survival have been consistently reported with TME.[2,3,5,15–17]

Circumferential resection margin and the role of preoperative radiotherapy

Rectal cancer spreads by local extension, via the lymphatics and via the bloodstream. Lymphatic drainage is associated with the arterial pedicle and is generally addressed by a combination of TME and high ligation of the inferior mesenteric artery. Local spread of a rectal cancer in the confines of the narrow pelvis results in a risk of involvement of the mesorectal fascia, the circumferential resection margin (CRM) in TME. Involvement of the CRM on the resected specimen appears to be the main determinant of an increased risk of local recurrence. A positive CRM, defined as tumour within 1 mm of the margin of the resected specimen, and depth of extramural invasion are independent predictors of local recurrence and poor prognosis.[9,18] These observations are supported by studies from Norway[19] and the Netherlands.[20]

The CRM may also be involved due to metastatic nodal disease. There is debate as to whether involved nodes, in their own right, increase local recurrence even if not directly involving the CRM. It has been reported that patients with positive lymph nodes have a higher risk of local recurrence.[21] However, others found that lymph node involvement was not associated with higher local recurrence, provided optimal TME is performed.[19,22] While other risk factors, such as vascular invasion, differentiation, etc., are undoubtedly major determinants of long-term survival, the single main factor that can be manipulated by optimal treatment is the CRM.

Debate persists as to the merits of routine, or selective, neoadjuvant therapy for patients with rectal cancer. However, there has been a recent shift towards selective use due to the adverse effects of radiotherapy and reports showing no long-term survival benefit in operable rectal cancer.[4,23] Indeed, many neoadjuvant trials have been conducted against an unacceptably high rate of local recurrence in the control arm.[24] There is also inconvenience and cost associated with radiotherapy.

Complications of preoperative radiotherapy

While a detailed discussion about radiotherapy is provided elsewhere (Chapter 7), a few issues with regard to early and later complications are noteworthy. Early complications include perineal wound breakdown, diarrhoea, proctitis, urinary tract infection, small bowel obstruction, leucopenia and venous thrombosis.

In addition, radiotherapy has been shown to have adverse effects on anal function and on the function and integrity of a coloanal anastomosis with, or without, formation of a colonic pouch.[25]

Comparing the pre- and postoperative situations, a German study[26] reported Grade 3 or 4 acute toxicity in 27% of patients with preoperative chemoradiotherapy versus 40% in the postoperative group ($P=0.001$); the corresponding rates of long-term toxic effects were 14% and 24%, respectively ($P=0.01$).

Downstaging rectal cancer with preoperative radiotherapy

The 15-cm rectum has been arbitrarily divided into three parts, with the lower rectum 0–6 cm, the middle rectum 7–11 cm and the upper rectum 12–15 cm from the anal verge. There is little debate as to whether a T3 middle or upper rectal cancer (that is, above 7 cm) is particularly at high risk of local recurrence, providing surgery is adequate and that a TME has resulted in an intact cover of mesorectal fat and fascia. However, in the lower rectum a T3 tumour has, by definition, gone through the wall of the bowel and commonly will have an involved margin at the level of the sphincter complex unless the rectum is excised en bloc with the sphincter. Endoanal ultrasound appears to be particularly good at estimating the T stage.[27] Correlations with pathology indicate accuracy of endorectal ultrasound (EUS), particularly in T staging, though less so in N staging.[27] EUS is particularly helpful in selecting patients who may be suitable for local excision, generally agreed to be those with early T1 tumours. However, the main determinant of local recurrence is undoubtedly a positive CRM, and EUS is poor at assessment of the CRM. Magnetic resonance imaging (MRI) has been particularly useful in the ability to visualise the CRM and to accurately predict either involved, threatened or clear margins and thus direct treatment strategy.[28,29] A patient with an obviously involved margin on MRI should be considered for neoadjuvant therapy to reduce margin involvement at subsequent surgery by 'downstaging' and perhaps 'downsizing' the tumour. All patients with a threatened margin (which really includes most very low tumours due to little surrounding mesorectum) should also be considered for preoperative treatment, whereas patients with clear margins can be treated by optimal surgery alone.

Increasingly, neoadjuvant therapy includes a combination of chemotherapy and radiotherapy. Frykholm et al.[30] published a small randomised controlled trial in 2001 in which patients with fixed rectal carcinomas were randomised to preoperative radiotherapy or chemo-radiotherapy (CRT). This trial showed a significant improvement in resectability and reduction in local failure with the use of CRT.[30] With preoperative irradiation of clinically mobile lesions, pathological complete response (pCR) rates of 10–20% have been reported, and with preoperative chemo-radiation, higher pCR rates of 30–35% have been reported.[31]

The delay following neoadjuvant treatment may be important. A dose of 25 Gy in five fractions (short-course radiotherapy) is usually combined with surgery within 1 week, with minimal downstaging or downsizing. Interim results from the ongoing

Stockholm-III trial, which compared outcomes of timing of surgery after short-course radiotherapy (SCRT) with immediate surgery, SCRT and surgery over 6 weeks later, and conventional long-course radiotherapy (RT), which traditionally has involved surgery over 6 weeks after completion of RT, have been reported.[32] SCRT was associated with more complications and more mortality in the elderly if surgery was delayed by more than 10 days after completion of RT, unless surgery was delayed for 6 weeks when results were comparable to those after conventional long-course radiotherapy (LCRT). The recommendation was that surgery after SCRT should be done either within 5 days or delayed for more than 4 weeks.

There has been debate as to the optimal delay even in long-course regimens. The Lyon R90-01 trial reported that long-course radiotherapy with a delay of 6–8 weeks for surgery results in a significantly better tumour response and pathological downstaging of rectal cancer compared to an interval of 3 weeks.[33]

MRI can predict T stage and CRM status

Recent reports suggest that a CRM at risk of tumour involvement can be reliably seen at preoperative MRI, with correlated histology of the resected specimen.[28,29,34] Data from the prospective, multicentre MRI and Rectal Cancer European Equivalence Study (MERCURY) confirm accurate prediction both of the T staging and CRM clearance of 1 mm from the resection margin. When the CRM was predicted free of tumour and the patient had surgery alone, a histologically clear CRM was achieved in 91%. Furthermore, the extramural depth of penetration was accurately predicted to within 0.5 mm in 95% of 295 patients who had surgery alone. Thus, it is possible to classify tumours preoperatively into mrT3a (extramural tumour extension less than 5 mm) and mrT3b (extramural tumour extension greater than 5 mm) subgroups and thus consider neoadjuvant therapy in advanced tumours. Vascular invasion and lymph node involvement can also be predicted, though sensitivity and specificity for nodal status remains problematic.

Previous studies reported a varying accuracy for T staging between 67% and 83%, with a considerable inter-observer variability.[34] However, it is the distance to the CRM that is the most powerful predictor of local recurrence, rather than T stage. In a large series of MRI evaluations of CRM, there was higher accuracy for predicting tumour-free resection margins (95%) than for prediction of T stage.[28]

Considerations for decision-making

The main purpose of imaging is to plan treatment and, as for any cancer, both tumour and patient factors have to be considered prior to decision-making. Tumour factors include the biological behaviour, site and extent/fixity of the tumour. Thus early T1 cancers may be suitable for local excision, with similar cancer-specific survival in favourable tumours compared with major excisional surgery.[35]

On imaging, important considerations include whether there is threat to the mesorectal fascia, evidence of extramural venous invasion (EMVI) or local invasion of the sphincter complex in the low rectum. Blomqivst has categorised rectal cancer into three distinct groups based on these prognostic features using the Mercury terminology of 'Good, Bad and Ugly'.[36] Other considerations include the depth and size of the pelvis, occasionally making an abdominal TME difficult due to lack of operating space (and hence a potential benefit in such cases from trans-anal TME).

EMVI is a marker of possible vascular metastases and, comparatively speaking, likely to have a larger detrimental impact on overall survival than involved lymph nodes. There is some evidence that patients with locally involved nodal disease, resected by optimal TME surgery, have a similar local recurrence rate to patients with non-involved nodes, but still high systemic recurrence, hence the need to consider adjuvant therapy.[37]

Patient factors in decision-making include local (pelvic) factors and systemic (general health) ones. Patients with previous radiotherapy, obstetric injury and a low anastomosis are likely to have poor function and consideration should be given to a permanent stoma in these circumstances and if oncological features allow, an intersphincteric abdominoperineal excision (APE) with a permanent end colostomy may be the safest and best option. Those with multiple comorbidities should be counselled about risk and sometimes a non-operative strategy may need to be employed (discussed at the end of the chapter).

Tumour disruption

Cutting into a primary tumour while mobilising the rectum results in a very high risk of spilling viable cancer cells. The occasions when this may happen in rectal cancer surgery include the following:

1. When an adherent loop of intestine is thought to be adherent to the tumour by 'inflammatory'

adhesions. The loop should be resected en bloc with the primary tumour rather than pinched off.[38]

2. Fragmentation of the mesorectal fascia. Heald has shown the importance of maintaining the integrity of the mesorectal envelope.[24] Rough traction, blunt dissection and failure to identify and follow the mesorectal fascia will contribute to disruption of the mesorectal envelope, which on removal will look ragged and shredded. Precise surgery using sharp or diathermy dissection under vision will reduce the incidence of this problem.

3. Injudicious exploration of the anterior plane in a man with an anterior encroaching tumour (see Fig. 6.1).

An anterior encroaching tumour in the male rarely penetrates through Denonvilliers' fascia to involve the seminal vesicles, prostate or base of bladder. However, all surgeons have experienced cases where this has occurred. Anterior tumours in females are less problematic as the uterus and vagina act as a barrier to involvement of the bladder and an en bloc hysterectomy, including part of the vagina, can be performed when the uterus or posterior vagina is involved.

An extensive anterior tumour may require neoadjuvant therapy and on occasions pelvic exenteration with total cystectomy, and may require cooperation with a urological team. Attention to detail and appropriate experience and radiological training result in very accurate MRI images clearly demonstrating the mesorectal fascia such that the need for a pelvic exenteration should have been visualized at imaging (**Fig. 6.1**).

Extent of excision – TME versus mesorectal transection, pelvic lymphadenectomy and level of vascular ligation

The extent of resection relates to the necessity for TME, the management of involved pelvic side-wall nodes and the role of lateral pelvic lymphadenectomy (LPLD),[39–41] and high versus low vascular ligation.[42,43]

TME

> ✅ It is now generally accepted that TME is optimal therapy for low or mid-rectal cancer.

The need for TME for upper rectal cancer is debatable and it is now considered unnecessary for oncological reasons. The key aspect is the extent of mesorectal spread distally, which has recently been reported to be up to 3 cm below the distal margin of the tumour.[44] Heald et al. described distal mesorectal deposits up to 4 cm.[45] Thus, a mesorectal clearance of 5 cm below the lower edge of the tumour by mesorectal transection (which should be carefully performed tangentially to the mesorectum and muscle tube) would seem adequate and thus would not always warrant TME for upper rectal cancer. The reasons to consider mesorectal transection revolve around a probable reduction in anastomotic leakage and better neorectal function when part of the mesorectum and some of the distal rectum is preserved.

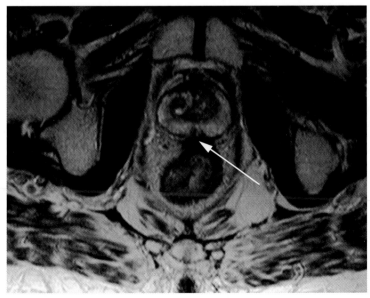

Figure 6.1 • An anterior tumour invading into the prostate can be seen (*arrow*).

Lateral pelvic lymph nodal involvement

There is ongoing debate as to the incidence, management and relevance of lateral pelvic side-wall nodes both in the East (in particular Japan) and the West, and a recent review provides an up-to-date analysis of many of the issues.[41] In essence, the incidence may be similar, mainly an issue with low rectal cancer and involved nodes are increasingly suspected at preoperative MRI.[41]

In a retrospective review by Ueno and colleagues of 237 patients with T3/4 low rectal cancer who underwent R0 resection, including lateral pelvic lymphadenectomy (LPLD), the incidence of lateral nodal involvement increased with decreasing tumour height.[46] Lateral nodes were involved in 17% when the tumour was 8 cm or less from the anal verge. On subset analysis this varied from 42% for tumours below 2 cm to 10.5% for tumours between 6 and 8 cm. A multicentre retrospective review from 12 leading Japanese hospitals of 2916 patients with T3/4 low rectal cancer reported lateral nodal involvement in 20.1% with tumours below the peritoneal reflection compared with 8.8% in those with upper rectal cancer.[47] Similarly, 20% involvement in low cancers has been reported in Brazil.[48]

Factors predicting an increased risk of involved lateral nodes include involved mesorectal nodes, female patients, advanced T stage, poor tumour differentiation, lymphovascular invasion and low rectal cancer.

There is undoubtedly a subset of patients with involved pelvic side-wall nodes who might benefit from LPLD, though it is of interest that neoadjuvant CRT may be as effective as nodal removal.[41] A more selective approach and modified surgical techniques such as pelvic autonomic nerve preserving dissection reduce the morbidity of LPLD.[41,49–51]

High versus low inferior mesenteric artery ligation

The inferior mesenteric artery (IMA) can be divided either flush on the aorta, although 1–2 cm distally from its origin is now recommended to reduce autonomic nerve injury (high ligation), or below the take-off of the ascending left colic artery (low ligation). There has been no reported difference in terms of cancer survival.[43]

General opinion has always supported using the descending colon instead of the sigmoid when performing an anastomosis to the anal canal. Not only does the sigmoid colon generate fairly high pressures, which could therefore lead to relatively poor function, but more importantly the marginal artery may be minimal, or absent, in the sigmoid, which is thus prone to ischaemia if used for anastomosis. However, the descending colon will not generally reach the anal canal unless the splenic flexure is mobilized in all cases, and there is a high tie of the inferior mesenteric artery, as the left colic artery is too short and will not permit the descending colon to reach (**Fig. 6.2**). Hence a low anastomosis will almost always need a high ligation, but for technical rather than cancer-specific reasons. A high anastomosis can usually be achieved quite easily with either a high or low ligation. A systematic review of published data in 2008 did not find any oncological or colonic perfusion differences in high ligation.[52]

However, in a randomised controlled trial comparing colonic pouches with straight coloanal anastomosis, the sigmoid was used in 42% of pouch anastomoses and this did not seem to have an overall negative effect on function.[53]

Implantation of viable cells

There is experimental evidence, supported by clinical observations, that colorectal cancer cells are shed into the bowel lumen and that viable cells can implant and grow.[54] A 'triple stapling' technique, where a linear stapler is placed below a cancer prior to peranal washout and a second linear stapler is placed distally across the washed muscle tube, facilitates distal washout and eliminates clamp slippage and faecal spillage and improves access to the distal rectum for ultra-low anastomosis.[55] A meta-analysis by Rondelli suggested that this was easy and worth doing and that colorectal surgeons were more likely to washout than general surgeons.[56]

Quality of life

Increasingly, quality of life (QoL) has been recognised as an important aspect of cancer care. In rectal cancer surgery QoL issues include preservation of continence, reasonable bowel frequency and avoidance, as far as possible, of permanent sexual and urinary disturbance.

Preservation of continence by restorative resection

Despite an increasing proportion of patients undergoing restorative resection, some still require an abdominoperineal excsion (APE) with a permanent stoma. An APE may be required for the following:

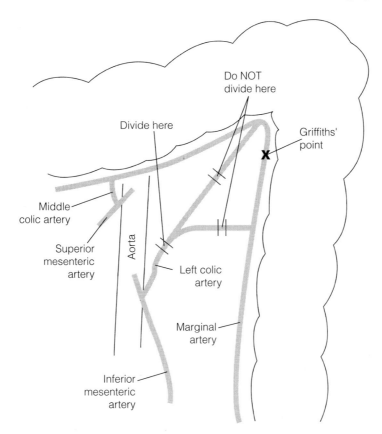

Figure 6.2 • When mobilising the vascular supply to the splenic flexure, do not divide the terminal branches of the left colic artery but rather leave them to support the marginal artery at the splenic flexure and divide the main trunk of the left colic as indicated. Frequently, the inferior mesenteric vein has to be mobilized below the inferior border of the pancreas to gain further length.

1. Cancer involving the sphincter or so close to the sphincter that attempts to preserve the sphincter complex are oncologically unsafe.
2. The functional result of restorative surgery is likely to be so poor that a colostomy would provide better QoL.
3. The potential complications of attempts to restore intestinal continuity are prohibitive, particularly in the frail and elderly.

Distal clearance margin

The literature is unclear on the definition of the distal margin. A distance of 5 cm of anorectal muscle tube at rigid sigmoidoscopy in a preoperative setting may expand to 8 cm after rectal mobilisation, and then shrink to 3 cm after specimen removal, simply because of contraction of the longitudinal muscle. If an attempt is then made to pin out the specimen, a margin of 4–5 cm may be achieved after fixation, but without pinning out, the final margin may measure only 2 cm.[57]

Against this background, it is very uncommon for rectal cancer to spread more than 1 cm below the distal palpable margin of the tumour. An exception is when the tumour is poorly differentiated, when distal spread up to 4.5 cm has occasionally been reported.[58] Of course, the preoperative biopsy may not accurately represent the final tumour histology, but given this caveat it is usually advised that a 5-cm distal clearance margin should still be considered for a poorly differentiated tumour, whereas a 2-cm margin should suffice otherwise. This distal muscle tube margin should not be confused with the recommended 5 cm of distal mesorectum recommended for higher tumours. For very low tumours the mesorectum has tapered out and is no longer an issue. In these cases, distal muscle tube excision is the issue.

For cancer in the lower third of the rectum (provided a tumour is not poorly differentiated), being able to apply a right-angled clamp, or staple line, below the lower margin of the tumour is generally considered sufficient clearance.[59] From time to time, the histology report will describe the tumour abutting the distal margin (i.e. being within 1 cm or less of the margin) but not involving it. Studies of resected specimens have shown that, as long as the margin itself is uninvolved the risk of recurrence is not increased,[38] provided that adequate circumferential clearance has been achieved.

Tumour height – the importance of rectal palpation (PR)

It is common to measure the height of the lower border of the tumour from the anal verge, which is often a variable point, for example being much further from the dentate line in patients with what has been described as a 'funnel' anus.

The dentate line can usually be felt with the examining finger. The mucosa above is more slippery to the examining finger than is the skin of the pecten. What actually matters in the critical case is not the measured height of the lower border of the tumour to the dentate line, but rather whether there is a sufficient margin either for a clamp, or stapler, to be placed below the tumour and above the dentate line or for the dentate line to be divided transanally without going too close to any palpably indurated tongue of tumour projecting downwards towards the dentate line. Added to this is a general assessment of the bulk of the tumour, surgical accessibility of the pelvis, the functional quality of the anus and the potential for improving tumour characteristics by preoperative radiotherapy.

Aspects of anal and neo-rectal function

A woman with a prior history of multiple vaginal deliveries, particularly if there has been a forceps delivery or a complication of episiotomy, has risks of an occult sphincter injury, detectable by anal ultrasonography. In practice, one is usually guided as to the quality of anal function by a history of flatus continence and an absence of episodes of faecal incontinence in the past. Of course, the tumour itself may have contributed to a sense of urgency in the more recent past and thereby may lead to unreasonable pessimism as to the true state of anal function.

Nevertheless, a patient with undoubtedly poor quality anal function will not be well served by an ultra-low anastomosis and is likely to be better off with an end colostomy. When the tumour itself is reasonably high in the rectum, then a low Hartmann operation or better still an intersphincteric resection of the short Hartmann stump will avoid the complications of a perineal wound. However, for a lower tumour, an abdominoperineal excision, excising part or all of the sphincter, may be the safest and most effective option.

Low rectal cancer and the English National Low Rectal Cancer Programme (LOREC)

Low rectal cancer is defined as 'an adenocarcinoma with its lower edge at, or below, the origin of the levators on the pelvic sidewall' and this usually corresponds to a tumour within 6 cm of the anal verge.[60] Cancers at this level commonly involve the levators and the sphincter complex and the concept of Extra Levator Abdomino Perineal Excision (ELAPE) has been a significant advance in improving outcomes in these patients with high risk tumours.[60] The LOREC programme aimed to improve outcome in low rectal cancer by optimal staging, selective neo-adjuvant therapy and appropriate surgical treatment ranging from restorative resection by coloanal anastomosis to intersphincteric APE and ELAPE in the most advanced tumours. ELAPE has been shown to reduce both CRM positivity and tumour perforation rates, thus reducing local recurrence and improving survival.

Abdominoperineal excision (APE)

Surgeons familiar with deep pelvic dissection and total mesorectal excision are now far less familiar with the bottom end of an abdominoperineal excision (APE), particularly in males. The scope for technical error is high as there is no clear anatomical plane from below, except anteriorly, where the plane, though present, can be exceedingly difficult. Pathologists report 'coning' or 'waisting' of the specimen, especially at the level of the levators (**Fig. 6.3**).

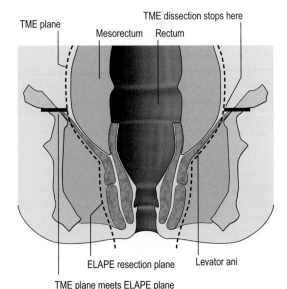

Figure 6.3 • TME and extralevator abdominoperineal (ELAPE) resection planes.

To some extent this is to be expected, as any cut voluntary muscle will contract and naturally give some impression of 'coning', but it is probable that surgeons are not excising the pelvic floor widely enough. Unless tumour is in the very distal anal canal, when there will be a threat of inguinal lymphatic spread, wide excision of ischiorectal fat is probably unnecessary. In contrast, it is important to excise widely at the level of the pelvic floor, particularly as this is the point where a low rectal cancer requiring an APE is likely to be situated (if it were not, then TME and restorative resection might be feasible).

> ✅ Extralevator APE (ELAPE) is recommended for advanced low rectal cancer and the prone position is increasingly favoured.[61]
> However, it is the concept of ELAPE that is crucial and patient position is optional provided the principle of operating on the inferior surface of the levator is followed.

The risk of local recurrence can be reduced by considering neoadjuvant therapy in all cases that require an APE. However, this risks over-treatment, with increased early and long-term complications. It is likely that a selective neoadjuvant policy, even for very low tumours, will be the norm in the future.

Reconstruction (colonic pouch, end-to-side or end-to-end anastomosis)

Straight coloanal anastomosis may result in poor function, certainly for a number of months and on occasion for a year or two. In a study of 84 cases treated at St Mark's Hospital by proctectomy with coloanal anastomosis, 8% went on to have a permanent colostomy constructed.[62] Increasingly, a neorectal reservoir is recommended, with most favouring a colonic 'J' pouch of 5–6 cm in length.[63] Several reports confirm that early function with a colonic pouch is superior to a straight coloanal anastomosis.[63–66] This is particularly important in elderly patients, in those with a slightly compromised anal function and in those with a relatively short life expectancy.

Additionally, a colonic pouch may result in a lower anastomotic leak rate compared with an end-to-end anastomosis.[53] General opinion now favours routine use of a pouch or a side-to-end anastomosis after TME.

Sexual and urinary disturbance

The pelvic autonomic nerves are responsible for normal urinary and sexual function (particularly in the male). The presacral nerves lie like a wishbone, joined at the sacral promontory and parting as they run distally on both pelvic side walls, and are responsible for ejaculation in the male. The nerves can be identified at the start of the posterior dissection and preserved in most cases.

The nervi erigentes lie anterolaterally in the angle between the seminal vesicles and the prostate and are responsible for male erection. Attempts to control bleeding by diathermy, clamping or suturing in this area may result in erectile failure, even when injury has been unilateral. Previously these neural structures were thought to be 'lateral ligaments' where the middle rectal artery enters, and traditionally many surgeons recommended clamping at this level. However, a significant middle rectal artery is uncommon and usually can be isolated and sealed by a light application of diathermy. Clamping here may damage the neural bundles and is no longer advocated.

With a posterior situated tumour and no evidence of disease in the anterior mesorectum on MRI, most surgeons would dissect immediately posterior to Denonvilliers' fascia/septum, to avoid potentially undue nerve injury. However in an anterior tumour, Denonvilliers's fascia/septum should be removed as it acts as a barrier to tumour penetration. In these circumstances, the nerves are at higher risk.

There have been suggestions that laparoscopic rectal mobilisation may be associated with more nerve injury, though this may be a learning curve phenomenon.[68,69]

> ✅ Patients should be warned that urinary and sexual dysfunction may follow rectal excision, whether for benign or malignant disease.

Temporary defunctioning stomas

Anastomotic leakage after a rectal anastomosis is common and the lower the anastomosis the higher the risk. Most reports suggest an incidence ranging from 10% to 28% after rectal cancer surgery.

> ✅✅ A recent excellent Swedish trial comparing patients after TME randomised to a defunctioning stoma, or no stoma, reported a reduction in leak rate from 28% to 10.3% in patients randomised to a stoma.[70] A meta-analysis and systematic review of the literature in 2008 also reported that a diverting stoma is associated with fewer clinical leaks and recommended a diverting stoma in all low rectal anastomoses.[71] Similar findings were reported from pooled data from major multicentre European trials.[72]

Alternative approaches to standard surgery for rectal cancer

Papillon/contact radiotherapy

Contact radiotherapy was first popularized by Jean Papillon in France in the early 1950s and is gaining popularity for selected patients. This strategy can be considered in patients with exophytic mobile cancers under 3 cm, and is a curative non-operative approach for some T1 cancers. The main indication continues to be elderly and/or frail patients unfit for major resectional surgery. A disadvantage is the lack of definitive histology and failure to treat the mesorectum, such that nodal metastases are a contraindication. It has been suggested that Papillon therapy can be combined with conventional external beam, or chemoradiotherapy, in selected unfit patients, or those who refuse surgery, in an effort to cure patients with more advanced tumours. Bleeding is the most common side-effect due to angiogenesis and neovascularisation.

Transanal endoscopic microsurgery (TEMS) and transanal minimally invasive surgery (TAMIS)

In the past, local excision could only be done transanally under direct vision. The equipment and technique of transanal endoscopy microsurgery (TEMS) was developed to allow transanal surgical access to virtually the entire rectum. This has been modified to adopt the transanal use of laparoscopic instruments (TAMIS).

TEMS has been shown to successfully treat selected early rectal cancers (ERC) with favourable pathology (pT1, <3 cm in diameter, well differentiated, no lymphovascular invasion).[35] If full-thickness histology shows adverse features, early completion surgery has been shown to provide similar cancer-specific survival to conventional upfront rectal excisional surgery.[35]

Advocates of TEMS for ERC (T1N0V0) argue that there is no difference in cancer-specific survival and the morbidity of major resectional surgery is avoided. The TREC trial is aiming to assess the combination of neoadjuvant therapy and TEMS compared with conventional rectal excisional surgery.

Laparoscopic surgery for rectal cancer

Laparoscopic colorectal cancer surgery was initially popularized in the 1990s, predominantly for colon cancer. Reports of laparoscopic resection to rectal cancer surgery reported favourable outcomes, similar to open surgery[73,74] with some criticism

that case selection meant that the results could not be extrapolated to routine practice. However, case selection is imperative, and laparoscopy should be an access technique applied to appropriate cases with a low threshold for converting to an open procedure if needed.

It is of interest that the latest data suggest that not only is there a learning curve for laparoscopic surgeons, but in terms of oncological outcome, the ALaCaRT[75] and ACOSOG Z6051[76] trials reported equivalence but failed to show 'non-inferiority' for laparoscopic rectal cancer surgery compared with open surgery. Advocates of laparoscopic surgery claim clear benefits in terms of reduction in adhesions, incisional hernia and a quicker return to work. However, it is clear that by whatever method rectal cancer surgery is performed, the 'decisions are more important than the incisions' and careful case selection and specimen-orientated TME surgery, in the correct anatomical planes, are the key to a good oncological outcome.

Robotic rectal cancer surgery

Robotic-assisted rectal cancer surgery is increasing in popularity and ongoing outcomes are emerging in randomised trials, particularly the ROLARR study with medium- to long-term results awaited.[77] Proposed advantages include articulating instruments and high-definition images that allow more precise dissection in the narrow male pelvis. Disadvantages include substantial cost differences, lack of training opportunities and increased operating times, especially in the early stages of a robotic programme. The concept of TME is crucial and specimen quality and feasibility should remain pivotal.

Transanal TME (TA-TME) for rectal cancer

The concept of transanal TME has evolved from aspects of TEMS and laparoscopic surgery. As for laparoscopic and robotic surgery, the transanal technique is an access technique to facilitate complex safe dissection utilising the shortest distance to the area of interest in the distal pelvis. TA-TME seeks to address the problem of low rectal dissection in the obese male with a narrow pelvis. Dissection is through the 'holy plane' of the mesorectal fascia, but approached through a rectotomy from below with an airseal system following purse-string closure of the rectum. An international registry has been established in the

UK and an initial report on early outcome in more than 800 patients is in press.

Non-operative approach for rectal cancer by 'watch and wait' after chemoradiotherapy

The Brazilian surgeon Angelita Habr-Gama has popularized the concept of 'watch and wait' for apparent complete clinical response of low rectal cancers following long-course chemoradiotherapy.[78]

Low tumours are more likely to respond for a number of reasons, including a more accurate target for delivery of radiation and a possible difference in behavior of low rectal cancer compared to cancer in the mid or upper rectum.[79]

The main contentious issue so far is that complete clinical response (CCR) may not equate to a pathological complete response (pCR) and current imaging modalities are not able to accurately predict complete pCR. However, patients who have achieved a CCR must be counselled about the possibility of a pCR in the specimen should they undergo surgery.

Our current recommendation is that long-course chemoradiotherapy is still reserved for appropriate cases (threatened CRM) and not in the hope of achieving a CCR in patients unfit for major resectional surgery.

Alternative non-surgical options in rectal cancer

In unfit patients, palliative options such as external beam radiotherapy for palliation of bleeding and consideration of a defunctioning stoma to treat, or avoid, obstruction should be considered. Liaison with experienced palliative care colleagues, the patient and the patient's family and carers can help to choose the most appropriate treatment for the individual.

Follow-up

There are three issues that need to be considered during follow-up:

1. Was a synchronous tumour overlooked preoperatively?
2. How should metachronous tumours be looked for?
3. Is there benefit in follow-up?

Synchronous tumours

There is approximately a 4% risk of a synchronous cancer at the time of the original resection and a 10–20% chance of a synchronous polyp. Preoperative optical complete colonoscopy is optimal and until recently barium enema was recommended to assess the colon completely prior to rectal cancer surgery. It seems likely that computerised tomography colonography (CTC) will replace barium enema in assessing the colon with the added advantage of additional abdominal imaging. Complete colonic assessment is crucial to identify cases where surgical management might involve more extensive, or even an additional, resection. If a complete preoperative colonic assessment was not performed, postoperative colonoscopy at about 6 months is recommended.

Metachronous tumours

The risk of a metachronous tumour is about 4%. It would seem sensible to screen the colon at intervals of 1, 3 and 5 years, and then every 5 years, with a final colonoscopy at the age of 75–80. This should protect the patient until at least the age of 80 years, when the risks of routine surveillance colonoscopy may start to outweigh benefit.

Surveillance for local and distant recurrence

Overall, 60–80% of recurrences of rectal cancer present within 2 years of surgery and more than 90% within 5 years. Recurrence is a misnomer as this represents progression of disease that was not detected initially while locoregional recurrence may be a result of inadequate local treatment.

A meta-analysis in 2007 concluded that intensive follow-up after curative resection of colorectal cancer improved overall survival and re-resection rates for recurrent disease.[80] A Cochrane review in 2008 came to the same conclusion, advocating intensive follow-up for patients after curative treatment for colorectal cancer.[81] Detection and resection of liver metastases is associated with 25–51% 5-year survival.[82] It is also generally agreed that chemotherapy for advanced unresectable disease may improve quality of life and is more effective when applied early.

✔✔ Two meta-analyses of all randomised trials of follow-up have shown improved survival with intensive follow-up.[81,83]

The way forward

Optimal imaging is crucial and may involve functional imaging such as PET-CT in combination with pelvic MRI; more accurate imaging will allow more selective use of neoadjuvant radiotherapy, which is a local treatment with little impact on systemic disease. Neoadjuvant chemotherapy (omitting radiotherapy) may improve outcome in patients detected at imaging to have a high risk of systemic metastases.

Key points

- MRI assesses the status of the mesorectal fascia (the potential CRM), aiding selection for neoadjuvant treatment.
- Optimal outcome for rectal cancer requires adequate TME.
- Consider defunctioning stoma in low anterior resection.
- Extralevator APE is optimal management of advanced low rectal cancer involving sphincters.
- Evidence suggests benefit of intensive follow-up.

⏵ Recommended videos:

Laparoscopic anterior resection with TME
- https://tinyurl.com/msyltoz

TaTME
- https://www.youtube.com/watch?v=P802mTMTIB8

TEMS
- https://www.youtube.com/watch?v=hyiJA9y1NwM

TAMIS
- https://www.youtube.com/watch?v=Vw8YqCZodP8

🌐 Full references available at **http://expertconsult.inkling.com**

Key references

70. Matthiessen P, Hallbook O, Rutegard J, et al. Defunctioning stoma reduces symptomatic anastomotic leakage after low anterior resection of the rectum for cancer: a randomized multicenter trial. Ann Surg 2007;246:207–14. PMID: 17667498.
A trial comparing patients after TME randomised to a defunctioning stoma, or no stoma, reported a reduction in leak rate from 28% to 10.3% in patients randomised to a stoma.

71. Huser N, Michalski CW, Erkan M, et al. Systematic review and meta-analysis of the role of defunctioning stoma in low rectal cancer surgery. Ann Surg 2008;248:52–60. PMID: 18580207.
A meta-analysis showing that a diverting stoma is associated with fewer clinical leaks.

81. Jeffery M, Hickey BE, Hider PN. Follow-up strategies for patients treated for non-metastatic colorectal cancer. Cochrane Database Syst Rev 2007;CD002200. PMID: 17253476.

83. Renehan AG, Egger M, Saunders MP, et al. Impact on survival of intensive follow up after curative resection for colorectal cancer: systematic review and meta-analysis of randomised trials. Br Med J 2002;324:813. PMID: 11934773.
Meta-analysis showing significant benefit for intensive follow-up.

7

Perioperative chemotherapy and radiotherapy for colorectal cancer

Simon Gollins
David Sebag-Montefiore

Introduction

Colorectal cancer is the third most common cancer in the UK, with approximately 41 000 cases diagnosed each year, of which about two-thirds arise in the colon and one-third in the rectum. Multidisciplinary management is of key importance to successfully integrate the various medical and surgical disciplines to improve patient outcome.

Recent statistics from Cancer Research UK[1] demonstrate a steady improvement in overall survival for bowel cancer. Between 1971 and 2011, age-standardised 5-year net survival increased from 24% to 59%. It is likely that improved staging, perioperative care, surgical technique and adjuvant therapy have all played a part in this improvement.

Adjuvant chemotherapy for colorectal cancer

Historically, high rates of local recurrence after rectal cancer resection meant that clinical trials could more easily determine the benefit of adjuvant chemotherapy (AC) on survival in colon cancer without the confounding effect of local recurrence that was present with rectal cancer.

Clinical trials performed in the 1980s convincingly demonstrated an improvement in disease-free and overall survival with the addition of 5-fluorouracil (5FU)-based chemotherapy after resection of stage III colon cancer and by the late 1990s a 6-month course of 5FU was standard.[2]

Oral forms of 5FU, namely uracil-tegafur (UFT) and capecitabine, have been shown to be as effective as intravenous (IV) 5FU and are licensed for adjuvant use.[3,4] The most commonly used oral agent is capecitabine and the toxicity profile differs, with capecitabine causing increased hand–foot syndrome compared to IV 5FU, and 5FU causing increased stomatitis and neutropenia compared to capecitabine.

✔✔ Oral capecitabine is at least equivalent to intravenous 5FU as adjuvant chemotherapy for colon cancer.[4]

Adding oxaliplatin to fluoropyrimidine chemotherapy in stage III patients reduces recurrence risk further (Table 7.1). Two randomised phase III trials (MOSAIC and NSABP C-07) examining the addition of oxaliplatin to 5FU[5,6] and a third (NO16968) the addition of oxaliplatin to capecitabine,[7] have consistently demonstrated an advantage. NICE has approved oxaliplatin for this indication.[8] Long-term follow-up data from the MOSAIC Trial have shown an 8.1% 10-year overall survival (OS) improvement in stage III (59.0% vs 67.1%, HR 0.80, $P=0.016$) but no difference in stage II patients (79.5% vs 78.4%, HR 1.00, $P=0.98$).[9]

✔✔ Three pivotal adjuvant chemotherapy trials demonstrated improved cancer-related outcome when oxaliplatin is added to fluoropyrimidine chemotherapy as adjuvant therapy of colon cancer.[5–7]

Table 7.1 • Disease-free and overall survival from trials testing the addition of oxaliplatin or irinotecan to fluoropyrimidine chemotherapy

	Oxaliplatin + 5FU	5FU	Irinotecan + 5FU	
MOSAIC				
All patients n = 2246				
5 yr DFS	73.3%	67.4%	–	HR 0.80 (0.68–0.93)
6 yr OS	78.5%	76.0%	–	HR 0.84 (0.71–1.00)
Stage III n = 1347				
5 yr DFS	66.4%	58.9%	–	HR 0.78 (0.65–0.93)
6 yr OS	72.9%	68.7%	–	HR 0.80 (0.65–0.97)
Stage II n = 899				
5 yr DFS	83.7%	79.9%	–	HR 0.84 (0.62–1.14)
5 yr OS	86.9%	86.8%	–	HR 1.00 (0.70–1.41)
NSABP C07				
All patients n = 2,409				
5 yr DFS	69.4%	64.2%	–	HR 0.82 (0.72–0.93)
5 yr OS	80.2%	78.4%	–	HR 0.88 (0.75–1.02)
Stage III				
5 yr DFS	64.4%	57.8%	–	Not stated
5 yr OS	76.5%	73.8%	–	Not stated
Stage II				
5 yr DFS	82.1%	80.1%	–	Not stated
5 yr OS	89.7%	89.6%	–	Not stated
NO16968				
n = 1886				
5 yr DFS	66.1%	59.8%	–	HR 0.80 (0.69–0.93)
5 yr OS*	77.6%	74.2%		Not stated
PETACC-03				
PETACC-03				
Stage III				
n = 2094				
5 yr DFS	–	54.3%	56.7%	HR 0.90 (0.79–1.02)
5 yr OS	–	71.3%	73.6%	P = 0.094
CALGB 8903				
n = 1264				
5 yr DFS	–	61%	59%	Not stated
5 yr OS	–	71%	68%	Not stated

DFS, disease-free survival; OS, overall survival; HR, hazard ratio.

*After 57 months follow-up only. Further longer-term follow-up data awaited.

Acute and long-term toxicity

Fluoropyrimidine chemotherapy is associated with lethargy, mucositis, diarrhoea and hand–foot syndrome. Watery eyes, minor nosebleeds and taste alterations are common but usually reversible. The risk of neutropenic sepsis is low, although a very small proportion of patients (<1%) are deficient in the enzyme dihydropyrimidine dehydrogenase and severe toxicity may be seen within the first 3 weeks of treatment.

The addition of oxaliplatin is associated with an increased risk of diarrhoea and neutropenia. The most significant toxicity, however, is neurotoxicity. This is seen during treatment, with paraesthesia and cold sensitivity of the extremities and larynx/upper oesophagus. Sensory neuropathy may develop either during or after completion of adjuvant chemotherapy. The incidence and severity of this peripheral sensory neuropathy (PSN) reduces over time. In the MOSAIC trial, grade 3 PNS (functional impairment) reduced from 12.5% during treatment to 0.7% by 10 months. The incidence of grade 3 PSN remained at 0.7% at 48 months post-treatment.[5]

The potential risks associated with the regimen should be weighed against the potential survival benefits of adding oxaliplatin. Generally, higher-risk patients of good performance status should be considered for an oxaliplatin-based combination.

The elderly

A lack of benefit in the elderly from the addition of oxaliplatin to 5FU has been suggested in meta-analysis.[10] However, data from the most recent XELOXA Trial suggest that the elderly benefit as much as younger patients.[7] However, because of increased toxicity in older patients, careful individual assessment must be made of the competing risks of toxicity, death from cancer and death other causes.

Stage II disease

There is less evidence supporting the use of AC in lymph node negative (stage II, Dukes' B) disease compared to stage III. The UK QUASAR 1 trial randomized 3239 patients (91% with stage II) to 5FU or observation. Use of chemotherapy reduced risk of recurrence by 22% (HR 0.78, $P = 0.008$) and improved OS by 3.6%.[11]

Oxaliplatin is not licensed or usually recommended for use in stage II cancers.[12] However, a number of features increase the risk of systemic recurrence in stage II disease to a level comparable with stage III, including stage pT4, extramural vascular invasion, obstructed or perforated cancers, poor or mucinous differentiation, and fewer than 12 lymph nodes assessed in the specimen. Oxaliplatin use can be considered in these patients.

Approximately 15% of stage II colon cancers have defects in the DNA mismatch repair system (dMMR) leading to microsatellite instability (MSI) and these tumours have a better overall prognosis compared to microsatellite-stable (MSS) tumours.[13] Meta-analysis suggested that patients with MSI tumours do not derive benefit from adjuvant chemotherapy using 5FU alone.[14] However, UK data from the QUASAR trial failed to demonstrate any effect of MMR status on adjuvant 5FU benefit.[15] Guidance from the UK Royal College of Pathologists recommends assessment of MSI either by immunohistochemistry or genetically for the four mismatch repair (MMR) proteins in stage II patients who are being considered for adjuvant therapy. Several commercial array-based assays have been developed to stratify stage II cancers into low versus high risk to attempt to inform patient discussion. Such tests add significantly to cost and thus far have not demonstrated an advantage in individual risk stratification over MSI.[16]

Addition of 'targeted' therapy to chemotherapy

Phase III trials have examined the addition of targeted agents in the adjuvant setting. No benefit for the addition of bevacizumab[17] or cetuximab[18] has been demonstrated.

✔✔ There is no evidence to support the addition of targeted therapy to adjuvant chemotherapy.

Likewise, there was no advantage for the addition of irinotecan to 5FU.[19]

Timing and duration of adjuvant chemotherapy

Most but not all clinical trials recommend a 6- to 8-week time point for the commencement of AC. A meta-analysis of 15 410 patients in 10 trials concluded that an increase of 4 weeks in the time to start AC was associated with a significant decrease in overall survival.[20] Chemotherapy should therefore start soon after surgery, although the authors acknowledge that a benefit for chemotherapy may still exist if a significant delay is needed.

Previous trials have demonstrated that 6 months of chemotherapy is as effective as a 12-month course of treatment. Six concurrent international trials including a total of 12,834 patients compared 6 versus 3 months of oxaliplatin-based adjuvant chemotherapy (either XELOX or FOLFOX). These were reported in abstract form at the American Society of Clinical Oncology Annual Meeting in June 2017 as a combined analysis through the IDEA collaboration. Grade 3 neurotoxicity was greater for 6 versus 3 months of treatment (16 v 3% for FOLFOX and 9 v 3% for XELOX, p<0.0001). Non-inferiority of 3 versus 6 months was not established for the overall cohort, or for patients treated with FOLFOX. However, non-inferiority of 3 versus 6 months was supported for XELOX (3 versus 6 months disease-free survival hazard ratio 0.95 [95% CI, 0.85–1.06]). As each individual trial treated varying proportions of patients with XELOX (0 to 75%), the regimen interaction likely produced the differential outcomes which were observed between individual studies. Certain substages (T1-3 N1) also showed non-inferiority for 3m v 6m. The data provide a framework for discussions on risks and benefits of individualized adjuvant therapy approaches.[21] The current UK FOxTROT trial (ISRCTN 87163246) in 1050 patients is examining whether introducing 6 weeks of preoperative chemotherapy will confer any benefit compared to standard postoperative therapy. Recruitment was completed in December 2016.

Adjuvant chemotherapy in rectal cancer

Current UK practice, supported by NICE guidance,[12] is to complete local treatment of the pelvis with surgery±radiotherapy before considering systemic AC. A systematic review of 9785 patients with rectal cancer in 21 randomised trials demonstrated modest improvements in both disease-free survival (DFS) (HR 0.75) and OS (0.83) with postoperative AC.[22] However, these trials pre-dated widespread use of total mesorectal excision (TME). Only one study tested AC following preoperative RT (EORTC 22921), and it notably failed to demonstrate significant benefit (HR 0.91, CI 0.77–1.08).[23] A recent meta-analysis of 1196 patients in four trials incorporating preoperative radiotherapy suggested limited or no benefit for AC (HR for DFS $0 \cdot 91$, CI 0.77–1.07; $P = 0 \cdot 230$).[24] However, a benefit was seen for tumours 10–15 cm from the anal verge (HR for DFS 0.59, CI 0.40–0.85, $P = 0.005$).

Several factors combine to reduce AC effectiveness in rectal cancer, including treatment delay and poor compliance. Morbidity from surgery and radiotherapy reduces patients' tolerance of AC. In addition, the presence of a temporary defunctioning ileostomy postoperatively can impair chemotherapy delivery because of diarrhoea. In EORTC 22921 and CHRONICLE less than half of patients (43% and 48%, respectively) completed all cycles of AC.[25,26] In EORTC 22921 and the I-CNR-RT trial 27% and 28% of patients, respectively, were unable to start AC.[25,27]

Currently there is a widespread lack of consensus in international guidelines with regard to the use of AC in rectal cancer, reflecting the evidence above. For example, UK NICE guidelines[12] recommend consideration of adjuvant chemotherapy for patients with high-risk stage II and all stage III rectal cancer, whereas ESMO guidelines are more circumspect following treatment with preoperative CRT.[28]

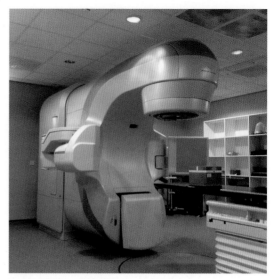

Figure 7.1 • A modern linear accelerator.

Radiotherapy

Radiotherapy is delivered with linear accelerators (**Fig. 7.1**) that can target tumours with accuracy (**Fig. 7.2**). Over the past three decades there has been a considerable effort to define the role of radiotherapy in rectal cancer. Until the mid-1990s randomised controlled trials included a standard arm of surgery alone.

The established indications for adjuvant radiation in rectal cancer include reducing the risk of local pelvic recurrence and to shrink locally advanced rectal cancer to facilitate successful resection.

There is considerable debate regarding the use of radiotherapy to increase the rate of sphincter-

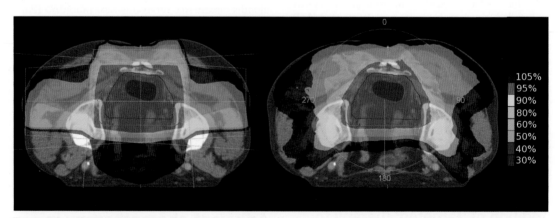

Figure 7.2 • Modem radiotherapy planning using 3-dimensional computerised tomography (3DCT) (*left*) and volumetric arc therapy (VMAT) (*right*). The dose intended to be delivered to the 'Planning Target Volume' (PTV), containing the tumour, is 100% and the dose delivered to various regions of the pelvis is illustrated by colour-wash. VMAT delivers a more conformal high-dose volume and less dose anteriorly to the small bowel and anterior part of the bladder. 3DCT treats a slightly smaller volume of tissue to a low-dose 'bath' outside the high-dose region.

preserving surgery or as organ conservation (to delay or avoid surgical resection altogether).

Evidence base for the use of adjuvant radiotherapy in resectable rectal cancer

A Cochrane overview[29] and other overviews[30,31] have all concluded that both preoperative and postoperative radiotherapy reduce the risk of local recurrence compared with surgery alone. However, although there is some evidence that cancer-specific survival was improved there was no definite evidence of any impact on overall survival. Both preoperative radiotherapy and the use of a biological equivalent dose of >30 Gy were associated with the greatest treatment effect.

In North America, clinical trials initially focused on the benefit of postoperative radiotherapy and its integration with systemic chemotherapy for patients with both stage II and stage III rectal cancer. The NIH consensus statement in 1990[32] recommended that patients with stage II and stage III rectal cancer should receive both systemic chemotherapy and concurrent chemoradiotherapy.

In contrast, clinical trials in northern Europe evaluated radiotherapy alone in the preoperative setting with a major interest in the use of a short accelerated schedule using 5 Gy per fraction. A sequence of randomised controlled trials, mainly in Scandinavia, refined the use of 'short-course radiotherapy' delivering 25 Gy in five daily fractions of 5 Gy with immediate surgery.[33–35] The Swedish Rectal Cancer Trial,[34] including 1168 patients, was the first to report an improvement in overall survival without the use of systemic chemotherapy. This trial also overcame the increase in early operative mortality that was seen in previous trials through the use of radiotherapy, by reducing the size of the radiotherapy fields and using a multifield (three- or four-field) technique.

However, lower local recurrence rates associated with the increasing use of TME[36,37] in individual surgical series and population-based studies required clinical trials to further evaluate the role of preoperative radiotherapy combined with TME.

Short-course radiotherapy and TME

Two trials, the Dutch TME and the MRC CR07 trials, then addressed the role of preoperative short-course radiotherapy followed by TME compared with a highly selective approach to postoperative radiotherapy restricted to patients with involvement of the circumferential resection margin. In the Dutch trial[38,39] highly selective postoperative treatment used radiotherapy alone and no systemic chemotherapy was allowed postoperatively. The CR07 trial[40] used concurrent 5FU chemoradiotherapy (CRT) when postoperative radiotherapy was indicated and a predetermined adjuvant systemic chemotherapy policy for each centre was applied to both treatment arms (Table 7.2).

The Dutch trial recruited 1861 and the MRC CR07 1350 patients. Both have demonstrated very similar findings where the risk of local recurrence was reduced from 11% with surgery first to 4–5% with the routine use of short-course preoperative radiotherapy. There was no evidence of a difference in operative mortality or anastomotic leak between the treatment arms.

No evidence of a difference in overall survival was seen between treatment arms in either trial. The reduction in local recurrence is seen across the subsites of the rectum and the absolute difference between the treatment arms is seen with increasing tumour and nodal stage.

✔️✔️ The Dutch TME and MRC CR07 trials both show that short-course radiotherapy halves the risk of local recurrence when combined with TME, but there is no difference in overall survival.[38-40]

CR07 demonstrated that good-quality surgery in the mesorectal fascial plane is vital to reducing the risk of local pelvic recurrence.[41]

Preoperative concurrent chemoradiotherapy

Two phase III trials tested the addition of concurrent 5FU/LV to radiotherapy compared to long-course radiotherapy alone. The EORTC 22921 trial[23] recruited 1011 patients and used a factorial 2×2 design to compare radiotherapy 45 Gy with or without concurrent 5FU/LV and a second randomisation of adjuvant postoperative 5FU/LV versus no chemotherapy. The FFCD 9203 trial[42] recruited 762 patients and compared radiotherapy 45 Gy with or without concurrent 5FU/LV with all patients recommended to receive postoperative adjuvant 5FU/LV.

The two trials reported very similar findings. The acute toxicity was increased but acceptable with the addition of concurrent chemotherapy and the risk of local recurrence was reduced from 15% to 8–10% in favour of chemoradiation (CRT). No evidence of a difference in disease-free or overall survival was seen.

✔️✔️ The addition of 5FU/LV to long-course radiotherapy halved the risk of local recurrence but had no impact on overall survival in two large European phase III trials.[23,42]

Table 7.2 • Key trials comparing outcomes following short-course preoperative radiotherapy and radiotherapy and chemoradiation

Trial	No. pts	Randomisation	N	1 endpoint	LR	OS	DFS
Short-course preoperative radiotherapy trials							
Dutch Trial CKVO 95-04 (2011) SCPRT	1861	25 Gy in 5 fractions + surgery	897	LR	10 years 5%	10 years 48%	Not stated
		Surgery + highly selective RT	908		11%	49%	
CR07 (2008) SCPRT	1350	25 Gy in 5 fractions + surgery	674	LR	3 years 5%	3 years 80%	3 years 78%
		Surgery + highly selective CRT	676		11%	79%	72%
Preop long-course RT ± chemotherapy trials							
EORTC 22921 (2006)	1011	45 Gy in 25 fractions vs	505	OS	5 years 17%	5 years 65%	5 years 54%
		5FU/FA + 45 Gy	506		vs 9%	vs 66%	vs 56%
FFCD 9203 (2006)	762	45 Gy in 25 fractions vs	367	OS	5 years 17%	5 years 68%	No data
		FUFA + 45 Gy	375		vs 8%	vs 67%	
Preop CRT vs postop CRT trial							
CAA/ARO/AIO-94 (2004)	823	Preop 50.4 Gy + 5FU vs	421	OS	5 years 6%	5 years 76%	5 years 68%
		Postop 55.8 Gy + 5FU	402		vs 13%	vs 74%	vs 65%

CRT, chemoradiotherapy; DFS, disease-free survival; FA, folinic acid; 5FU, 5-fluorouracil; LR, local recurrence; OS, overall survival; RT, radiotherapy; SCPRT, short-course preoperative radiotherapy.

The German Rectal Cancer Group,[43] at a similar time, compared preoperative CRT versus postoperative CRT, recruiting 823 patients. This trial demonstrated a lower rate of local recurrence (6% vs 12%), reduced acute and late toxicity in favour of preoperative CRT, but without any evidence of a difference in disease-free or overall survival (Table 7.2).

The three trials were highly influential and led to a significant shift from the use of postoperative CRT to preoperative CRT.

Non-inferiority of capecitabine to infusional 5FU in preoperative CRT regimes has been demonstrated in two randomized trials.[44,45]

Short-course radiotherapy versus preoperative CRT

Two trials have directly compared short-course radiotherapy with preoperative CRT. The Polish trial[46] was designed to test whether preoperative CRT would increase the rate of sphincter-preserving surgery and randomised 312 patients.

The comparison of local recurrence and toxicity were secondary end-points and the trial was not statistically powered for these specific questions. The Trans Tasman Radiation Oncology Group[47] randomised 326 patients with local recurrence as the primary end-point. In both trials there is no evidence of a difference in local recurrence or survival.

Short-course radiotherapy and delay to surgery

Although there is clear evidence that short-course preoperative radiotherapy (SCPRT) reduces the risk of local recurrence, there is limited information regarding its efficacy in downstaging locally advanced disease where a delay prior to surgery is required. However, evidence is now emerging. Small series of patients[48,49] have reported acceptable toxicity and a complete pathological response (pCR) rate of 8–15% when this approach is used in elderly and poor performance status patients. The Stockholm III trial (accrual completed) compares SCPRT and immediate surgery with SCPRT and delay with long-course radiotherapy prior to surgery. An interim analysis of 120 patients treated with SCPRT and delay reported a pCR rate of 12.5%.[50] This strategy warrants wider evaluation, offers an alternative treatment when preoperative CRT is not feasible (comorbidity, relative contraindications to 5FU) and has been incorporated into three randomised trials described in the section 'Neoadjuvant Chemotherapy' below.

Late toxicity and second malignancy

Although preoperative radiotherapy and CRT reduce the risk of local recurrence, there is no evidence of an improvement in survival. The benefit in the reduction in local recurrence must be compared with the risks of late toxicity. Long-term side-effects of pelvic radiotherapy for rectal cancer include bowel, sexual and urinary dysfunction and sterility.[51–53] An initial Swedish report using wide field radiotherapy suggested an increased risk of second malignancy.[52] However, more recent analysis of Dutch[54] and Swedish[55] trials failed to confirm this.

Quality-of-life data from the CR07 trial demonstrate a significant impairment in sexual function attributable to surgery and a further detriment due to radiotherapy.[53] Both the Dutch and CR07 trials show a similar pattern for faecal incontinence.[51,53] The Polish and TROG trials[46,47] have not shown a difference in clinician-assessed late toxicity when short-course radiotherapy was compared with preoperative CRT. A systematic review of randomised controlled trials in rectal cancer showed that patient-reported outcomes demonstrated consistently higher toxicity than clinician-reported outcomes and that there was variable quality between studies.[56]

Patient selection

The routine use of preoperative radiotherapy is difficult to justify if good quality TME alone reduces the risk of local recurrence to low levels and a more selective approach is needed.

The MERCURY international phase II observational study established the role of pelvic magnetic resonance imaging (MRI) in the staging of rectal cancer.[57] This study demonstrated equivalence between the measured extramural spread of tumour seen on high-resolution MRI and the same measurement on histopathology whole mounts after surgery alone. Further reports have described a good prognosis group of patients in whom the risk of local recurrence is very low without radiotherapy.[58] MRI can also identify when the primary tumour extends to or within 1 mm of the mesorectal fascia[59] (**Fig. 7.3**), a situation where downstaging with preoperative CRT is indicated (**Fig. 7.4**). The recent MERCURY II prospective observational study has suggested that MRI scanning for low rectal cancers can identify tumours in which there is a 'safe' resection plane and preoperative radiotherapy is not indicated.[60]

Many centres have adopted a risk-stratified approach. The 2011 UK NICE guidelines[12] defined three risk groups for local recurrence. In the low-risk group, radiotherapy is not given and preoperative CRT is recommended in the high-risk, margin-threatened group (Table 7.3). In the

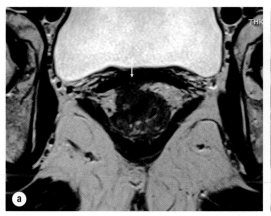
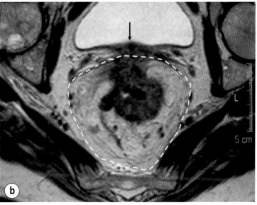

Figure 7.3 • MRI is now a standard preoperative technique to identify rectal cancer that threatens, involves or breaches mesorectal fascia. Such patients can then be selected for more aggressive preoperative treatment to try to downsize the tumour and facilitate complete resection. In **(a)** a low rectal tumour threatens the mesorectal fascia anteriorly (*white arrow*) and also sits very close to the right levator ani at 8 o'clock. In **(b)** a mid-rectal cancer breaches the mesorectal fascia (*white dashed line*) to involve the bladder wall anteriorly (*black arrow*).

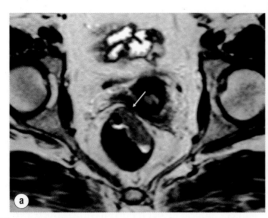

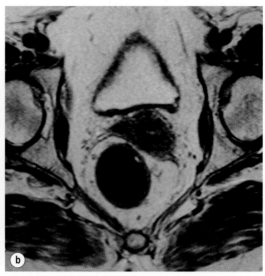

Figure 7.4 • Response to neoadjuvant chemoradiotherapy. **(a)** A bulky mid-rectal tumour threatens the expected CRM anteriorly (*white arrow*). **(b)** Following an excellent response to neoadjuvant CRT, the CRM is no longer threatened.

Table 7.3 • NICE stratification of rectal cancer according to risk of local pelvic recurrence

Risk of local pelvic recurrence	Characteristics of rectal tumours predicted by MRI
Low (resectable)	cT1 or cT2 or cT3a **and** no lymph node involvement
Moderate (resectable)	any cT3b or greater, in which the potential surgical margin is not threatened **or** any suspicious lymph node not threatening the surgical resection margin **or** the presence of extramural vascular invasion
High (borderline resectable or unresectable, i.e. threatened or involved CRM)	a threatened (<1 mm) or breached resection margin **or** low tumours encroaching onto the intersphincteric plane or with levator involvement

NICE Guideline CG131; 2011.[12]

tumours. Surgical quality based on TME gradually improved during the Dutch and CR07 trials but has also continued to improve since. These advances have markedly improved outcomes using surgery alone, resulting in low rates of local recurrence. A Norwegian population-based series of 15 193 rectal cancer patients from 1993 to 2010 showed that local recurrence rates following surgery alone were initially high, at 14.1% (1993–1997), but a decade later had fallen dramatically to 5.3% (2007–2010).[61] Patients who received preoperative radiotherapy between 2007 and 2010 had only a marginally lower recurrence rate of 4.3%.

For lower rectal cancers extra-levator abdomino-perineal excision has been reported to reduce risks of resection margin involvement and specimen perforation and an increasing use of this technique may in time reduce the use of preoperative radiotherapy.[62,63]

However wide variation in radiotherapy usage exists. In a recent report, among 9201 patients who had a rectal cancer resection (all disease stages), across 148 English NHS Trusts, the proportion of rectal cancer patients managed with surgery alone varied from as little as 22% to 95%.[64]

medium-risk group either SCPRT or preoperative CRT may be used as there is evidence to support both approaches and no clear evidence that one is superior to the other. ESMO guidelines advocate a similar approach.[28] The choice between SCPRT and CRT remains controversial, particularly because neither has been shown to increase overall survival.

There is increasing evidence that modern preoperative staging, combined with adoption of best-quality TME surgery, produces low recurrence rates using surgery alone in patients with non-margin-threatened

Sphincter preservation

There is very little evidence to support the view that preoperative CRT increases the chance of a sphincter-preserving resection. In the majority of patients with a mid or upper rectal cancer, an anterior resection is feasible without tumour shrinkage. Very low tumours less than 4 cm from the anal verge require an abdominoperineal excision. Therefore, it is only in a very small group of patients whose distal tumour extent is 4–6 cm from the anal verge where preoperative CRT may play a role in achieving a sphincter-preserving procedure.[65]

Organ preservation

There is increasing interest in the role of non-surgical therapy to avoid major resectional surgery. This approach has been pioneered by Habr; patients with complete clinical response after chemoradiotherapy undergo intensive follow-up, with surgery reserved for locoregional failure. Approximately 20–30% of patients have sustained local control without radical surgery.[66–68]

A Dutch publication describes similar results.[69] However, only 10% of the patients treated with CRT achieved a complete clinical response (CCR) and entered the study. The definition of CCR was rigorous, consisting of negative biopsy, complete clinical resolution, no suspicious findings on flexible sigmoidoscopy and no evidence of residual tumour on pelvic MRI.

In a recent UK report, 129 rectal cancer patients achieving a complete clinical response to CRT were managed by a watch-and-wait approach. A substantial proportion avoided major surgery, with 44 (34%) experiencing local regrowths and 36 (88%) of 41 patients with non-metastatic local regrowths being salvaged.[70] There was no difference in overall survival compared to a matched cohort undergoing surgery, although the watch-and-wait group had superior 3-year colostomy-free survival (74% vs 47%, $P=0.0001$).

An alternative strategy is to use transanal endoscopic microsurgery (TEMS)[71] to accurately assess the impact of a good clinical response to preoperative treatment to determine which patients can undergo intensive follow-up and those who require a formal resection based on histopathological findings. Such a strategy has recently been described for a cohort of 62 patients from four regional UK centres with cT1–2 N0 rectal cancers, staged using high-quality MRI and endorectal ultrasonography. Following SCRT and TEMS, 60 patients achieved an R0 resection, 20 resected specimens were ypT0 and only in four patients were there intraluminal local recurrences.[72]

Prospective multicentre studies are required to determine the benefits of both of the above strategies. It is likely that the patients most likely to benefit from a non-surgical approach are those with early stage disease. In the UK, this group of patients is not normally treated with preoperative radiotherapy at all. Therefore, prospective studies are essential to determine the value of this approach. The UK phase II TREC trial (ISRCTN14422743) examined the feasibility of randomising patients between standard TME versus SCRT followed by TEMS (results awaited).

Modern radiotherapy techniques, including intensity-modulated radiotherapy (IMRT) and volumetric arc therapy (VMAT) (Fig. 7.2), allow increased conformality of treated volumes. This potentially allows delivery of increased dose to the tumour without excessive morbidity to surrounding normal tissues, thereby reducing short- and long-term toxicity compared to conventional 3DCT planning. This may have relevance to an organ-sparing approach although prospective studies are needed to prove clinical benefit.[73]

Low-energy contact X-ray brachytherapy (CXB, the Papillon technique) involves insertion of an X-ray tube through the anus and placing it in close contact with the tumour.[74] Recent NICE Interventional Procedures Guidance (IPG532)[75] indicates that CXB is an option for patients with early rectal cancer in whom surgery is not considered suitable. Further evidence is required regarding the benefit of CXB in addition to CRT.

Future directions: intensification of neoadjuvant treatment

Reduction of rectal cancer local recurrence has not had any significant impact on distant metastatic relapse and this is now the major cause of death.[24,40,76] Features on histological examination of resected specimens predict increased risk of postoperative systemic recurrence, including more than 5 mm invasion of disease through the muscularis propria into the mesorectum (≥T3c), extramural vascular invasion (EMVI) and lymph node involvement. For patients with such features, with optimum surgery and selective use of preoperative radiotherapy, distant metastatic relapse is about sixfold greater than local recurrence (about 30% vs 5%).[40,76,77] MRI scanning is the pre-treatment investigation that can most reliably identify such features.[78]

Potential strategies to improve neoadjuvant therapy include adding a second drug to preoperative CRT and the introduction of neoadjuvant chemotherapy (NAC) prior to LCCRT or SCRT.[79]

Addition of a second concurrent chemotherapy agent during LCCRT

Five randomised phase III trials have added oxaliplatin to either 5FU or capecitabine during CRT, with variable results. Two have thus far published long-term outcomes in full-length reports, The ACCORD 12 trial compared 45 Gy capecitabine CRT with 50 Gy oxaliplatin and capecitabine in 598 patients and reported no difference in the rate of pCR (the primary end-point) or 3-year disease-free survival (DFS) or overall survival.[80] The German CAO/ARO/AIO-04 trial randomised 1265 patients to LCCRT using concurrent 5FU then 16 weeks of postoperative 5FU-based chemotherapy, with or without oxaliplatin. DFS was increased from 71.2 to 75.9% (HR 0.79,

$P = 0.03$).[77] However, because oxaliplatin was added to both the concurrent and adjuvant chemotherapy components and different 5FU dose intensities were used between treatment arms, the benefit of oxaliplatin-intensified CRT is not known. The NSABP R-04,[81] PETTAC 6[82] and STAR 1[83] trials, reported in abstract form, do not describe any improvement in cancer outcomes for their primary end-point (local recurrence, DFS and overall survival respectively). Concurrent single agent fluoropyrimidine (5FU or capecitabine) CRT remains the standard of care. The currently recruiting UK phase III ARISTOTLE trial (ISRCTN09351447) compares capecitabine-based CRT with or without additional irinotecan.

Neoadjuvant chemotherapy

Administering systemic neoadjuvant chemotherapy (NAC) before local pelvic treatment is attractive because treatment delivery is potentially improved and micrometastases receive full-dose chemotherapy months earlier than with postoperative adjuvant chemotherapy. NAC can improve pelvic tumour-related symptoms[84] and also allows earlier defunctioning stoma reversal, with potential quality of life and health economic benefits. However, theoretical disadvantages to the use of NAC include delayed time to surgery and disease progression and decreased effectiveness of subsequent radiotherapy due to emergence of radio-resistant clones.

Several phase II trials of NAC have suggested acceptable toxicity, low rates of progression whilst on NAC and promising response rates.[84-86] One phase III randomised trial from Poland[87] compared standard LCCRT followed by surgery, with SCPRT then 6 weeks of FOLFOX chemotherapy then surgery. A total of 541 patients with fixed T3 or T4 tumours were included, although staging MRI was not mandated. Oxaliplatin was included initially in both standard and experimental arms but later allowed to be omitted. There was no difference between the arms in R0 resection rate (the primary end-point), local failure, distant failure or DFS. A marginally statistically significant difference in overall survival was reported (73% vs 65%, $P = 0.046$), although this significance disappeared once patients with recurrent tumours were removed from the analysis.

Two other trials have a similar design, the Dutch-Scandinavian RAPIDO trial (NCT01558921), which completed accrual of 920 patients in June 2016, and the Chinese 552-patient STELLAR trial (NCT02533271), currently recruiting. Recruitment continues in the 460-patient French PRODIGE 23 trial (NCT01804790), comparing standard preoperative LCCRT including capecitabine, with 12 weeks of FOLFIRINOX prior to LCCRT. The US PROSPECT trial (NCT01515787) in 1060 patients compares NAC with preoperative LCCRT in early tumours (T2–3 N1 or T3N0) not intended for abdominoperineal excision. In the experimental arm LCCRT is used only if there is a poor response with NAC.

Key points

- Between 1971 and 2011, age-standardised 5-year bowel cancer survival increased from 24% to 59%. It is likely that improved staging, perioperative care, surgical technique and adjuvant therapy have all had a role in this improvement.
- Oxaliplatin-fluoropyrimidine adjuvant chemotherapy improves survival and is standard for stage III colon cancer and is commonly used for high-risk stage II colon cancer.
- Adjuvant chemotherapy is used in rectal cancer by extrapolation from colon cancer but the evidence to support its use following high-quality TME surgery and preoperative (chemo)radiotherapy is weak.
- There is no evidence to support the use of targeted agents as adjuvant therapy.
- There is a strong evidence base demonstrating that preoperative radiotherapy reduces the risk of local recurrence after resection of rectal cancer, although it does not improve overall survival.
- The addition of concurrent 5FU to long-course radiotherapy reduces the risk of local recurrence.
- A risk-adapted policy for the use of preoperative radiotherapy based on optimum preoperative staging including pelvic MRI scanning, balances the benefit and risks.
- Earlier stage tumours have a greater chance of achieving a complete response to pelvic chemoradiation, thereby potentially avoiding radical surgery. However, different potential strategies to achieve organ preservation require further prospective multicentre study.
- Strategies incorporating neoadjuvant preoperative chemotherapy in rectal cancer are attractive because micrometastatic disease (the main cause of rectal cancer death), is treated earlier than with current standard postoperative chemotherapy. However, further prospective evidence is required to confirm the benefit of this approach.

🌐 Full references available at **http://expertconsult.inkling.com**

Key references

4. Twelves C, Wong A, Nowacki MP, et al. Capecitabine as adjuvant treatment for stage III colon cancer. N Engl J Med 2005;352(26):2696–704. PMID: 15987918.
   The X-ACT study showed equivalence between bolus 5FU and folinic acid and oral fluoropyrimidine capecitabine after 6.9 years of follow-up.

5. Andre T, Boni C, Mounedji-Boudiaf L, et al. Oxaliplatin, fluorouracil, and leucovorin as adjuvant treatment for colon cancer. N Engl J Med 2004;350:2343–51. PMID: 15175436.

6. Yothers G, O'Connell MJ, Allegra CJ, et al. Oxaliplatin as adjuvant therapy for colon cancer: updated results of NSABP C-07 trial, including survival and subset analyses. J Clin Oncol 2011;29:3768–74. PMID: 21859995.
   The NSABP C07 study demonstrated that the addition of oxaliplatin to infusional 5FU/LV resulted in a better 5-year disease-free survival and overall survival. This benefit was at the expense of increased acute toxicity, including neurotoxicity.

7. Haller DG, Tabernero J, Maroun J, et al. Capecitabine plus oxaliplatin compared with fluorouracil and folinic acid as adjuvant therapy for stage III colon cancer. J Clin Oncol 2011;29:1465–71. PMID: 21383294.

23. Bosset JF, Collette L, Calais G, et al. Chemotherapy with preoperative radiotherapy in rectal cancer. N Engl J Med 2006;355:1114–23. PMID: 16971718.
    The EORTC 22921 trial showed that the addition of 5FU/LV to long-course radiotherapy halved the risk of local recurrence but without any difference in overall survival.

38. Kapiteijn E, Marijnen CA, Nagtegaal ID, et al. Preoperative radiotherapy combined with total mesorectal excision for resectable rectal cancer. N Engl J Med 2001;345:638–46. PMID: 11547717.

39. van Gijn W, Marijnen CA, Nagtegaal ID, et al. Preoperative radiotherapy combined with total mesorectal excision for resectable rectal cancer: 12-year follow-up of the multicentre, randomised controlled TME trial. Lancet Oncol 2011;12:575–82. PMID: 21596621.
    The Dutch TME trial demonstrated that the addition of short-course preoperative radiotherapy halved the risk of local recurrence but with no evidence of an effect on overall survival.

40. Sebag-Montefiore D, Stephens RJ, Steele R, et al. Preoperative radiotherapy versus selective postoperative chemoradiotherapy in patients with rectal cancer (MRC CR07 and NCIC-CTG C016): a multicentre, randomised trial. Lancet 2009;373:811–20. PMID: 19269519.
    The MRC CR07 trial demonstrated that the addition of short-course preoperative radiotherapy halved the risk of local recurrence but with no evidence of an effect on overall survival.

42. Gérard JP, Conroy T, Bonnetain F, et al. Preoperative radiotherapy with or without concurrent fluorouracil and leucovorin in T3–4 rectal cancers: results of FFCD 9203. J Clin Oncol 2006;24:4620–5. PMID: 17008704.
    The FFCD 9203 trial showed that the addition of 5-FU/LV to long-course radiotherapy halved the risk of local recurrence but without any difference in overall survival.

8

Advanced and recurrent colorectal cancer

Omer Aziz

Introduction

The treatment of advanced and recurrent colorectal cancer represents a significant challenge to oncologists and surgeons, requiring a multimodality treatment approach. As a result, these patients are best managed in specialist centres by an advanced colorectal cancer multidisciplinary team (MDT).

For the purposes of this chapter, *advanced primary colon and rectal cancer* is defined as any or all of the following:

- Tumours that locally invade into adjacent organs or structures (T4a and T4b lesions according to AJCC TNM classification 7th edition). In the case of rectal cancer, these are tumours that have grown beyond the facial plane removed in a total mesorectal excision (beyond-TME).
- Tumours that have spread to lymph nodes outside their regional lymphatic drainage area (AJCC TNM classification 7th edition, stage 4 disease).
- Tumours that present with systemic (e.g. liver or lung) or peritoneal (e.g. ovaries or omentum) metastases (AJCC TNM classification 7th edition, stage 4 disease).

Recurrent colorectal cancer is defined as any or all of the following:

- Local recurrence at site of previous surgery.
- Peritoneal recurrence (colon or rectal peritoneal metastases – CRPM).
- Systemic recurrence (non-locoregional nodal or solid organ metastases).

Incidence

Despite improved access to screening, colorectal cancer still presents as advanced primary or recurrent disease. Population-based studies suggest surgery with curative intent for all-stage disease has a 5-year local recurrence cumulative incidence of 13% (23% for rectal cancer), and systemic metastasis cumulative incidence of 26%.[1,2] The timing and sites of distant metastases are important to consider:

- **Liver metastases:** Synchronous liver metastases are found in 15% of presenting colorectal cancers. Metachronous liver metastases within 5 years of diagnosis occur in 13% of cases.[3]
- **Lung metastases:** Synchronous lung metastases are found in 11% of presenting colorectal cancers. Metachronous lung metastases within 5 years of diagnosis occur in 6% of cases.[4]
- **Colorectal peritoneal metastases** (CRPM) are found in 10.3% of primary right-sided cancers and 6.2% of left-sided cancers.[5] They are found in up to 27% of primary rectal cancers.[6]
- **Bone metastases:** The 5-year incidence is 10%.[7]
- **Brain metastases:** The 5-year incidence is 2%.[8]

Survival from surgery for advanced and recurrent colorectal cancer can be presented as *relative survival* (RS). This is the ratio of observed survival rate to the expected survival rate in a comparable population of patients without colorectal cancer. Longitudinal studies looking at Western populations over the last 40 years have suggested that the volume of surgery taking place for locally recurrent colorectal cancer with curative intent has risen from 16% of cases to 58%, with a 5-year RS of 36%. In the same population over the same time period, the volume of surgery with curative intent for metastatic colorectal cancer has risen from 7% to 24% of cases, with a 5-year RS of 24%.[9] The median overall survival for patients being treated for metastatic colorectal cancer reported in phase III oncology trials and large observational series is 30 months.[10]

Diagnosis and staging of advanced and recurrent CRC

Histological confirmation and biomarkers

✅ Histological confirmation through biopsy is important before treatment. DNA- and RNA-based biomarker testing such as *RAS* and *BRAF* mutation analysis not only guides epidermal derived growth factor (EGFR)-based antibody therapy (cetuximab and panitumumab), but also has prognostic significance:[10]
    Extended *RAS* analysis to include *KRAS* exons 2, 3 and 4, and *NRAS* exons 2, 3 and 4 is recommended. Tumours harbouring any of these RAS mutations respond poorly to EGFR antibody therapy.
    BRAF should accompany *RAS* analysis, as this is a significant negative prognostic indicator with regard to overall survival (OS) and may also predict EGFR antibody therapy response.
    DNA mismatch repair (MMR) status (by microsatellite instability or MMR- immunohistochemistry) can assist genetic counselling and have prognostic importance.

In patients with advanced disease and those with local recurrence, colonoscopy may be used to obtain these samples. Other options include radiological biopsy or in selected cases of CRPM, laparoscopic assessment.

✅ The serial enlargement of a lesion accompanied by either positive PET–CT or rising CEA level may be accepted for tumour diagnosis.[11]

In cases where biopsy is not possible, biomarker analysis of the original archived specimen has reasonable concordance rates.

Radiology

Computed tomography
Computed tomography (CT) scanning of the thorax, abdomen and pelvis with oral and intravenous

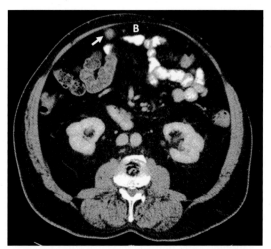

Figure 8.1 • CT scan with oral and intravenous contrast demonstrating CRPM in the omentum (*arrow*) of a patient who previously had a right hemicolectomy for a T4N1M0 adenocarcinoma of the hepatic flexure. The distinction between this and the adjacent loop of small bowel (*B*), which has been opacified with oral contrast, can easily be made.

contrast is the gold standard for disease staging. Oral contrast opacifies small bowel and identifies sites of extraluminal disease (**Fig. 8.1**). CT also plays an important role in image-guided biopsy.[11]

Magnetic resonance imaging
Magnetic resonance imaging (MRI) is a discriminatory test to stage tumours in the pelvis. In locally advanced/recurrent rectal cancer and CRPM involving the pelvis, MRI helps identify the planes of dissection and structures that require removal to achieve complete tumour clearance. Pelvic examination under anaesthesia is used alongside MRI to determine R0 resectability. MRI liver is more sensitive for lesions <10 mm in diameter than CT. Its diagnostic accuracy for liver lesions may be improved through contrast enhancers (gadoxetate).[11]

Positron emission tomography
Positron emission tomography (PET) CT is an investigation for the detection of extrahepatic metastases and local recurrence, and has been shown to change management in 8–30% of cases. Its role is limited to selected cases, with no consensus on its routine use.[11]

Ultrasonography
Ultrasonography (US) may include endorectal ultrasonography (ERUS) for targeted biopsy and assessement of sphincter involvement, and contrast-enhanced US for characterisation of liver lesions, surgical planning and biopsy.

The advanced colorectal cancer MDT

Advanced colorectal cancer MDTs should include appropriately experienced colorectal surgeons, clinical and medical oncologists, radiologists, pathologists and clinical nurse specialists. In centres undertaking pelvic clearance (exenteration) surgery for locally advanced and recurrent rectal cancer, the MDT should be supported by urologists, gynaecological oncologists and plastic (reconstructive) surgeons. Units undertaking sacrectomy and pelvic bony excisions will need spinal and orthopaedic surgeons. For CRPM, liver and lung metastases there should also be a defined pathway to discuss patients with peritoneal tumour, hepatobiliary and thoracic specialist MDTs.

The advanced colorectal cancer MDT plans appropriate diagnostic work-up and establishes goals of treatment. A personalised approach accounting for previous treatment is required. If the disease is not potentially resectable with 'R0' margins (complete resection with clear margins of at least 1 mm and no microscopic residual disease) then neoadjuvant treatment such as chemo- and/or radiotherapy should be considered for downstaging. If an R0 resection cannot be obtained, then the goal of treatment is to strike a balance between quality of life and duration of disease control. For chemotherapy this involves taking into account toxicity, and for surgery, the procedural morbidity. Symptom control is important, and centres should have access to specialist palliative care teams. Data on interventions and patient outcome should be collected prospectively with a view to obtaining long-term follow-up data.

Patients with oligometastatic disease (more than one distant metastatic site) should be considered for systemic chemotherapy versus synchronous or staged R0 resection of the sites. In the case of staged resections, the order in which these are undertaken is important. Despite the absence of high-quality data, patients with resectable oligometastatic disease are increasingly being considered for staged surgery. Finally, there is a role for local ablative techniques in treating lung and liver metastases. These include thermal devices (radiofrequency, cryo-, or microwave ablation), non-thermal devices (brachytherapy and external beam high precision radiotherapy), embolisation (radioembolisation with selective internal radiation therapy or transarterial chemoembolisation) and locally delivered chemotherapy.

Locally advanced primary and recurrent rectal cancer

'Locally advanced primary rectal cancers' are defined in this chapter as primary rectal cancers beyond the total mesorectal excision plane (PRCbTME), a term coined by the 'Beyond TME Collaborative'.[11] These lesions range from being just beyond the circumferential resection margin of a TME (T4a) to infiltrating adjacent organs (T4b). 'Recurrent rectal cancer' in this chapter is defined as local recurrence following previous mesorectal excision. Whilst both groups potentially require multivisceral surgery beyond the traditional mesorectal excision (TME) planes to achieve an R0 resection, it should be noted that only 50% of recurrent rectal cancer cases are selected for surgery, either because an R0 margin cannot be obtained, the patient is unfit for multivisceral resectional surgery, or the morbidity is unacceptable to the patient.[12] It is therefore very important to appropriately counsel the patient and set realistic expectations. Data on outcomes from specialist centres suggest that in selected cases, R0 rates of around 86% can be achieved for locally advanced primary rectal cancer, with 5-year overall survival rates of 62%.[13] For recurrent rectal cancer these figures are lower, with R0 rates of over 60% and 55% 3-year disease-free survival. R1 and R2 resections are associated with a very poor prognosis.[14]

Radiotherapy

✓✓ Patients should be considered for neoadjuvant chemoradiotherapy prior to surgery.[15]

An established regime is 45 Gy in 25 fractions with concurrent fluoropyrimadine-based chemotherapy. The optimal timing of subsequent re-staging and surgery after completion is debatable. Whilst some have suggested re-staging at 6–8 weeks,[11] it is recognised that tumour regression can occur up to 12 weeks.

✓ A number of established groups including the author's institution re-stage at 10 weeks, with surgery undertaken at 12–14 weeks.[12]

Localised radiotherapy may have a role in the treatment of recurrent rectal cancer, although outcome data are scarce. Options include:

- Intraoperative radiotherapy at the time of surgery as either intraoperative electron beam radiotherapy or high-dose-rate brachytherapy at surgical sites where the resection margin is threatened.[12]
- Stereotactic body irradiation therapy (CyberKnife system) delivering multiple beams to well-defined targets in few fractions. Indications include irresectable pelvic sidewall and pre-sacral recurrences.[16]

Perineal excision

For low rectal cancers, the concept of 'extralevator abdominoperineal excision' (ELAPE) with a cylindrical specimen has gained acceptance. However, it is important to note that in the context of locally advanced primary low rectal cancers, there may be a need for an extended excision of the ischio-anal fat akin to 'salvage' surgery for recurrent anal cancers after chemoradiotherapy. **Figure 8.2** illustrates the difference in these two procedures.

Pelvic multivisceral exenteration

Organs that may require removal with the rectum in locally advanced primary and recurrent rectal cancers include anterior structures (bladder, prostate, seminal vesicles, urethra, uterus, vagina), posterior structures (pre-sacral fascia and sacrum) and lateral structures (ovaries and associated structures, ureters and pelvic sidewall vessels, nerves and musculoskeletal tissue).

Patterns of rectal cancer recurrence

Classification systems describing the patterns of recurrence in rectal cancer have been proposed, but standardisation of this nomenclature has not been achieved. A simplified version has been described by Renehan[12] as:

- Central recurrence (**Fig. 8.3**) most commonly arising at a previous rectal anastomotic site or in the residual mesorectum. These can go on to involve the anterior urogenital structures and can also extend posteriorly up to the sacral fascia or

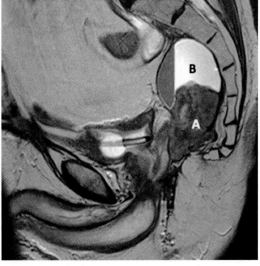

Figure 8.3 • MRI demonstrating central recurrence in a rectal stump following previous Hartmann's procedure (A) with associated cystic cavity (B).

periosteum but not the bone. Both may be resected en bloc for an R0 resection without sacrectomy.
- Sacral recurrence (**Fig. 8.4**) where bony invasion is present and an R0 resection is only possible with a sacral resection through a two-stage combined abdominosacral approach.
- Lateral recurrence (**Fig. 8.5**) involves the lateral pelvic sidewall, encasing iliac vessels, pelvic autonomic nerves and ureter and can extend through the greater sciatic foramen with or without invasion of the sciatic nerve. Of all the types of recurrence, this is the most difficult

Extralevator (ELAPE)

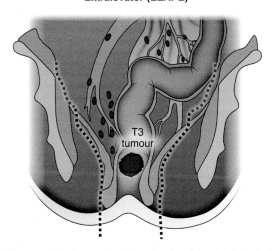

Ischio-anal resection

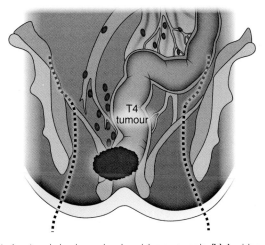

Figure 8.2 • Approaches to perineal excision. **(a)** Standard extralevator abdominoperineal excision approach. **(b)** A wider ischio-anal approach for low, locally advanced T4 rectal cancers.

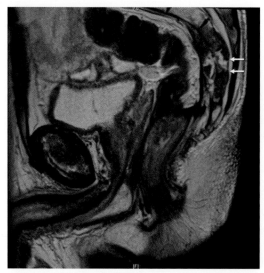

Figure 8.4 • MRI demonstrating sacral recurrence (*arrows*) extending up to the level of S3.

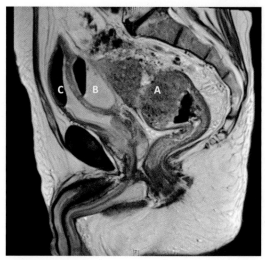

Figure 8.6 • MRI demonstrating locally advanced rectal cancer (*A*) with anterior perforation and associated abscess cavity (*B*) adjacent to bladder (*C*). The patient required total pelvic clearance.

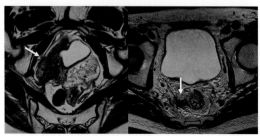

Figure 8.5 • Lateral recurrences of the left pelvic sidewall involving left internal iliac vessels and ureter (left scan, *arrow*) or abutting left internal iliac artery branches (right scan, *arrow*).

in which to achieve an R0 resection, and is therefore associated with the poorest prognosis. Techniques to achieve clear lateral margins involving en bloc resection of the iliac vessels and other sidewall structures[17] and extended lateral pelvic sidewall excision[18] have been described in order to achieve an R0 resection with promising early results.

Types of pelvic clearance

Pelvic clearance (exenteration) surgery needs to be tailored to include:

• Total pelvic clearance (TPC) involves removal of the rectum, sigmoid colon, bladder, draining lymph nodes, pelvic peritoneum and lower ureters. In males the prostate and seminal vesicles are also excised (**Fig. 8.6**). In females the uterus, ovaries, fallopian tubes and required part of the vagina can be removed. The patient

has an end colostomy and an ileal conduit as the most common urinary reconstruction technique.

• Anterior pelvic clearance involves removal of the distal ureters, bladder, prostate and seminal vesicles in a male, and in females also the uterus, ovaries, fallopian tubes and vagina as required. It is not a commonly performed operation for rectal cancer and reserved mainly for tumours of the upper rectum and rectosigmoid that invade into anterior structures. This operation is more commonly used for the treatment of advanced urological and gynaecological tumours. The distal rectum is spared and may be re-anastomosed. An ileal conduit is required for urinary reconstruction.

• Posterior pelvic clearance is a procedure performed in women, involving the removal of the rectum and uterus, required part of the vagina, ovaries and fallopian tubes. This may be with or without removal of the anus (perineal excision). The bladder is spared.

In the lateral dissection of the pelvic sidewall, surgery may be undertaken in three planes of dissection to get R0 clearance (**Fig. 8.7**):

• Mesorectal fascial plane – a continuation of the standard TME plane.

• Ureteric plane – deep to the lateral peritoneum where the ureter lies.

• Bony plane – lateral to internal iliac vessels along the obturator internus and piriformis muscles in the lateral pelvic compartments.

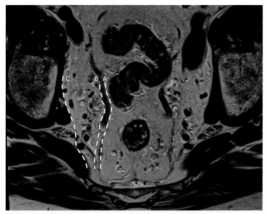

Figure 8.7 • MRI demonstrating planes of the right pelvic side-wall: mesorectal plane (*A*), ureteric plane (*B*) and bony plane lateral to internal iliac vessels (*C*).

Sacrectomy

> ✅ Resection of the sacrum at S3 or below has acceptable morbidity and established oncological and functional benefit.[19]

S1 and S2 involvement is challenging due to the need for pelvic reconstruction and stabilisation as well as the resulting sensory and motor neurological deficit (the procedure involves ligation of the cauda equina and freeing the sacrum with sacrifice of sacral nerve roots below the level of resection). A recent series reporting on high sacrectomy with preservation of S1 and avoidance of pelvic stabilisation procedures has demonstrated an R0 resection rate of over 70% with a major complication rate of 43%.[20] Not surprisingly, patients undergoing high sacrectomy had a higher rate of postoperative neurological (motor and sensory) deficit and neuropathic bladder dysfunction. Otherwise there was minimal increased morbidity with the high sacrectomy. New techniques such as unilateral sacral compartment excision also offer the prospect of high sacral resection without the need for pelvic stabilisation, but more data on these are awaited.[21]

Perineal reconstruction

This may be required due to the size of the defect and impaired wound healing after previous chemoradiotherapy. Omentoplasty to the pelvis should be attempted where possible. Biological mesh reconstruction of the pelvic floor has been described for ELAPE; however, it is usually not appropriate in exenterative surgery due to the size of the defect and the fact that it also requires a flap of skin for closure. Pedicled flaps are most commonly used and include:

- Rectus abdominis myocutaneous flaps (unilateral with reconstruction of the abdominal harvest site often using mesh).
- Gracilis myocutaneous flaps (bilateral as they offer the least coverage).
- Gluteal myocutaneous rotational or advancement flaps (usually both sides).
- Inferior gluteal artery perforator flap (usually both sides).

Where pedicled flaps are not an option, free flaps can be considered. The decision should be made with a plastic surgeon, and tailored to patient factors (comorbidity, tissue quality and perfusion) as well as previous surgery (abdominal and perineal incisions).[12] Vaginal reconstruction can be achieved and intercourse is feasible after this.[22]

Colorectal peritoneal metastases (CRPM)

CRPM (**Fig. 8.8**) can present synchronously (10.3% of primary right colon cancers, 6.2% of left colon cancers, and 27% of rectal cancers)[5,6] and metachronously (20% of colorectal cancers).[23]

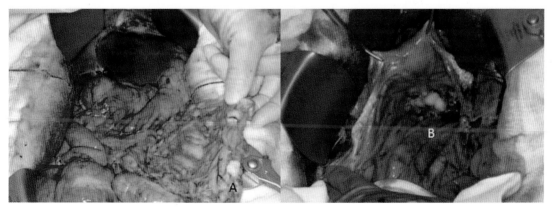

Figure 8.8 • CRPM involving the omentum (*A*) and recto-uterine pouch of Douglas (*B*).

✅✅ Systemic chemotherapy and palliative support used to be the mainstay of treatment, with surgery restricted to relieving obstruction. In the past decade, however, compelling data on outcomes from cytoreductive surgery with hyperthermic intraperitoneal chemotherapy (CRS/HIPEC) from several specialist centres have emerged.[24] These studies have shown a median survival of 63 months and a 5-year survival of 51% is achievable with CRS/HIPEC, compared to 24 months and 13% for matched patients receiving systemic chemotherapy alone (**Fig. 8.9**).[25]

✅ CRS/HIPEC is now a recommended treatment for selected cases of CRPM.[10]

CRS/HIPEC

This is an established treatment for peritoneal tumours (appendix neoplasms and pseudomyxoma peritonei [PMP]). PMP is a rare syndrome that arises from a low-grade appendiceal mucinous neoplasm (LAMN) that perforates, with leakage of mucin and cells into the peritoneal cavity, resulting in abdominal distension and organ compression.[26] The principle is to remove all visible tumour followed by administration of HIPEC using a cytotoxic drug with depth of penetration of approximately 3 mm. Hyperthermia itself also has a direct cytotoxic effect, probably through

formation of heat shock proteins.[27] **Figure 8.10** shows the 'Coliseum' technique (see also Video 1).

CRS can include peritonectomy, omentectomy, umbilectomy, excision of falciform ligament and ligamentum teres, cholecystectomy and any other required visceral resections. These may include segmental small- and/or large-bowel resections, splenectomy, total abdominal hysterectomy, bilateral salpingo-oophoerctomy and gastrectomy. HIPEC at 42 degrees is administered for 60–90 minutes with either mitomycin C or oxaloplatin and intravenous 5FU. (See Video 2 for an outline of the CRS procedure.)

Scoring systems

There are currently two main systems used to stratify outcomes from CRS/HIPEC, namely the Peritoneal Cancer Index (PCI) Sugarbaker, and the Completeness of Cytoreduction (CC) score developed by Sugarbaker.[28]

PCI is an intraoperative score accounting for both size and distribution of lesions (**Fig. 8.11**). Thirteen regions are each given a score of 0–3 based on lesion size, with final score ranging from 0 to 39. A higher PCI is associated with poorer short- and long-term outcomes.[27]

CC score is calculated at the end of the operation. CC = 0 indicates no residual disease, CC = 1 indicates nodules less than 2.5 mm in size remained, CC = 2 indicates nodules between 2.5 mm and 2.5 cm, and CC = 3 indicates that nodules over 2.5 cm remained.

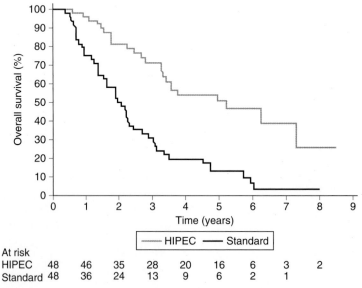

Figure 8.9 • Overall survival of group receiving CRS/HIPEC (labelled 'HIPEC') versus those on systemic chemotherapy (labelled 'Standard').[25]

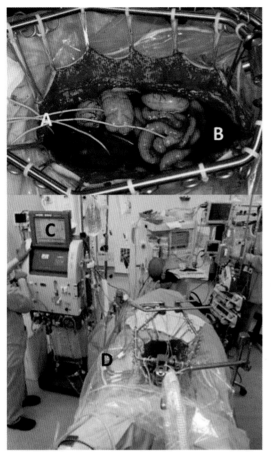

Figure 8.10 • Open 'Coliseum' technique for HIPEC with temperature probes (*A*), circulating intraperitoneal chemotherapy solution (*B*), HIPEC circulation and delivery system (*C*) and HIPEC inflow and outflow ports (*D*).

Patient Selection

In England, CRS/HIPEC is a procedure that remains restricted to specialised units. Specialist peritoneal tumour MDTs in these centres take into account the patient's full treatment history, tumour type and biology, previous chemotherapy, prior surgery and future options. Patients are carefully selected and counselled for surgery. Laparoscopy plays a role in some cases (see Video 3 for a diagnostic laparoscopy for CRPM). Annually audited results demonstrate a major morbidity rate of less than 30% and mortality of less than 1%.

Colorectal liver metastases

Certain 'technical criteria' have to be fulfilled in order for liver metastases to be considered resectable, as outlined in Table 8.1. In a proportion of patients resection is made possible through portal vein embolisation, two-stage hepatectomy or hepatectomy combined with ablation. The finding that despite being technically resectable, approximately half of patients develop widespread systemic disease within 3 years, has led to 'oncological criteria' that should also be considered when selecting patients (Table 8.1).[10]

✔✔ If a patient fulfils these criteria to undergo surgical resection, there is the option of either upfront surgery or perioperative (pre- and postoperative) chemotherapy. The best available data from the EPOC study are not conclusive on whether perioperative chemotherapy improves outcome. The study reported a 5-year OS rate of 51% (95% CI 45–58) in the perioperative chemotherapy group versus 48% (95% CI 40–55) in the surgery-only group.[29] It would therefore not be unreasonable to consider upfront surgery for easily technically resectable liver metastases with favourable oncological criteria, but choose perioperative chemotherapy for patients with favourable technical criteria, but unfavourable oncological criteria as outlined in Table 8.1. Data from the EPOC group also suggest that perioperative chemotherapy should comprise 3 months chemotherapy before surgery and 3 months' chemotherapy post-surgery with FOLFOX or alternatively capecitabine with oxaliplatin – CAPOX.

Two further groups of patients with colorectal liver metastases should be considered.

The first is patients with primary colorectal tumours and synchronous liver metastases. In these patients consideration should be given to synchronous versus staged resections, although the former is generally reserved for small isolated lesions. Ultimately the combined morbidity of both procedures needs to be considered. In the case of staged resections, surgery for the primary tumour and liver metastases does not necessarily need to be interrupted with systemic chemotherapy.[30] Ultimately these decisions need to be taken in consultation with a hepatobiliary MDT.

The second is patients with unresectable colorectal liver metastases in whom systemic chemotherapy renders the disease resectable. This has led to the introduction of the concept of 'conversion chemotherapy' into clinical practice. It is an area where data on long-term outcome from surgery after conversion versus continuation of chemotherapy are required.

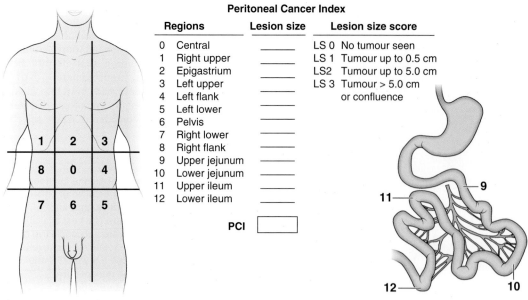

Peritoneal Cancer Index

Regions	Lesion size	Lesion size score
0 Central	_____	LS 0 No tumour seen
1 Right upper	_____	LS 1 Tumour up to 0.5 cm
2 Epigastrium	_____	LS2 Tumour up to 5.0 cm
3 Left upper	_____	LS 3 Tumour > 5.0 cm
4 Left flank	_____	or confluence
5 Left lower	_____	
6 Pelvis	_____	
7 Right lower	_____	
8 Right flank	_____	
9 Upper jejunum	_____	
10 Lower jejunum	_____	
11 Upper ileum	_____	
12 Lower ileum	_____	

PCI [   ]

Figure 8.11 • Peritoneal Cancer Index (PCI).

Table 8.1 • Technical and oncological criteria considered in surgery for colorectal liver metastases

Technical criteria	Oncological criteria
1. R0 resection possible	1. 5 or fewer lesions
2. Maintenance of 30% of future liver remnant (FLR) or a remnant liver-to-body-weight ratio >0.5 (e.g. >350 g of liver per 70 kg patient)	2. Presence (or suspicion) of extrahepatic disease
3. R0 resection possible only with complex procedures (portal vein embolisation, two-stage hepatectomy or hepatectomy combined with ablation).	3. The resectability of extrahepatic disease
	4. Evidence of tumour progression

Key points

- Advanced and recurrent colorectal cancers should be managed in specialist centres with the required multidisciplinary teams.
- Histological confirmation, biomarker (extended *RAS, BRAF*) and DNA mismatch repair testing should be undertaken at the outset where possible.
- CT thorax, abdomen and pelvis with oral and intravenous contrast and MRI for pelvic tumours is the minimal recommendation for staging advanced and recurrent colorectal cancers.
- Radiotherapy should be considered for patients with locally advanced and recurrent rectal cancer prior to surgery.
- Locally advanced and recurrent rectal cancers require surgery beyond the TME plane through exenterative surgery that must be tailored to the patient.
- Sacrectomy should be undertaken in units with the required expertise and access to spinal orthopaedic or neurosurgeons.
- Perineal reconstruction should be planned with a plastic surgeon and the type of flap used tailored to the patient.

- CRS/HIPEC is an established treatment for CRPM and is undertaken in specialist centres in the UK with the required decision-making and operative experience.
- All units treating advanced and recurrent colorectal cancer should collect, audit and present their long-term outcome data.
- Treatment of liver metastases should be planned with a specialist hepatobiliary MDT and based on both technical and oncological criteria.

▶ Recommended videos:

1. HIPEC: the 'Coliseum' technique – https://youtu.be/UB4Lxypd0Kw
2. Cytoreductive surgery procedure – https://youtu.be/_WT8grwjzoQ
3. Diagnostic laparoscopy for CRPM – https://youtu.be/aEHgQubDKNw

🌐 Full references available at **http://expertconsult.inkling.com**

Key references

15. McCarthy K, Pearson K, Fulton R, et al. Pre-operative chemoradiation for non-metastatic locally advanced rectal cancer. The Cochrane Database of systematic reviews 2012 Dec 12;12:. CD008368. PMID: 23235660.

A meta-analysis of six randomised controlled trials comparing the efficacy of preoperative chemoradiation to radiotherapy alone before surgery in the treatment of T3–4, node-positive (locally advanced) rectal cancer. While there was no difference in overall survival, chemoradiotherapy was significantly associated with less local recurrence.

25. Elias D, Lefevre JH, Chevalier J, et al. Complete cytoreductive surgery plus intraperitoneal chemohyperthermia with oxaliplatin for peritoneal carcinomatosis of colorectal origin. J Clin Oncol 2009;27:681–5. PMID: 19103728.

A case-control study comparing the long-term survival of matched groups of patients with isolated and resectable peritoneal metastases from colorectal cancer treated with systemic chemotherapy including oxaliplatin or irinotecan versus cytoreductive surgery with hyperthermic intraperitoneal chemotherapy and systemic chemotherapy. Patients with isolated, resectable peritoneal cancer achieved a median survival of 24 months with modern chemotherapies, but only surgical cytoreduction plus HIPEC was able to prolong median survival to 63 months, with a 5-year survival rate of 51%.

29. Nordlinger B, Sorbye H, Glimelius B, et al. Perioperative FOLFOX4 chemotherapy and surgery versus surgery alone for resectable liver metastases from colorectal cancer (EORTC 40983): long-term results of a randomised, controlled, phase 3 trial. Lancet Oncol 2013;14:1208–15. PMID: 24120480.

A randomised controlled trial that found no difference in overall survival with the addition of perioperative chemotherapy with FOLFOX4 compared with surgery alone for patients with resectable liver metastases from colorectal cancer.

9

Anal cancer

David J. Humes
John H. Scholefield

Introduction

Anal cancer is rare, accounting for approximately 2–4% of large bowel malignancies; however, there is some evidence that its incidence is increasing. Most anal cancers arise from the squamous epithelium of the anal margin or anal canal, although a few arise from anal glands and ducts.

Traditionally, the anal region is divided into the anal canal and the anal margin or verge. The natural history, demography and surgical management of anal cancer differ between these areas. There is controversy regarding the exact definition of the anal canal. Anatomists see it as lying between the dentate line and the anal verge, whereas surgically it is defined as lying between the anorectal ring and the anal verge. For pathologists, the canal has been defined as corresponding to the longitudinal extent of the internal anal sphincter. The canal above the dentate line is lined by rectal mucosa, except for a small zone immediately above the dentate line called the transitional or junctional zone. Inferiorly, the canal is covered by stratified squamous epithelium. Further confusion relates to the definition of the anal canal and anal margin as sites for cancer. The anal margin is variously described as the visible area external to the anal verge, or as the area below the dentate line. Anal margin tumours are said to be within a 5-cm radius of the anal orifice. This argument has become less important as surgery plays a lesser role in treatment, but reports of surgical results from past decades are confused by this variation in definition.

Over 80% of anal cancers are of squamous origin, arising from the squamous epithelium of the anal canal and perianal area; 10% are adenocarcinomas arising from the glandular mucosa of the upper anal canal, the anal glands and ducts. A very rare and particularly aggressive tumour is anal melanoma. Lymphomas and sarcomas of the anus are even less common but have increased in incidence in recent years, particularly among patients with human immunodeficiency virus (HIV) infection. There has also been a rise in the incidence of other anal epidermoid tumours among patients with HIV.

Epidermoid tumours

Aetiology and pathogenesis

Anal squamous carcinomas are relatively uncommon tumours; there are just over 1300 cases of anal cancer diagnosed each year in the United Kingdom (UK).[1] Based on these figures, each consultant colorectal surgeon might expect to see one or two anal cancers every year or so. However, anal cancers are probably under-reported, since some anal canal tumours are misclassified as rectal tumours and some perianal tumours as squamous carcinomas of the skin.

A recent study using English data from the National Cancer Data Repository reported an incidence of 0.73 and 1.13 per 100 000 population, respectively, for men and women from 2006 to 2010. These figures represented a 69% and 126% increase in incidence when compared to rates from 1990 to 1994.[2] This increase in incidence has also been confirmed in studies in the USA using data from the Surveillance, Epidemiology and End Results (SEER) Program, in France using cancer registry data and in Norway.[3-5] The median age at diagnosis is 60 years. There is wide geographical variation in the incidence of anal cancers around the world. Areas with a high incidence of anal cancer usually also have a high incidence of cervical, vulval and penile tumours (reflecting the common aetiological agent – papillomaviruses).

The increasing incidence of HIV infection has resulted in a rise in the incidence of anal cancer; this has been seen particularly in areas such as San Francisco, with a large homosexual population, reportedly seeing a large increase but part of this increase in recent times may be due to detection of more in situ lesions among men who have been targeted for screening.[6] Daling et al.[7] identified risk factors for the development of squamous cell carcinoma of the anus: a history of receptive anal intercourse in males increased the relative risk of developing anal cancer by 33 times compared with controls with colon cancer, and a history of genital warts also increased the relative risk of developing anal cancer (27-fold in men and 22-fold in women). This reflects the likely aetiological link to human papillomaviruses in anal squamous cell carcinoma.

✓✓ The incidence of anal cancer is increasing in both males and females with a greater increase in females.[2]

Epidemiological and molecular biological data have shown an association with human papillomavirus (HPV) type 16 DNA, and less commonly types 18, 31 and 33 and their DNA was consistently found to be integrated into the genome in cervical, vulval and penile squamous cell carcinomas. The same HPV DNA types have also been identified in a similar proportion of anal squamous cell carcinomas.[8]

There are more than 60 types of HPV (a DNA virus), capable of causing a wide variety of lesions in squamous epithelium. Common warts can be found on the hands and feet of children and young adults, and are caused by the relatively infectious but otherwise innocuous HPV types 1 and 2. Anogenital papillomaviruses are less infective than HPV types 1 and 2 and are exclusively sexually transmitted. The epidemiology of genital papillomavirus infection is poorly understood, largely due to the social and moral taboos surrounding sexually transmissible infections. Anogenital papillomavirus-associated lesions range from condylomas through intraepithelial neoplasias to invasive carcinomas. The most common HPV types causing genital warts are types 6 and 11, which may also be isolated from

low-grade intraepithelial neoplasia. HPV types 16, 18, 31 and 33 are much less commonly associated with genital condylomas but are more commonly found in high-grade intraepithelial neoplasias and invasive carcinomas, with the most frequently isolated being HPV 16 (84%) and the next most frequent HPV18.[9] Once one area of the anogenital epithelium is infected, spread of papillomavirus infection throughout the rest of the anogenital area probably follows, but remains occult in the majority of individuals. Although there is a commonly held belief that anal cancer occurs only in individuals who practise anal intercourse, this is unfounded.

✓ Anal and genital papillomavirus-associated lesions may be identified clinically either by naked eye inspection or with high-resolution anoscopy with the application of acetic acid to the epithelium, resulting in an 'aceto-white' lesion. This technique permits targeted biopsy of a lesion, but histological examination remains the diagnostic standard. The natural history of anal papillomavirus infection and intraepithelial neoplasia is in large part dependent on the infecting viral type and on the host immune state. In immunocompetent individuals the risk of malignant conversion from AIN III to invasive cancer is around 10% over 10 years, but in HIV patients the risk is nearer 30% in 10 years.[10]

Premalignant lesions

Anogenital intraepithelial neoplasia of the cervix (CIN), vulva (VIN), vagina (VAIN) and anus (AIN) is graded from I to III, according to the number of thirds of epithelial depth that appear dysplastic on histological section. Thus, in grade III the cells of the whole thickness of the epithelium appear dysplastic, being synonymous with carcinoma in situ.

High-grade anal intraepithelial (AIN III) lesions may be characterised by hyperkeratosis or changes in the pigmentation of the epithelium. Thus, carcinoma in situ may appear white, red or brown, the pigmentation commonly being irregular. The lesions may be flat or raised, but ulceration is suggestive of invasive disease. It is important that any suspicious area is biopsied and examined histologically. The terms 'Bowen's disease of the anus' and 'leucoplakia' are best avoided as they are confusing and convey no specific information, the malignant potential of leucoplakia being very uncertain.

At present, multifocal genital intraepithelial neoplasia represents a difficult clinical problem, which may be further complicated by the occurrence of synchronous or metachronous AIN.[11]

Histological types

Included within the category of epidermoid tumours are squamous cell, basaloid (or cloacogenic) carcinomas and muco-epidermoid cancers. The different morphological types of anal cancer do not appear to have different prognoses. Tumours arising at the anal margin tend to be well differentiated and keratinising, occurring more in men, whereas those arising in the canal are more commonly poorly differentiated and are commoner in women. Basaloid tumours arise in the transitional zone around the dentate line and form 30–50% of all anal canal tumours.

Patterns of spread

Anal canal cancer spreads locally, mainly in a cephalad direction, so that the tumour may appear to have arisen in the rectum. The tumour also spreads outwards into the anal sphincters and into the rectovaginal septum, perineal body, scrotum or vagina in more advanced cases (**Fig. 9.1**). Lymph node metastases occur frequently, especially in tumours of the anal canal. Spread occurs initially to the perirectal group of nodes and thereafter to inguinal, haemorrhoidal and lateral pelvic lymph nodes. The frequency of nodal involvement is related to the size of the primary tumour together with its depth of penetration. Approximately 14% of patients will present with inguinal lymph node involvement, but this rises to approximately 30% when the primary tumour is greater than 5 cm in diameter. Only 50% of enlarged nodes at presentation will subsequently be shown to contain tumour. Synchronously involved nodes carry a particularly poor prognosis, whereas when metachronous spread develops the salvage rate is much higher.

Haematogenous spread tends to occur late and is usually associated with advanced local disease. The principal sites of metastases are the liver, lung, para-aortic nodes and bones. However, metastases have been described in the kidneys, adrenals and brain.

Clinical presentation

The predominant symptoms of epidermoid anal cancer are pain and bleeding, which are present in about 50% of cases. The presence of a mass is noted by a minority of patients, around 25%. Pruritus and discharge occur in a similar proportion. Advanced tumours may involve the sphincter mechanism, causing faecal incontinence. Invasion of the posterior vaginal wall may cause a fistula.

Cancer of the anal margin usually has the appearance of a malignant ulcer, with a raised, everted, indurated edge. Lesions within the canal may not be visible, though extensive lesions spread to the anal verge, or can extend via the ischiorectal fossa to the skin of the buttock. Digital examination of the anal canal is usually painful, and may reveal the distortion produced by the tumour. Since anal cancer tends to spread upwards, there may be involvement of the distal rectum, giving the impression that the lesion has arisen there. Involvement of the perirectal lymph nodes may be palpable on digital examination. If the tumour has extended into the sphincter muscles, the characteristic induration of a spreading malignancy may be felt around the anal canal.

Patients should be assessed for other risk factors such as HIV and all patients should be considered for testing and referred to an HIV clinic if found to be positive. Female patients should also have a referral for cervical cancer screening if not up to date.

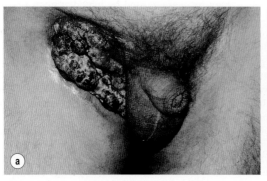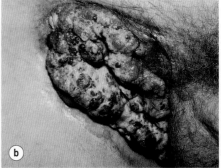

Figure 9.1 • Locally advanced anal cancer involving the anal canal, perianal skin, perineal skin and base of scrotum. Treatment with chemo-irradiation failed to control the disease and the patient underwent a salvage abdominoperineal excision.

✅ Although up to one-third of patients will have inguinal lymph nodes that are enlarged, biopsy will confirm metastatic spread in only 50% of these; the rest are due to secondary infection. Biopsy or fine-needle aspiration is recommended to confirm involvement of the groin nodes if radical block dissection is contemplated.[12] Distant spread is unusual in anal cancer, so hepatomegaly, though it must be looked for, is very uncommon. Frequently, other benign perianal conditions will exist in association with anal cancer, such as fistulas, condylomas or leucoplakia.

Investigation

The most important investigation in the management of anal cancer is a detailed clinical examination under anaesthetic. Examination under anaesthesia permits optimum assessment of the tumour in terms of size, involvement of adjacent structures and nodal involvement, and also provides the best opportunity to obtain a biopsy for histological confirmation.

All patients should be staged with magnetic resonance imaging (MRI) of the pelvis and computed tomography (CT) of the chest, abdomen and pelvis. The MRI allows locoregional staging whilst the CT stages for metastatic disease. The use of 18 F-FDG positron emission tomography (PET)/CT has been suggested for staging. It may help with planning of radiotherapy and improve assessment of locoregional lymph node involvement.[13] However, it is not currently mandated in all cases as part of the European or US National Comprehensive Cancer Network (NCCN) guidelines as it has not been fully assessed.[12] Endoanal ultrasound has been suggested but may only be useful in small tumours as more information is usually available from MRI, particularly on spread beyond the anal canal.

Enlarged inguinal lymph nodes can be characterised by clinical and radiological features as to whether they may be reactive or metastatic. In cases where there is doubt, fine-needle aspiration can be performed, although this may not be required in those who have had a PET/CT that shows avid uptake. Serum tumour markers are unhelpful as they do not provide reliable information.

Clinical staging

No one system of staging for anal tumours has been adopted universally. However, the current 7th edition of the American Joint Committee on Cancer (AJCC) and Union for International Cancer Control (UICC) staging is the most widely used and follows the TNM classification (Table 9.1).

Table 9.1 • AJCC TNM staging of anal cancer, 7th edition

T stage	N stage	M stage
T1 – <2 cm	N1 – Mesorectal nodes	M0 – No metastasis
T2 – >2 to 5 cm	N2 –Unilateral internal iliac or inguinal nodes	M1 – Distant metastasis
T3 – >5 cm	N3 – Perirectal and inguinal lymph nodes or bilateral internal iliac and/or inguinal lymph nodes	
T4 – Invasion into adjacent organs (e.g. vagina, urethra)		

Treatment

Historical
Traditionally, anal cancer was treated as a 'surgical' disease. Anal canal tumours were treated by radical abdominoperineal excision and colostomy, whereas anal margin lesions were treated by local excision. Over the past 30 years, non-surgical radical treatments, i.e. radiotherapy with or without chemotherapy, have taken over as primary treatments of choice in most cases.

Abdominoperineal excision (APE) for anal canal cancer differs little from the procedure used for rectal cancer, but particular care is taken to clear the space below the pelvic floor. Around 20% of cases are incurable surgically at presentation.

Around 75% of cancers at the anal margin have been treated in the past by local excision. The rationale for this was based on the perception that margin lesions rarely metastasise, though this has not always been confirmed by prolonged follow-up.

Current

✅✅ The current standard of care for anal cancer is chemoradiotherapy with 50.4 Gy radiotherapy in 28 daily fractions with mitomycin C and 5FU in all cases except those where local excision is complete or there are contraindications to radiotherapy. This achieves equivalent survival rates to surgery but with the advantage of stoma avoidance in the majority of cases.[12,14,15]

Radiation-alone therapy
The initial treatment for anal cancer was radiotherapy because the mortality and morbidity of surgical

treatment of anal carcinoma were unacceptable. By the 1930s, however, it was recognised that the low-voltage radiotherapy used frequently produced severe radionecrosis. As surgery became safer, APE for invading lesions, and local excision for small growths, became the standard treatment for the next four decades.

The development in the 1950s of equipment that could deliver high-energy irradiation by the cobalt source generator or, more recently, by linear accelerators, enabled radiotherapists to deliver higher penetrating doses to deeper placed structures with less superficial scatter of energy. Radiation damage to surrounding tissues was consequently reduced while simultaneously delivering an enhanced tumouricidal effect.

Chemo-irradiation therapy (combined modality therapy)

Combined modality therapy for anal cancer was championed by Norman Nigro. Nigro chose to use 5-fluorouracil (5FU) and mitomycin C empirically as a preoperative regimen aimed at improving the results of radical surgery.[16] The radiotherapy then consisted of 30 Gy of external beam irradiation over a period of 3 weeks. A bolus of mitomycin C was given on the first day of treatment, and 5FU was delivered in a synchronous continuous 4-day infusion during the first week of radiotherapy. After completion of radiotherapy, a further infusion of 5FU was administered and patients later proceeded to APE. It was evident to Nigro that the majority had quite

dramatic tumour shrinkage: in his 1974 publication the tumour was reported to have disappeared completely in all three patients. No tumour was found in the surgical specimen in either of the patients who underwent APE; the third refused surgery.

A variety of similar techniques have subsequently been described. With wider experience, it became clear that higher doses of radiotherapy (45–60 Gy) could be applied, usually split into two courses to minimise morbidity; however, recent RCT results have now shown no need to have a break in radiotherapy treatment.

All the reported series describe excellent results, but there was a debate about whether chemotherapy added any advantage over radiotherapy alone.

The UK Coordinating Committee on Cancer Research (UKCCCR ACT I) compared chemo-irradiation with radiotherapy alone in a randomised multicentre study.[15] This study randomised 585 patients. The trial showed that combined modality therapy gave superior local control of disease compared with radiotherapy alone. Only 36% of patients receiving combined therapy had 'local failure' compared with 59% of those receiving radiotherapy alone. Although there was no significant overall survival advantage for either treatment regimen, the risk of death from anal cancer was significantly less in the group receiving combined modality therapy (**Fig. 9.2**). As a result of this trial it seems that the standard treatment for anal squamous carcinoma should be a combination of radiotherapy and intravenous 5FU with mitomycin, which remains the gold standard.

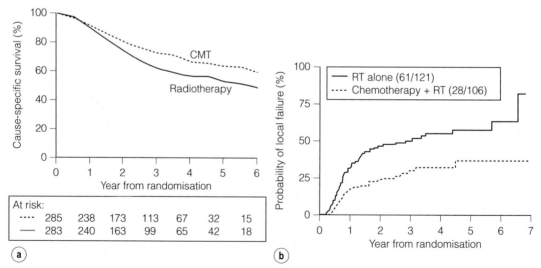

Figure 9.2 • (a) Deaths from anal cancer. Number of events: radiotherapy (RT) 105, combined modality therapy (CMT) 77 (RR=0.71, 95% CI 0.53–0.95, P=0.02). Number at risk=number alive. **(b)** UKCCCR Anal Cancer Trial: risk of local failure (T1–2 and N0).
Panel **(a)**: UKCCCR Anal Cancer Trial Working Party. Lancet 1996;348:1055, Figure 5. With permission from Elsevier.
Panel **(b)**: Northover J, Meadows A, Ryan C et al., on behalf of UKCCCR Anal Cancer Trial Working Party. Lancet 1996;349:206. With permission from Elsevier.

Mitomycin causes much of the toxicity of chemoradiation (a problem particularly in elderly patients) and thus trials of the use of cisplatin as an alternative to mitomycin have been performed (RTOG, 2006).[17] This trial randomised 682 patients but showed that cisplatin had no advantage over mitomycin and may be inferior. The UK ACT II trial randomised 940 patients in a 2×2 design comparing CRT using cisplatin/5FU versus mitomycin/5FU, with or without two cycles of adjuvant cisplatin/5FU. It reported 3-year progression-free survival of 74% (maintenance arm) versus 73% (no maintenance arm). This trial confirmed the current standard regime used in the UK of 5FU with mitomycin with 50.4 Gy radiotherapy in 28 daily fractions. The mitomycin is given on day 1 with 5FU infusions given days 1–4 and 29–32.[14] The personalising anal cancer radiotherapy trial (PLATO) will aim to optimise radiotherapy dose for low-, intermediate- and high-risk anal cancers and will incorporate the ACT 3, 4 and 5 studies.

Complications of chemoradiation for anal carcinoma include diarrhoea, mucositis, myelosuppression, skin erythema and desquamation. Late complications include anal stenosis and fistula formation. Many oncologists prefer to defunction anterior tumours in women as there is a high incidence of rectovaginal fistula formation in this group during radiotherapy treatment.

HIV patients with anal epidermoid cancers are probably best treated with chemoradiation, but have increased toxicity.[18]

Role of surgery today

Although surgeons no longer play the central therapeutic role, they nevertheless have important contributions to make.

Initial diagnosis
Most patients present to surgeons, who are best suited to perform examination under anaesthesia (EUA) to confirm diagnosis and assess local extent.

Lesions at the anal margin

✅ Small T1 (<2 cm) lesions at the anal margin may still be treated by local excision alone, obviating the need for protracted courses of chemoradiation. The lesion needs to be excised with a clear margin of skin and deeper tissue (of at least 5 mm), it is accepted that this may mandate excision of part of the distal sphincter complex. The specimen and excision margins should be discussed at a specialist anal cancer multidisciplinary team (MDT). There is some evidence that the risk of regional lymph node metastasis is not related to primary tumour size,

which may explain the disappointing results sometimes reported after local excision; this conflicts with the view that tumour size is related to stage, which explains the excellent results of local excision in small tumours.[12]

Due to the risk of incontinence associated with obtaining adequate margins of clearance, lesions of the anal canal should not be considered for local resection, but biopsy only. APE is no longer a first-line treatment for anal cancer and should only be considered if the patient has contraindication to primary chemoradiotherapy or has declined it.

Surgery may be required for a defunctioning stoma prior to oncological treatment, with definitive indications being incontinence, obstruction, perianal sepsis and fistulation. Defunctioning for local symptoms such as tenesmus or pain may be considered to prevent breaks in treatment. Patients should be warned that only 50% of these stomas are eventually reversed and that upon reversal bowel function may be poor.[19]

Treatment complications and disease relapse
Surgeons retain an important role in the treatment of anal cancer after failure of primary non-surgical therapy, either early or late. Four situations may require surgery after chemoradiation for anal cancer treatment: residual tumour, complications of treatment, incontinence or fistula after tumour resolution, and subsequent tumour recurrence.

1. The appearance of the primary site is often misleading after radiotherapy. In most patients complete remission is indicated by the tumour disappearing completely. In some, however, an ulcer remains, occasionally looking like an unchanged primary tumour. Only generous biopsy will reveal whether the residual ulcer contains tumour or consists merely of inflammatory tissue. Histological proof of residual disease is essential before radical surgery is recommended to the patient. For patients with proven residual disease, a salvage APE may be the only option. In fit patients with extensive pelvic disease extending around the vagina or bladder, pelvic exenteration may need to be considered. This type of surgery carries a high morbidity with impaired wound healing due to the radiotherapy. A primary reconstruction of the perineal area using a myocutaneous flap is strongly recommended in salvage APE for anal cancer.

2. Complications of non-surgical treatment for anal cancer do occur in a proportion of patients, including radionecrosis, fistula and incontinence. Severe anal pain due to radionecrosis of the anal lining may necessitate either a colostomy, in the hope that the lesion may heal after faecal diversion, or radical anorectal excision with a flap used to reconstruct the perineum.

3. Occasionally, a tumour is so locally extensive that the patient will be rendered incontinent as a consequence of primary tumour shrinkage. Although rectovaginal fistula may be amenable to repair, sphincter damage is unlikely to improve with local surgery, necessitating APE of the anorectum. APE of the rectum under these circumstances is usually best undertaken in conjunction with a myocutaneous flap to aid perineal wound healing.

4. When there is recurrent disease developing after initial resolution, biopsy is mandatory before surgical intervention. These biopsies need to be of reasonable size, number and depth as the histological appearances following radiotherapy can make histopathological interpretation difficult. If high-dose radiotherapy was used for primary treatment, further non-surgical therapy for recurrence is usually contraindicated, making radical surgical removal necessary.

Inguinal metastases

There is a concern that irradiation of the groins as part of the radiotherapy protocol for anal squamous tumours may overtreat some patients. However, prophylactic low-dose radiotherapy to clinically uninvolved inguinal nodes is currently advised for all T2–4 tumours of the anal canal and margin due to the high risk of recurrence. CT and MRI are not sensitive enough to discriminate between involved and uninvolved nodes. CT/PET as outlined above may help, but inguinal sentinel node biopsy may provide an alternative to imaging-based staging for these nodes. As yet the data available are from small series only and the results are inconsistent.[20,21]

✅ Inguinal lymph nodes are enlarged in up to a third of patients with anal cancers. Inguinal lymph node involvement is now treated by chemoradiotherapy; if this is contraindicated then block dissection may be undertaken at APE.[12] However, histological or cytological confirmation is mandatory before radical groin dissection, as up to 50% of cases of inguinal lymphadenopathy may be due to inflammation alone.

Enlargement of groin nodes sometime after primary therapy is most likely to be due to recurrent tumour; radical groin dissection is indicated in this situation, with up to 50% 5-year survival.

Long-term outcomes

Whilst the prospect of clinical cure has been the focus of outcome reporting for patients treated by chemoradiotherapy, it is now becoming evident that following treatment patients suffer a significant number of long-term consequences directly related to treatment. In a follow-up study of 84 patients from Denmark treated with chemoradiotherapy for anal cancer with a median follow-up of 33 months, faecal and urinary incontinence were reported on a monthly basis in 40% and 43% of patients, respectively.[22] Only 24% of those responding were satisfied with their sexual function. Further efforts should be made to minimise the side-effects of treatment and to improve patients' quality of life following treatment.

Treatment of intraepithelial neoplasia

HPV infection of the anogenital area is very common; it is reported that over 70% of sexually active adults have at some time had occult or overt genital HPV infection. In most individuals the infection remains occult, but in a minority the infection manifests itself as either condylomas or intraepithelial neoplasia. As with other viral infections, it is impossible to eradicate HPV infection by surgical excision; for this reason, surgical excision of condylomas is effectively performed more for relief of symptoms and cosmesis.

If AIN is suspected patients should undergo an examination under anaesthesia with excision of discrete lesions which are small enough not to risk anal stenosis, biopsy of larger suspicious areas and anal mapping (clock face biopsies with a skin punch) to exclude field change. A recent systematic review highlighted the poor evidence base on which current guidelines for the management of AIN are based.[10] Those patients with AIN I/II have a low risk of progression to AIN III and cancer so can be discharged with appropriate advice and reassurance. Patients with AIN III require regular 6-monthly follow-up with clinical examination, which may include anal colposcopy/ high resolution anoscopy (HRA) and photographic documentation of the area with biopsy of any suspicious or bleeding area. Those with immune-compromise require regular follow-up as their risk of progression to invasive disease is greater. Reported treatments for AIN vary from targeted destruction using electrocautery, infrared coagulation or surgical excision to immunomodulation using topical agents such as 5FU and imiquimod. It is the author's opinion that ablation makes histological assessment difficult and risks early recurrence of the disease from hair shafts and pilosebaceous units. There is, however, a lack of robust evidence to support these treatments and the side-effects such as local reactions and anal stenosis are significant. Aggressive surgical excision of the whole perianal skin and anal canal and resurfacing with split skin with a defunctioning colostomy has been used to treat wide areas of AIN III. This sort of surgery necessitates multiple procedures and carries significant morbidity, which for a condition of uncertain malignant potential may make the treatment worse than the disease.

Rarer tumours

Adenocarcinoma

Adenocarcinoma in the anal canal is usually a very low rectal cancer that has spread downwards to involve the canal; however, true adenocarcinoma of the anal canal does occur, probably arising from the anal glands, which arise around the dentate line and pass radially outwards into the sphincter muscles.

This is a very rare tumour, quite radiosensitive, and is increasingly being treated by chemoradiation.

Malignant melanoma

This is another very rare tumour, accounting for just 1% of anal canal malignant tumours with an incidence of 0.34 per 1 million population in the USA.[23] The lesion may mimic a thrombosed external pile due to its colour, although amelanotic tumours also occur. Anal melanomas have a dismal prognosis; the literature suggests a median survival of around 18 months after diagnosis and only 10–20% 5-year survival irrespective of treatment option.[23,24] A recent systematic review based mainly on retrospective studies of surgical treatments concluded that APE conferred no survival benefit over local excision but did confer some advantage in local control. Therefore the authors suggested local excision in the first instance to minimise morbidity and improve quality of life and only to proceed if this fails.[25] Liver and lung metastases are common. As the chances of cure are minimal, radical surgery as primary treatment should be avoided, but local excision may provide useful palliation.[26] Novel systemic therapies for metastatic melanoma hold some promise for the future.

Key points

- The incidence of anal cancer is increasing.
- HPV is an aetiological factor in anal squamous cell carcinomas. Women with previous gynaecological lesions on the cervix and vulva and the immunosuppressed (transplant recipients and HIV patients) are at risk of AIN. These premalignant lesions may be rapidly progressive in immunocompromised patients.
- The management of anal squamous carcinoma has changed dramatically in the last few years. Chemo-irradiation is the treatment of first choice for most lesions.
- Surgery may be the primary treatment modality for small perianal lesions that can be locally excised.
- Melanoma of the anus is very rare and has a dismal prognosis. Radical surgery, chemotherapy and radiotherapy are of little benefit. Local excision may provide some useful palliation.

🌐 Full references available at **http://expertconsult. inkling.com**

Key references

2. Wilkinson JR, Morris EJ, Downing A, et al. The rising incidence of anal cancer in England 1990–2010: a population-based study. Colorectal Dis 2014;16(7):O234–9. PMID: 24410872.

A large population-based study of the incidence of anal cancer using English National Cancer Data Repository data between 1990 and 2010. Reporting a rise in incidence in both males and females.

12. Goh V, Peiffert D, Cervantes A, et al. Anal cancer: ESMO-ESSO-ESTRO Clinical Practice Guidelines for diagnosis, treatment and follow-up. Ann Oncol 2014;25(Suppl 3:iii):10–20. PMID: 25001200.

European clinical guidelines on the diagnosis, treatment and follow-up of patients with anal cancer.

14. James RD, Glynne-Jones R, Meadows HM, et al. Mitomycin or cisplatin chemoradiation with or without maintenance chemotherapy for treatment of squamous-cell carcinoma of the anus (ACT II): a randomised, phase 3, open-label, 2×2 factorial trial. Lancet Oncol 2013;14(6):516–24. PMID: 23578724. Randomised controlled trial of mitomycin or cisplatin chemoradiation with or without maintenance chemotherapy for anal cancer (ACT II); 940 patients enrolled and confirmed fluorouracil and mitomycin with 50.4 Gy radiotherapy in 28 daily fractions as the standard practice in the UK.

15. Epidermoid anal cancer: results from the UKCCCR randomised trial of radiotherapy alone versus radiotherapy, 5-fluorouracil, and mitomycin. UKCCCR Anal Cancer Trial Working Party. UK Co-ordinating Committee on Cancer Research. Lancet 1996;348(9034):1049–54. PMID: 8874455. Randomised trial of radiotherapy alone versus radiotherapy, 5-fluorouracil, and mitomycin with 585 patients randomised. Confirmed the standard treatment for anal cancer should be a combination of radiotherapy and infused 5-fluorouracil and mitomycin.

10

Diverticular disease

Des Winter
Eanna Ryan

Historical perspectives

Colonic diverticulosis is a common anatomical disorder characterised by acquired, sac-like mucosal protrusions (diverticula) through the muscle wall.[1] They are false diverticula because they do not involve all colonic layers. The term 'diverticulum' ('divertikel' in German) was originally used to describe what was an anatomical curiosity in the early 1800s and was not in widespread use until the recognition of 'perisigmoiditis' and related colovesical fistulas by the latter half of the 19th century.[2] It was Lord Berkeley Moynihan (1865–1936 Leeds) who propagated the term 'diverticulitis' at the turn of the 20th century[3] while more latterly diverticulosis was proposed as an umbrella term for asymptomatic individuals as well as symptomatic patients.[4] For decades much of what was written was based on erroneous assumption; a lack of evidence created a knowledge vacuum that was filled with the dogma of the era. We were left with variable terminology and a multiplicity of management protocols.

Terminology

According to existing guidelines,[5–9] the terminology set out in Box 10.1 is used in defining the different clinical pictures with which colonic diverticula may be associated.

Anatomical and physiological perspectives

Colonic diverticulosis and related disorders are traditionally thought to be a Western world,

industrialised country, mature age-group phenomenon with clearly defined origins in meat-rich, fibre-poor diets. Some of the earliest descriptions date only to the early 20th century[10] and the scientific basis for our current understanding is still limited. Parks described his findings on diverticula based on 300 cadaveric dissections in 1968.[1] He noted that diverticula tended to form rows in the lateral intertaenial (rather than antimesenteric) areas, that they were mainly in the sigmoid but could be scattered throughout the colon, and that frequently a blood vessel pierced the wall at the neck of the diverticulum. Much of what was determined about the incidence of diverticulosis was from this and other mid-20th century post-mortem studies.[11–13] Population-based studies confirm diverticula are rare before the age of 30, more common after 40, found in one-third after 60 and in more than 50% of those older than 70 years of age. The age-related phenomenon gives clues to the aetiology and points to general ageing processes, including declining collagen strength or repair.

Incidence and geographical differences

Race and geography

Geographic disparities in the incidence of diverticulosis imply that it is predominantly a disease of industrialised societies associated with an ageing population and Western diet. Moreover, the incidence of diverticular disease has increased in North America by up to 50% in the past two decades, and more so in younger people.[14,15] In contrast, diverticular

Box 10.1 • Terminology

Diverticulosis: the presence of colonic diverticula.

Diverticular disease: clinically significant and symptomatic diverticulosis which may be due to –
Diverticulitis or
Other less well-described manifestations (e.g. visceral hypersensitivity without evidence of inflammation).

Symptomatic uncomplicated diverticular disease (SUDD): persistent abdominal symptoms attributed to diverticula without colitis or diverticulitis.

Diverticulitis: acute or chronic abdominal symptoms in the presence of inflamed diverticula.
Uncomplicated – CT shows only colonic wall thickening with fat stranding.
Complicated –abscess, peritonitis, stricture, fistula or haemorrhage.

Segmental colitis associated with diverticulosis (SCAD): inflammation resembling inflammatory bowel disease isolated to areas marked by diverticulosis.

disease is extremely rare in Asia and Africa compared to Europe and the USA[16] with a reported prevalence as low as 0.5–1.7% in China and Korea.[17,18] Industrialisation or immigration to Western countries results in an increase in the incidence of diverticular disease.[19,20] This has been best described in Japanese immigrants to Hawaii where necropsy studies demonstrate a dramatic increase in diverticulosis compared to age-matched mainland Japanese controls (52% vs 0.5–1%).[20] Similarly, the rates of diverticular disease have risen among the urban, industrialised, black population in South Africa compared with their rural counterparts.[21]

However, the increasing incidence of diverticular disease is not solely due to adoption of a Western lifestyle, and genetic factors may play a role. There are distinct differences in diverticulosis prevalence within ethnic groups living in the same region. For example, studies of ethnic groups living in Israel demonstrate differences in Ashkenazi Jews (16.2%), Sephardic Jews (3.8%) and Arabs (0.7%).[22,23] Aside from variances in prevalence between different ethnicities, anatomical variations also exist with a reported frequency of right-sided diverticulosis of 20% in patients <40 years increasing to 40% in patients >60 years old in Asian populations.[24,25] Furthermore, while the incidence of diverticular disease increases as these countries become more Westernised, the anatomical location (right colon) remains the same.[26,27]

Age and gender

Recent studies point towards age- and gender-related differences in patients presenting with diverticulitis. Males are more likely to develop diverticulitis

at a younger age whereas there is a female predominance in older patients.[28,29] In Western populations, approximately one-fifth of patients with diverticulitis are under the age of 50 (reported incidence 18–34%).[30–32] There was a trend towards a more aggressive surgical approach in younger patients based on the hypothesis that the disease was more virulent in this subgroup.[33,34] Emerging evidence would suggest that younger age is a risk factor for recurrent disease rather than an indication for early intervention in the acute setting, as these patients are just as likely to settle with conservative management.[35,36]

Diet

Painter and Burkitt[2] described diverticular disease as a deficiency of dietary fibre, proposing that consumption of a refined Western diet led to longer colonic transit times, decreased stool volume and increased intraluminal pressures.[36] Although a role for dietary fibre in the pathogenesis of diverticular disease is plausible, there is little evidence to support this hypothesis. Conclusions are drawn from several randomised controlled trials with small patient numbers producing conflicting results[37,38] and do not demonstrate an improvement in symptoms or diverticulitis recurrence overall. In addition, controversy exists as to whether low-residue diets may improve symptoms. Residue refers to any indigestible food substance that remains in the intestinal tract and contributes to stool bulk.[39] Historically, low-residue diets were recommended because indigestible remnants were thought to clog in diverticula leading to diverticulitis or perforation.[40] These concerns were dismissed by conclusive evidence from the health professionals follow-up study.[41]

✔ Low-fibre diet has an epidemiological association with the development of diverticular disease. However, recommending fibre as a treatment for diverticulosis is largely based on outdated, poorly controlled studies.

✔ Young patients (<50 years) may be more likely to suffer from recurrent diverticulitis. At present there is no evidence to support aggressive surgical intervention in cases of uncomplicated diverticular disease.

Aetiology and pathogenesis

There are several theories as to the pathogenesis of diverticular disease. Aside from luminal trauma, potential aetiological factors include elevated colonic pressures, compromised colon wall integrity and altered bacterial flora.[42–48] Colonic wall abnormalities (specifically colonic wall thickening, increased collagen cross-linking,[49] muscle atrophy[50] and shortening of taeniae coli[13]) are thought to produce a 'stiffer', less compliant colon predisposing to diverticular herniation. In addition, abnormalities in cholinergic smooth muscle excitation and neuro-humoral signalling (serotonin, nitric oxide, VIP) may contribute to disordered contractions and increased intraluminal pressures.[51–54]

Lifestyle

Both the health professionals follow-up study (47 228 men) and the Swedish mammography cohort study demonstrate a positive correlation between obesity and diverticular-associated complications.[55,56] Indeed, according to the American taskforce, obesity is recognised as a risk factor for diverticular disease.[57] This may be due to obesity-associated inflammation (cytokine secretion from metabolically active visceral fat).[58]

Smoking

There is evidence for an association between diverticular disease and smoking. Pathological examination suggests a higher incidence of strictures and perforation in smokers compared to non-smokers.[59] There may be a gender difference, with a higher likelihood of abscess or perforation in female smokers compared to males.[60]

NSAIDs

It is hypothesised that NSAIDs (non-steroidal anti-inflammatory drugs) may cause colonic injury via direct topical injury and/or impaired prostaglandin synthesis compromising mucosal integrity, increasing permeability and enabling the influx of bacteria and other toxins.[48] Data from the health professionals follow-up study showed an increased incidence of uncomplicated diverticular disease in patients who used NSAIDs compared with their counterparts who did not.[60] In addition, NSAID use is associated with diverticular complications, including bleeding and perforation.[61,62]

Diverticulitis

The extent of the problem

It was misquoted for many years that about 25% of patients with diverticulosis will develop an acute inflammatory condition characterised by left iliac fossa or suprapubic pain, malaise and fever (diverticulitis), a figure that was rarely challenged although the basis for it is unclear. The origin of this overestimate may have been the misquoting of the proportion re-presenting following an episode of diverticular symptoms,[1] rather than the actual prevalence of diverticulitis. A modern (1986–2004) population-based study found 1.7% of male healthcare professionals aged between 40 and 75 years developed diverticulitis, giving a crude annual incidence of 1/1000 (801 events in 47 228 persons over 18 years).[41] This figure has been confirmed as an accurate representation of the USA population in whom there was an age-adjusted hospitalisation rate of 75/100 000 in 2005[63] or 1/1000 in the present decade at the projected trajectory. The population trends seen in this national inpatient sample (1998–2005) reflect the worldwide finding of male predominance aged under 45 but female predominance in those older, as well as an increasing incidence in the under-45 age group. Fascinatingly, there was a large difference in the rates of diverticulitis admissions between the West (50.4/100 000) versus the other sectors of the USA (>70/100 000). The west of the USA also has a higher fibre intake and relatively lower colorectal cancer incidence than the rest of the country.[64] While this supports the historical assumption that high dietary fibre protects against the development of both disorders, the association is speculative until cofactors (hereditary, ethnic, socioeconomic, dietary, smoking, alcohol, etc.) are excluded.

Classification

It is now widely accepted that diverticulitis encompasses a wide spectrum of pathologies, ranging from acute uncomplicated diverticulitis to perforation with peritonitis. Although the underlying pathophysiology may be similar in all cases, the clinical manifestation of the disease differs greatly between individuals. It is helpful to further classify patients according to those who have 'moderate diverticulitis' and those with 'severe diverticulitis'[65] (see Table 10.1). The adult prevalence of perforated diverticulitis is

Table 10.1 • CT classification of acute diverticulitis

Moderate diverticulitis	Severe diverticulitis
Localised sigmoid colon wall thickening (>5 mm) Inflammation localised to pericolic fat	Moderate diverticulitis plus any of: Abdominopelvic abscess Free extraluminal gas Extraluminal contrast extravasation

Source: Ambrosetti P, Grossholz M, Becker C, et al. Computed tomography in acute left colonic diverticulitis. Br J Surg 1997;84(4):532–4.

Table 10.2 • Classification systems for diverticulitis

	Hinchey classification[71]	Köhler modification[72]	Modified Hinchey[73]	Hansen/Stock[74]
Stage I	Pericolic abscess confined by the mesocolon	Pericolic abscess	0 Mild clinical diverticulitis I Pericolic abscess or phlegmon Ia Colonic wall thickening/confined pericolic inflammation Ib Confined small (<5 cm) pericolic abscess	0 Diverticulosis I Acute uncomplicated diverticulitis
Stage II	Pelvic abscess, distant from area of inflammation	IIa Distant abscess amenable to percutaneous drainage IIb Complex abscess with/without associated fistula	II Pelvic, distant intra-abdominal, or retroperitoneal abscess	Acute complicated diverticulitis IIa Phlegmon, peridiverticulitis IIb Abscess, sealed perforation IIc Free perforation
Stage III	Generalised peritonitis resulting from pericolic/pelvic abscess rupture into peritoneal cavity	Generalised purulent peritonitis	III Generalised purulent peritonitis	Recurrent diverticulitis
Stage IV	Faecal peritonitis resulting from free perforation of colonic diverticulum	Faecal peritonitis	IV Generalised faecal peritonitis	N/A

approximately 3.5 per 100 000 and the incidence has more than doubled in the last two decades.[66–69] Reasons why this may be are speculative, including NSAIDs, opioids, corticosteroids and smoking.[59,61,70]

Table 10.2 compares the different classification systems for diverticulitis.

Segmental colitis-associated diverticulosis

Segmental colitis associated with diverticulosis (SCAD) is found in less than 1% of colonoscopy procedures.[75,76] The majority of these patients have simply bleeding per rectum rather than any significant change in bowel habit or constitutional symptoms. Many resolve without therapy such that medical treatment should be reserved for those with troublesome symptoms.[77,78]

Diagnosis and imaging

The diagnosis of diverticulitis is largely based on clinical impression.[79] Confirmatory imaging is helpful in determining the extent, degree and local consequences of the inflammatory process as well as excluding other disorders.[80,81] Ultrasound is adequate, with reasonable sensitivity and specificity using graded compression and other tricks of waveform

distortion that may not be readily available in every emergency room environment.[82,83] Although a relatively inexpensive, easily reproducible and safe modality, sonographic imaging displays reduced acoustic acuity in gas-distended or obese patients. Historically, a water-soluble (rather than barium-based) contrast enema with fluoroscopic images was used to confirm diverticulitis but the test was an unpleasant, messy, time-consuming endurance for patients and radiologists.[65]

Not surprisingly, CT in rapid, multiple slice scanners capable of variable plane reconstruction became the gold standard in determining the diagnosis and staging of diverticulitis[83,84] (**Figs 10.1** and **10.2**). Downsides include the allergic and nephrotoxic risks of intravenous contrast so assessment of relevant history and biochemistry is essential. Widespread and repeated CT exposure to radiation is estimated to potentially harm individuals[85] so patient age and exposure history are factors. A pragmatic approach might be to use ultrasound initially, reserving CT for unclear cases or those in whom crisp anatomical definition is required (e.g. abscess needing drainage, suspicion of malignancy, unexpected or atypical sonographic findings etc.) (**Figs 10.3** and **10.4**).

Colonic imaging (either colonoscopy or CT colonography) is still performed routinely following an episode of diverticulitis to rule out neoplasia (either coexistent or mimicking an inflammatory

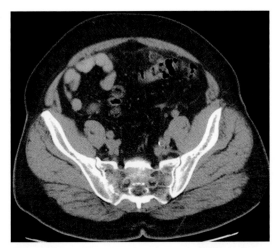

Figure 10.1 • CT image of moderate sigmoid diverticulitis.

process). The utility of these procedures has been questioned by authors from the Antipodes.[86,87] Where there has been good-quality cross-sectional imaging of relatively mild diverticulitis in an otherwise asymptomatic young patient with no premorbid reasons to screen, then diverticulitis is a soft indication for colonoscopy. Conversely, where there are atypical imaging features (i.e. localised lymphadenopathy, relative absence of diverticula, focal mass effect, more than one site of 'fat stranding') or complicated diverticulitis then early colonoscopy is very much indicated. While tradition considered that endoscopic insufflation would be too dangerous within 6 weeks of assumed diverticulitis[88] there is little substance to this dogma and careful colonoscopy can be performed after an interval of 1–2 weeks where there is clinical suspicion of neoplasia (e.g. unresolved or progressive symptoms).

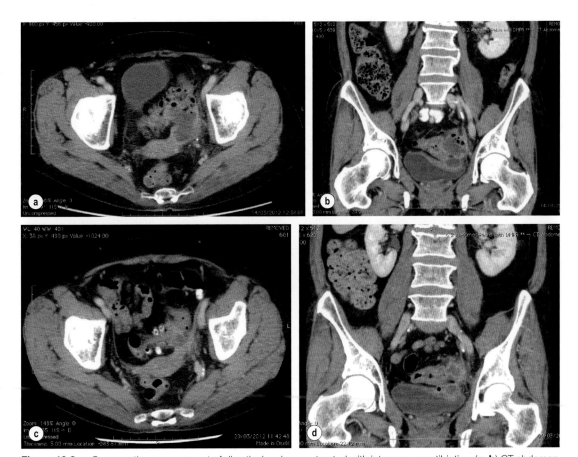

Figure 10.2 • Conservative management of diverticular abscess treated with intravenous antibiotics. (**a, b**) CT abdomen on presentation demonstrates a perisigmoid abscess (Hinchey II diverticulitis). (**c, d**) CT abdomen on day 7 following treatment with i.v. cefuroxime, ciprofloxacin and metronidazole demonstrates resolution of abscess.

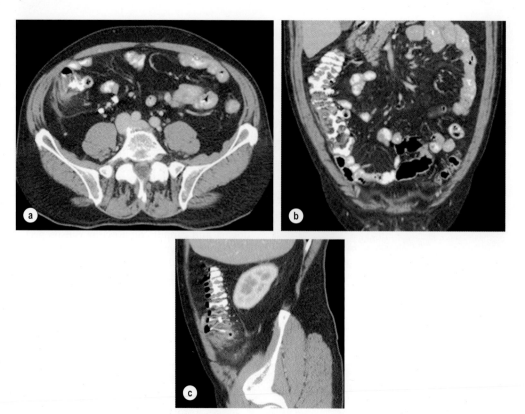

Figure 10.3 • Right-sided diverticulitis. CT may be useful in patients with atypical clinical findings. The images demonstrate caecal diverticulitis as a cause for right iliac fossa pain in a 60-year-old male.

Magnetic resonance imaging (MRI) is of immense value in intestinal disorders because soft-tissue delineation exceeds that of ultrasound or CT and additional benefits include fistulography, multiphase component separation and an absence of ionising radiation.[89–91] MRI is expensive, requires expert interpretation and scan platforms are claustrophobic, noisy places that patients must endure for prolonged periods. Open scanners have gone a long way to address the problem but they are few in number as yet.

> ✅ CT is the gold standard in diagnosing and staging the severity of diverticulitis.[92]
>
> Recent evidence suggests that routine follow-up colonoscopy may not be warranted in every patient and should be determined on a case-by-case basis depending on the level of clinical concern.[86,87]

Treatment

Conservative and medical options

Asymptomatic patients with diverticulosis do not require treatment. There was a historical vogue (until very recently) for advising patients to avoid nuts and seeds based on the misguided assumption that they precipitated symptomatic events by local trauma or obstruction. In keeping with the folklore of diverticular management in the 20th century, this was without scientific basis or fact.[41] Furthermore, although it seems unlikely to harm and may help prevent development of diverticula, there is scant proof that changing to a higher fibre intake can change the course of symptomatic diverticular problems.[38] Even when combined with non-absorbable antibiotics (rifaxamin), any perceived benefit is small and not much better than placebo.[93] Lifestyle optimisation (i.e. high freshly sourced fibre intake, low animal fat/processed diet, smoking cessation, exercise, minimal anti-inflammatory drug intake etc.) are central to primary disease prevention and are sensible in all populations regardless of the presence of diverticula.

There are limited medical options for patients with recurrent or persistent symptoms deemed attributable to diverticulitis (or 'diverticular disease'). There is modest benefit to a prolonged course of 5-aminosalicylates or probiotics in short-term, small trials.[94,95] There is a relatively small side-effect profile to these agents due to their relatively specific intestinal drug delivery mechanism. However, the numbers needed to treat are probably high, the compliance poor and the overall applicability of the approach is low.

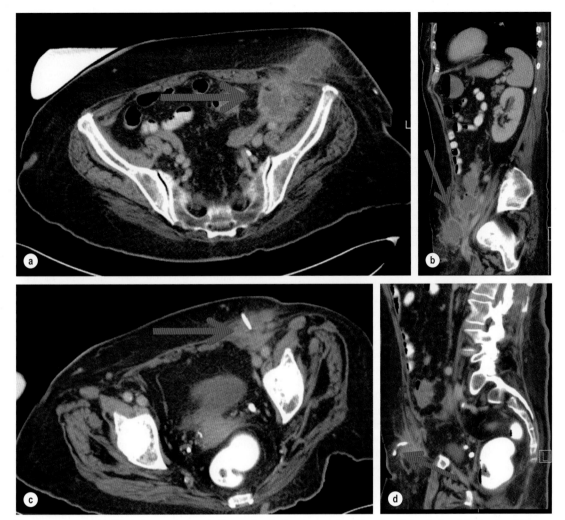

Figure 10.4 • **(a, b)** CT abdomen demonstrating a diverticular abscess involving the abdominal wall (*red arrow*; history of right hemicolectomy and end ileostomy). **(c, d)** The abscess was drained percutaneously with resolution of symptoms. *Red arrow* demonstrates placement of drain.

☑☑ As the aetiology is unknown, diverticulitis may be an inflammatory condition rather than an infective/bacterial problem. Two randomised trials[84,96] have found that antibiotic treatment for acute uncomplicated diverticulitis neither accelerates recovery nor prevents complications or recurrence. As such, observational treatment without antibiotics can be considered appropriate in non-septic patients.

☑ When antibiotics are indicated there is currently no consensus on the most appropriate antibiotic regimen or route (oral/intravenous) for diverticulitis; however, broad-spectrum agents covering Gram-negative and anaerobic organisms are advised.

Emergency surgery

Historical perspectives

Henri Albert Hartmann (1860–1952 Paris, France) first described an alternative to abdominoperineal excision of the sigmoid and rectum for carcinoma at the French Surgical Association in 1921.[97,98] The dissection extended below the peritoneal reflection with transection of the lower rectum, closure of the remaining short rectal stump and peritoneum, with formation of an end colostomy. Of course, this is not what was performed for acute diverticulitis in the 20th century but, amazingly, the eponymous term has endured regardless of the historical inaccuracy.

This was due to the absence of a suitable alternative to describe what was, in essence, a non-restorative subtotal sigmoid colectomy with a long, intraperitoneal, closed rectosigmoid stump and end colostomy. This operation triumphed over previously performed three-stage procedures whereby an initial defunctioning loop colostomy was performed with subsequent resection and anastomosis (if and when the patient recovered), and eventually, colostomy closure. The mortality of this latter approach was unacceptably high and, while that of a 'Hartmann's procedure' is still 10–15% in the present era, a one-stage non-restorative operation was thought safer. Short-term complications include persistent sepsis (often in the residual sigmoid stump due to persistent diverticulitis or opening of the staple line), stoma problems (necrosis, retraction, stenosis etc.), and wound complications (including dehiscence). In the longer term, as many as half the patients are left with a permanent stoma due to the reluctance of the surgeon (or indeed the patient) to submit to the perils of another operation for anastomosis.

Does perforated diverticulitis require resection in all cases? Carl Eggers (1879–1956 New York, USA), a German-American surgeon, described a series of patients with diverticulitis of whom those with generalised peritonitis he had managed with drainage alone.[99] Two randomised clinical trials (Denmark and France) in the 1980s and 1990s dealt with this question. Although both were underpowered, the data did support an organ-preserving approach. Patients in whom a drainage procedure (with or without a defunctioning stoma) alone was performed for purulent peritonitis had a lower mortality than those resected.[100,101] There may have been more short-term septic issues with an organ-preserving operation but this was in an age with fewer broad-spectrum antibiotics and less widespread availability of interventional radiology drainage of abscesses than now.

Laparoscopic peritoneal lavage for generalised purulent peritonitis

Alas, the trials were not enough to change practice at the time. They did give food for thought to another pioneering surgeon, Gerry O'Sullivan (1946–2012 Cork, Ireland), who considered it feasible to laparoscope a patient in whom there was generalised peritonitis and pneumoperitoneum on CT or plain radiography (erect chest or abdominal X-ray) due to perforated diverticulitis. By simply performing laparoscopic peritoneal lavage (LPL) the initial results championed a stoma-free, low morbidity approach[102] (**Fig. 10.5**). The utility and low mortality (~5%) of the approach to generalised peritonitis due to perforated, purulent diverticulitis were confirmed in several series.

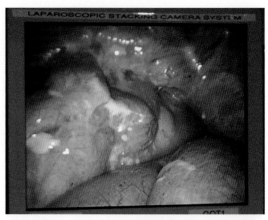

Figure 10.5 • Laparoscopic image of Hinchey III purulent diverticulitis.

The natural selection bias inherent in non-randomised studies meant that more robust data were necessary. This led to a number of multicentre, randomised trials comparing laparoscopic lavage with colonic resection (usually with a stoma) for acute perforated non-faeculant diverticulitis. To date, four randomised trials (LADIES, SCANDIV, DILALA and LapLAND) have been registered[103–106] (see Table 10.3). Three of these trials have published results.[107–109] The SCANDIV trial randomised patients with suspected perforated diverticulitis and free air on CT scan to laparoscopic lavage ($n = 101$) or colonic resection ($n = 98$) with or without primary anastomosis, as 'determined by surgeon preference and local practices'. While the reintervention rate was higher in the lavage group, morbidity and mortality (13.9% vs 11.5%) were not significantly different. The LOLA arm of the LADIES trial randomised patients with Hinchey III diverticulitis to laparoscopic lavage ($n = 46$) or sigmoid resection ($n = 40$) but was closed due to a higher reintervention rate in the lavage group, although there were fewer stomas and lower mortality (9% vs 14%). The DILALA trial randomised patients ($n = 65$) with Hinchey III (purulent peritonitis) diverticulitis at laparoscopy to laparoscopic lavage ($n = 39$) or an open resection ($n = 36$). Lavage was shorter with faster recovery and lower mortality (7.7% vs 11.4%). Notably, the crude aggregated data from these trials show fewer stomas and lower mortality with laparoscopic lavage but possibly higher postoperative intervention (e.g. abscess drainage). Subsequent cost analyses from two of these randomised trials provide evidence that laparoscopic lavage is more cost-effective than sigmoid resection.[110,111]

Shock, requirements for inotropes and infirm patients or those on immunosuppressants are contra-indications to laparoscopic lavage for generalised, diverticular-related peritonitis. Furthermore, if faecal peritonitis or a visible colonic wall breach

Table 10.3 • Randomised trials comparing laparoscopic lavage with resection

Name	Study	Objective	Inclusion criteria	Recruitment	Study number
LADIES The Netherlands	Multicentre two-armed randomised trial: LOLA arm – laparoscopic lavage, Hartmann's or resection and anastomosis (2:1:1); DIVA arm – for faeculent peritonitis Hartmann's or resection and anastomosis (1:1)	To assess the superiority of laparoscopic lavage compared with sigmoidectomy in patients with purulent perforated diverticulitis, with respect to overall long-term morbidity and mortality	Patients with signs of general peritonitis and suspected perforated diverticulitis. Radiological examination by radiography or a CT abdomen with diffuse-free intraperitoneal air or fluid for patients to be classified as having perforated diverticulitis	Recruitment commenced 2009	LOLA arm: 264 DIVA arm: 212
DILALA Scandinavia	Multicentre randomised trial comparing laparoscopic lavage to Hartmann's procedure as treatment for acute perforated diverticulitis (1:1)	To compare laparoscopic lavage to Hartmann's procedure as treatment for acute perforated diverticulitis	Clinical symptoms, elevated inflammatory markers, CT abdomen showing signs of free gas and/or intra-abdominal fluid. Emergency surgery decided by the attending surgeon	Recruitment commenced 2011	Laparoscopic lavage: 39 Hartmann's procedure: 36
SCANDIV Scandinavia	Multicentre randomised clinical superiority trial (centre-stratified block randomisation).	To determine whether laparoscopic lavage changes the rate of severe complications in patients with acute perforated diverticulitis who traditionally are treated with primary resection	Clinical suspicion of perforated diverticulitis with indication for urgent surgery. CT abdomen with free air and findings suggesting diverticulitis. Patients randomised after diagnostic laparoscopy	Recruitment commenced 2010	Laparoscopic lavage: 101 Hartmann's procedure: 98
LapLAND Ireland	Multicentre randomised trial comparing Hartmann's procedure or resection/anastomosis (1:1)	To compare outcomes following Hartmann's or resection with anastomosis and defunctioning stoma and laparoscopic lavage alone for the treatment of acute perforated non-faeculant diverticulitis	Clinical evidence of generalised peritonitis. Free air on erect chest X-ray or CT abdomen suggestive of perforated diverticulitis. Laparoscopy to confirm diagnosis and exclude faecal peritonitis	Recruitment commenced 2010	300 Still recruiting

is identified at laparoscopy then resection is indicated. Many cases show features of stercoral rather than diverticular perforation (i.e. history of prolonged constipation, minimal or absent diverticula, large hole with focal necrosis not inflammation). It should be considered routine to perform gas-leak testing during laparoscopy (transanal carbon dioxide or air insufflation of the sigmoid submerged in saline lavage) to exclude a hole before considering lavage alone. Ongoing sepsis (peritonitis should resolve within 24 hours) following seemingly successful lavage suggests source control was not achieved and re-intervention should be considered.

Resection with primary anastomosis

Primary resection and anastomosis (PRA) with or without a defunctioning ileostomy has emerged as a worthy alternative to Hartmann's procedure (HP) in the setting of peritonitis secondary to diverticular perforation.[112] Indeed, some studies demonstrate superior outcomes compared to Hartmann's procedure, quoting mortality rates of 5% for PRA versus 15% for HP.[113] Furthermore, PRA compares favourably in terms of postoperative morbidity, including wound and stoma complications and sepsis. In the most recent systematic review, anastomotic leak rates were in the order of 6%,[114] notably lower than the reported anastomotic leak rate in Hartmann's reversal (8%). The ongoing DIVA arm of the LADIES trial is the first randomised trial comparing Hartmann's procedure with sigmoidectomy plus primary anastomosis.

A treatment algorithm is shown in **Fig. 10.6.**

> ✅ Aggregated data from randomised trials testing laparoscopic lavage for perforated, non-faeculant diverticulitis suggest it is feasible in patients wishing to avoid a stoma. Those with ongoing sepsis due to a failure of source control may need timely re-intervention to avoid mortality risks.[107–109]

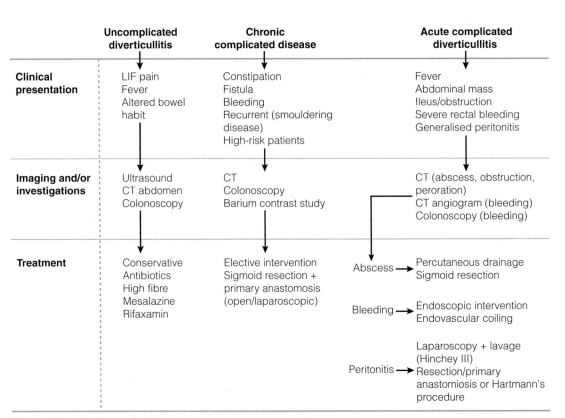

Figure 10.6 • Treatment algorithm.
Based on Klarenbeek BR, de Korte N, van der Peet DL, et al. Review of current classifications for diverticular disease and a translation into clinical practice. Int J Colorectal Dis 2012; 27(2):207–14. With permission from Springer Science + Business Media.

Elective resection – facts, fiction and functional outcome

Elective resection for recurrent diverticulitis was once practised commonly after the second or third episode. However, the practice is risky, with reports of 1% mortality, 30–50% morbidity and as many as 10% receiving a stoma (at least in the short term).[115-117] The natural history of diverticulitis is such that one in six patients undergo surgery at presentation while approximately 20–25% re-present, with a similar proportion requiring surgery, such that less than 5% have more than two episodes.[118] In that series, six of the 78 patients readmitted with diverticulitis a second time died, a proportion commented to be twice that of those presenting for the first time. Parks did not suggest elective resection to improve this statistic although many have used his data to support the premise of a 'prophylactic' operation. Indeed, he pointed out that several patients died in their first admission from suspected diverticulitis in which radiology or necropsy tests were not performed so that they could not be classed as diverticular deaths in the paper. Had they been, the mortality was likely much higher for the first episode than reported for the second. The principles on which this outdated and flawed concept was founded predate modern cross-sectional imaging such that the diagnosis was clinical and inferred from subsequent barium enema.[119-121] Some patients had ongoing symptoms and others came to emergency surgery for diverticulitis, so it was extrapolated that elective surgery was indicated to prevent a life-threatening event. We now know that diverticulitis follows a predictable course in the majority, such that recurrence runs at 2% per year while the risk of requiring emergency surgery following diverticulitis is calculated to be only one event in 2000 patient-years.[66] Furthermore, Mayo Clinic data suggest that diverticulitis is not a progressive disease in terms of severity or mortality risk.[122] Indeed, as it has been throughout the last century, the highest risk of extreme sepsis and death is with the first episode. The overwhelming majority of these patients have no history of diverticulitis and had no premorbid diagnosis of diverticulosis.[67,122-126] For these reasons successfully treated acute uncomplicated diverticulitis is no longer deemed an indication for elective surgery,[126,127] and both the American Society of Colon and Rectal Surgeons, and the Association of Coloproctology of Great Britain and Ireland advocate that the decision to undergo elective resection should be made on an individualised basis.[92,128]

There are certain diverticular-associated phenomena that are relative or absolute indications for elective surgery. These include fistula (e.g. colovesical, colovaginal, colocutaneous), obstruction from a stricture and persisting diverticulitis ('smouldering diverticulitis') unresponsive to medical therapy. The latter is an uncommon event characterised by symptoms matched with a persistent subtle, tender mass in the left iliac fossa, persistently elevated markers of inflammation (e.g. C-reactive protein), and no other abnormality on colonoscopy and cross-sectional imaging.

Are there circumstances where a patient should consider elective resection for recurring episodes of diverticulitis each of which resolve fully? After four defined episodes the risk of further episodes requiring admission and surgery is particularly high in the younger (<50 years of age) population.[129] Therefore, in young patients eager to avoid further morbidity and time off work in whom an elective operation can be performed with a mortality risk of <1%[32] elective sigmoid resection is reasonable. However, the preoperative discussion should include the fact that recurrent diverticulitis may arise, that a stoma may be required (at least in the short term), that coexisting functional symptoms will persist, and that over 20% complain of urgency and even incontinence episodes.[130] The laparoscopic approach is attractive to patient and surgeon as there are short-term advantages with smaller wounds, less morbidity and less time dependent on supportive care.[131]

> ✔ Indications for elective resection include: fistula, diverticular stricture and disease refractory to conservative management.
>
> Sigmoid resection may be considered in patients who have undergone abscess drainage or laparoscopic lavage, but there is no evidence to support surgical intervention in these cases.

Diverticular haemorrhage

The proportion of patients with diverticulosis presenting with bleeding was originally thought to be as high as 3–5%.[132] However, this was based on a somewhat oversimplified quotient (number bleeding divided by number presenting to hospital with a diagnosis of diverticulosis) that would have hugely overestimated the prevalence. Modern population-based data would suggest less than one event in 2000 person-years (383 bleeds with only 70 requiring transfusion or intervention in 730 446 person-years of follow-up).[41] One group found no inflammation but non-uniform intimal thickening in the vasa recta of bleeding diverticula.[133,134] The majority of diverticular haemorrhages cease spontaneously. A requirement of more than four units of red cell concentrate may indicate patients at risk of ongoing bleeding.[135] Visceral angiography with embolisation[136–138] is preferable to blind colectomy, with which morbidity and mortality risks are high. One of the challenges to the surgeon faced with operating on an (all too often) elderly patient with lower gastrointestinal bleeding is what to remove? Many a young surgeon was caught out doing a left colectomy on the assumption that the sigmoid was the culprit only to find ongoing bleeding: 'diverticular' haemorrhage is right-sided in over 50% and a proportion are due to angiodysplasia.

Key points

- The spectrum of diverticular disease encompasses asymptomatic diverticulosis, uncomplicated diverticulitis, complicated diverticular disease (abscess, perforation, stricture, fistula), diverticular bleeding and SCAD (segmental colitis-associated diverticulosis).
- The annual incidence of diverticulitis is approximately 1/1000 in Western populations.
- There is a male predominance in younger patients while females are more likely to develop diverticulitis at an older age.
- The aetiology remains unknown but genetics/ethnicity, geographical location and lifestyle factors (smoking and obesity) all play a role.
- There is a tenuous link between lack of dietary fibre and the development of diverticulosis.
- Computed tomography is the ideal investigation for symptomatic diverticular issues. A colonoscopy may not be necessary if CT findings are consistent with diverticulitis and there is a low clinical concern for other pathologies (i.e. cancer).
- Antibiotics do not influence outcomes of uncomplicated diverticulitis in non-septic patients and can be safely omitted.
- Perforated diverticulitis with purulent (not faeculant) peritonitis may be managed with laparoscopic lavage or resection depending on the clinical circumstances and patient wishes. The optimal strategy depends on the physiological status of the patient, the extent of contamination (Hinchey grade) and the experience of the surgeon.
- Elective sigmoid resection after diverticulitis is unwarranted in the majority unless there are good disease-specific (e.g. colovesical fistula) or patient-related indications (e.g. after multiple admissions in a young patient).

🌐 Full references available at **http://expertconsult. inkling.com**

Key references

84. Unlu C, de Korte N, Daniels L, et al. A multicenter randomized clinical trial investigating the cost-effectiveness of treatment strategies with or without antibiotics for uncomplicated acute diverticulitis (DIABOLO trial). BMC Surg 2010;10:23. PMID: 20646266.

The DIABOLO trial randomised patients (*n* = 528) to observation or antibiotics for uncomplicated acute diverticulitis. No significant differences were found for time for recovery, disease progression, recurrent diverticulitis, sigmoid resection, readmission, adverse events or mortality. Hospital stay was significantly shorter in the observation group (2 vs 3 days; *P* <0.00).

92. Feingold D, Steele S, Lee S, et al. Practice parameters for sigmoid diverticulitis. Clinical Practice Guideline Task Force of the American Society of Colon and Rectal Surgeons. Dis Colon Rectum 2014;57(3):284–94. PMID: 24509449.

The ASCRS continue to recommend antibiotics to cover Gram-negative and anaerobic organisms for acute diverticulitis (level I evidence, grade C). Whilst the recent randomised trial and meta-analysis data are acknowledged, they state that 'further research is required before adopting an antibiotic-free treatment strategy'.

96. Chabok A, Pahlman L, Hjern F, et al. Randomized clinical trial of antibiotics in acute uncomplicated diverticulitis. Br J Surg 2012;99(4):532–9. PMID: 22290281.

The AVOD trial randomised patients (*n* = 669) to symptomatic treatment and antibiotics compared to symptomatic treatment alone for uncomplicated diverticulitis. There was no significant difference in complication rate, length of stay or recurrent diverticulitis between the groups.

11

Ulcerative colitis

Scott R. Kelley
Eric J. Dozois

Introduction

Ulcerative colitis (UC) is an idiopathic relapsing inflammatory bowel disease (IBD) involving the mucosa and lamina propria of the rectum and variable extent of the proximal colon. Characterised by remissions and exacerbations, the clinical spectrum of disease can range from inactive to fulminant. Medical management is generally effective in controlling ulcerative colitis, but ultimately 30–40% of patients will require surgical intervention. Criteria for the management of acute and chronic disease are well established, with surgery playing a fundamental role, as removal of the colon and rectum is essentially curative.

Epidemiology

Ulcerative colitis is an uncommon disease with varying incidence rates (0.5–24.5/100 000) and discernible differences are seen between different geographic and ethnic regions of the world.[1] Less common in Asia, Africa, South America and Southeastern Europe, UC has a varied incidence of between 2 and 15 cases per 100 000 persons per year in developed and industrialised Western countries of North America, Northwestern Europe and the UK. A significant trend of increasing incidence and prevalence rates has been reported in underdeveloped parts of the world as they become more industrialised, thus supporting the importance of environmental factors in the development of UC.

The onset of symptoms typically plateaus around the fourth decade of life, remaining fairly constant thereafter. A second peak of onset around the sixth to seventh decade has been described, though there is uncertainty as to whether this is truly a subsequent peak or merely difficulty in differentiating it from other colitides.[2]

Ulcerative colitis is seen with near equal frequency in males and females.[1] Caucasians and African Americans have a nearly equivalent incidence, while the Jewish populace experiences the highest documented rates. Hispanic, Native American, African and Asian populations have the lowest incidence.[2]

Aetiopathogenesis

The pathogenesis of UC remains enigmatic, though multiple factors have been described as potential causative or protective agents in its occurrence and include: diet, alcohol and tobacco consumption, socioeconomic status, hygiene, urban living conditions, antibiotic usage, gut flora dysbiosis, probiotic use, non-steroidal anti-inflammatory agents, appendicectomy, breastfeeding, oral contraceptive use, stress, and familial and genetic causes.

Though a significant number of dietary factors have been evaluated as potential causative agents for UC, no consensus has emerged.[2,3] A decreased risk has been associated with alcohol consumption, and the risk declined as daily alcohol consumption increased.[4]

Evidence demonstrates that smoking is protective against disease activity, and it has been shown that those who quit smoking are more likely to have a relapse. Ex-smokers are 70% more likely to develop ulcerative colitis when compared to those who have never smoked, though the causation remains unclear. Supplemental nicotine therapy has not consistently been shown to be more effective than placebo or conventional therapy (steroids/5-aminosalicylic acid), and has a significant side-effect profile.[2,3]

The hygiene hypothesis contends that cleaner living environments reduce the amount of organisms one is exposed to early in life, thus reducing the ability of the immune system to become tolerant, and subsequently causing an aberrant response when thus exposed.[5] Ulcerative colitis is more common among urban populations, is associated with indoor living, smaller families, and individuals of middle and upper socioeconomic status, who primarily reside in more sanitary surroundings.[6]

Antibiotic usage and the resulting gut flora dysbiosis are commonplace in developed countries, and hypothetically a potential cause of UC when taking into consideration that higher rates of utilisation are seen in industrialised and developed nations, though this is yet to be proven.[3] A correlation has been demonstrated in children with UC, who are more likely to have received antibiotics during their first year of life.[7]

A predisposition for UC has been reported to be as high as 29% in those with a positive family history, and between 10% and 20% of affected individuals have a first-degree relative with IBD. Twin studies have consistently shown a higher concordant disease rate in monozygotic compared to dizygotic pairs (approximately 50% versus nearly 0%), where the concordance among ordinary siblings was found to be around 5%.[8]

Clinical presentation

Colonic involvement at presentation can vary widely between different geographic regions, though proctosigmoiditis is the most common. In the USA 46% presented with proctosigmoiditis, 37% pancolitis and 17% with left-sided colitis.

Common symptoms associated with UC include urgency, diarrhoea, tenesmus and haematochezia. Constipation, a complaint in 15–20% of patients, is related to incomplete evacuation of the rectum. Symptoms correlate with severity of disease, and increasing severity leads to worsening nausea, emesis, abdominal distension and weight loss. Protein-losing enteropathy may lead to loss of lean body mass and anaemia, and growth retardation in children. Haemodynamically significant haemorrhage is an uncommon complication, but is responsible for 10% of emergency colectomies. Severity can also have systemic manifestations, including tachycardia, pyrexia, leucocytosis and increased fluid requirements, indicating toxicity.

Approximately 5–15% of patients with UC develop acute severe colitis, and up to 50% present initially with fulminant disease. Intense medical treatment has a high chance of inducing remission but when unsuccessful, urgent surgery will be necessary in up to 20% of patients. Perforation is a rare but serious occurrence, with a mortality approaching 60%.

Extraintestinal manifestations

Upwards of 20% of patients with UC will develop extra-alimentary manifestations during the course of illness including, but not limited to, musculoskeletal (the most common), hepatopancreatobiliary, dermatological, thromboembolic and ophthalmological derangements.[9] Most extraintestinal manifestations present after an exacerbation of colonic inflammation, but they can also occur at the time of the acute flair. Colectomy is beneficial in inducing remission of peripheral arthropathy, erythema nodosum and iritis. Pyoderma gangrenosum does not universally respond, and axial arthropathy, primary sclerosing cholangitis, uveitis and episcleritis proceed independently of surgical intervention.

Musculoskeletal

Peripheral arthropathy asymmetrically involves numerous small and large joints (knees being the most common), affecting up to 20% of patients, with severity paralleling disease activity. The arthropathy is typically fleeting, rheumatoid factor negative (seronegative) and non-deforming. It disappears when medical treatment induces remission or after proctocolectomy, although it has been documented in patients with pouchitis after restorative proctocolectomy.[10]

Axial arthropathy (ankylosing spondylitis) involving the sacroiliac joints and one or more vertebrae occurs in up to 5% of patients. The majority of cases are HLA-B27 positive, unrelated to the activity of colitis and predominantly unresponsive to treatment. Asymptomatic sacroileitis is limited to the sacroiliac joint, is HLA-B27 negative, largely unaffected by treatment and is radiographically detected in 24% of patients. Although both ankylosing spondylitis and asymptomatic sacroileitis have an overall poor response to treatment, antitumour necrosis factor (TNF)-α agents have recently shown promise.[10]

Hepatopancreatobiliary

Primary sclerosing cholangitis (PSC) is an idiopathic chronic and progressive disorder manifesting as stricturing, inflammation, and fibrosis of intra- and extrahepatic bile ducts. It is one of the most serious complications of UC. Patients with coexisting PSC and UC are at a markedly increased risk of colonic neoplasia (five times), necessitating close colonoscopic surveillance with extensive biopsy sampling. Around 5% of patients with UC will develop PSC, whereas upwards of 75% of patients with PSC are found to have concurrent UC.[11] The clinical course of PSC does not parallel underlying bowel disease and may present independently of colonic symptoms. An increased risk of development has been demonstrated in patients with HLA B8, DR2, DR3 or DR6 haplotype positivity. Treatment of PSC with steroids, colectomy or antibiotics is ineffectual. Patients undergoing restorative proctocolectomy have a higher subsequent incidence of pouchitis and dysplasia in the ileal pouch mucosa.[12] Ultimately, the disease progresses to liver cirrhosis and eventual failure, which may prompt consideration for liver transplantation.

> ✅ The cumulative risk of pouchitis at 1, 2, 5 and 10 years after ileal pouch–anal anastomosis was 15.5%, 22.5%, 36% and 45.5% for the patients without PSC, and 22%, 43%, 61% and 79% for the patients with PSC.[12]

Cholangiocarcinoma is a rare association with UC, and PSC is the greatest risk factor for its development. The prognosis is dismal, with a median survival of 9 months after diagnosis, and 12–15% of patients transplanted for PSC have cholangiocarcinoma.[13]

Dermatological

Erythema nodosum (EN) classically presents as tender, inflamed, red nodules mainly on the anterior surfaces of the lower extremities. The most common cutaneous lesion, it is seen in 10–20% of patients with UC. Exacerbations often parallel disease activity and frequently resolve after colonic disease subsides, although EN can precede bowel occurrence.[10]

Pyoderma gangrenosum (PG) occurs in 1–10% of patients with UC, and presents as plaques or pustules that break down and form painful ulcerations with undermined borders and necrotic centres. Legs are the most commonly affected area, though it can occur anywhere, including peristomally. Occurrences do not always parallel colonic disease activity.[10]

Thromboembolic

The incidence of deep venous thrombosis and pulmonary embolism in UC is threefold higher than the general population and associated with morbidity and mortality.[14] Though unproven, a hypercoagulable state in UC is hypothetically related to corticosteroid usage, activation of the coagulation cascade during a systemic inflammatory state, or up-regulation of acute phase reactants with flares.

Though rare, cerebral venous and dural sinus thrombosis can occur and results in a potentially devastating stroke. More commonly seen in patients with active disease, cases have been reported up to 10 years after a proctocolectomy.

Ophthalmological

Manifestations of episcleritis, uveitis and scleritis can occur in up to 5% of patients. Ocular symptoms often present concurrently with peripheral arthritis and erythema nodosum. Episcleritis, the most common ophthalmopathy, presents with pain, burning and scleral injection. It usually occurs in parallel, as well as resolves with the treatment of colonic disease. Uveitis presents with pain, blurred vision, photophobia and headaches. Classically, the redness is most prominent centrally and dissipates radially. Uveitis does not typically coincide with flares, and prompt treatment is necessary to decrease the risk of visual impairment. Scleritis presents similarly to episcleritis, though it is more severe and necessitates aggressive treatment in order to minimise retinal detachment and optic nerve impairment. In scleritis, unlike episcleritis, the sclera will appear pink or violet between the dilated surface vessels.[10]

Diagnosis and evaluation

With an extensive differential and no one exclusive pathognomonic test, a firm diagnosis of UC is dependent on several factors, including the clinical presentation, radiological work-up, endoscopic evaluation and histopathological determination of tissue biopsies. The differential diagnosis can include infectious (viral, bacterial, protozoal) as well as non-infectious causes (Crohn's disease, indeterminate colitis, collagenous colitis, ischaemic colitis, radiation colitis, diversion colitis, pharmacotherapy-induced colitis), and obtaining a detailed history and physical examination is imperative.

Microbiology

Colitides that can mimic UC include *Clostridium difficile*, *Escherichia coli* (serotype 0157:H7), *Salmonella*, *Shigella*, *Entamoeba* and *Campylobacter* infections. Stool studies for bacteria, ova and parasites should be obtained to confirm the true diagnosis and direct appropriate treatment. An increasing incidence of *Clostridium difficile* colitis in patients with IBD complicates their management and all patients with IBD hospitalised with an acute exacerbation should be assessed for synchronous infection.

Endoscopy

Endoscopy plays a pivotal role in the evaluation and diagnosis of UC, allowing for direct mucosal visualisation as well as providing an avenue for obtaining tissue biopsies. Other important indications include evaluating the proximal extent of colonic involvement, determining severity, differentiating from Crohn's disease, as well as monitoring responsiveness to medical management and surveillance.

During an acute attack, complete colonoscopy is generally avoided to decrease the risk of a potential perforation, while flexible or rigid proctoscopy is often utilised. Since inflammatory changes begin just above the anorectal junction and spread proximally, proctoscopy provides easy access to the lower rectum where biopsies can be obtained below the peritoneal reflection, minimising the risk of free perforation.

There is an overall lack of specific endoscopic features related to UC, though characteristic patterns of inflammation are appreciated. In the quiescent phase the mucosa will appear relatively normal, with the exception of neovascular changes. Oedema, erythema and an abnormal mucosal vascular pattern are endoscopically observed findings with mild inflammation. Loss of the vascular pattern (the submucosal vessels seen through the transparent mucosa) is a result of mucosal oedema, which makes it appear opaque. Oedema can also cause fine granularity in which there is a delicate regular stippled appearance of the mucosal surface. As the disease activity progresses to a moderate stage, superficial erosions, ulcerations and contact bleeding secondary to scope trauma are observed. Inflamed and regenerated mucosa surrounded by ulcerations lead to the development of pseudopolyps and a cobblestone appearance, which can also be appreciated during more severe conditions. Long-standing chronic inflammatory changes can give rise to a 'featureless microcolon' with mucosal atrophy, muscular hypertrophy, a decreased luminal diameter and loss of haustral folds.[15]

Histopathology

Inflammation in UC is confined to the rectum and colon. The mucosal columnar glandular epithelium extends into the anal canal to the level of the anal transitional zone. Segmental or skip areas do not occur, rather the inflammation in the colon and rectum is diffuse without intervening normal mucosa. The rectum is always involved, although the appearance of relative rectal sparing can occur in patients receiving transanally applied anti-inflammatory agents. A spared rectum not associated with local treatment should raise the suspicion of Crohn's disease. Backwash ileitis occurs only in cases with colonic extension to the ileocaecal junction.

Microscopic examination of a biopsy in early disease will demonstrate mucosal inflammation, goblet cell depletion, crypt of Lieberkuhn distortion, and vascular congestion. Mucin within goblet cells is expectorated, making them appear less evident or absent (goblet cell depletion). Branching of crypts may also be evident owing to regeneration following crypt epithelial damage. As severity progresses the lamina propria will exhibit infiltration by neutrophils, plasma cells, lymphocytes, eosinophils and mast cells. Neutrophils present within the epithelium of crypts (cryptitis) can aggregate in the crypt lumen, forming abscesses. Mucosal destruction, ulceration and subsequent atrophy are partly the result of rupturing of crypt abscesses. In advanced or late forms of UC, crypt destruction and loss occur as a result of damage to the crypt basal epithelium. Deeper submucosal or transmural inflammation with ulceration can also be observed, leaving large areas of exposed muscularis propria covered with granulation tissue giving the appearance of pseudopolyps. In the more chronic and quiescent phase a distorted architectural pattern with crypt distortion, branching and foreshortening can be identified.

Imaging

Although the reference standard for the diagnosis and follow-up of patients with UC is endoscopy, multiple traditional and emerging imaging modalities can also be utilised to assess patients with UC.

Conventional supine and upright abdominal X-rays are used to evaluate complications, including obstruction, dilatation or perforation. Dilatation of the transverse colon to greater than 6 cm is often seen in the face of toxic megacolon, and with imminent perforation is an indication for emergency surgical intervention.[16]

There has been a movement away from contrast X-rays as endoscopic evaluation has become more commonplace. The earliest finding on double-contrast barium enema consists of a fine granular appearance in the rectosigmoid region as a result of mucosal oedema and hyperaemia. Advanced disease is characterised by the absence of haustral folds, narrowing and shortening of the colon, and diffuse ulceration. More chronic forms will present with colonic shortening, luminal narrowing, loss of haustral folds and widening of the presacral space.

In comparison to Crohn's disease, computed tomographic (CT) and magnetic resonance imaging studies for evaluating UC are less commonly obtained. CT is a relatively poor test for detecting the mucosal abnormalities of early disease, though more advanced UC often has a hallmark finding of diffuse colonic wall thickening. The benefit of CT lies in the ability to evaluate intraluminal and extraluminal disease, guide and monitor response to treatment, as well as detect complications.[16]

Serology and microbiome

Serologic markers sensitive for inflammation, but not specific, include white blood cell (WBC) count, C-reactive protein (CRP) and erythrocyte sedimentation rate (ESR). Anti-saccharomyces cervisiae antibodies (ASCS) are more specific for Crohn's disease and perinuclear anti-neutrophil cytoplasmic antibody (p-ANCA) for chronic UC. The Prometheus antigen testing panel can be used to rule out IBD, but lacks the specificity to differentiate between Crohn's disease and UC.

Decreasing faecal calprotectin levels have been shown to correlate with mucosal healing when used in conjunction with ESR and CRP. Profiling the intestinal microbiome has shown promise that IBD results from alterations between the intestinal microbes and mucosal immunity, though significant research still needs to be completed.

Colorectal cancer and surveillance

Prolonged duration, continuously active disease, severity of inflammation, PSC and diffuse involvement (pancolitis) are cumulative risk factors for the development of colorectal cancer in the setting of UC. Incidence rates for the development of cancer correspond to cumulative probabilities of 2% by 10 years, 8% by 20 years and 18% by 30 years.[17] As a general rule, beginning 10 years after the diagnosis of UC, the incidence of colorectal cancer increases by approximately 1% per year as long as the patient has their colon. The relative risk for cancer in relation to ulcerative proctitis has been estimated to be 1.7, left-sided colitis 2.8 and pancolitis 14.8. In relation to the general population, there is an overall eightfold higher risk of colorectal cancer, with a 19-fold higher risk in

patients with extensive colitis. It has been shown that roughly 17% of all deaths in UC are a result of colorectal cancer.

Dysplasia-associated lesion or mass (DALM) refers to a visibly raised dysplastic lesion within an area of inflammation, and confers a high risk of malignant potential. DALMs have been subdivided into adenoma-like (similar to sporadic adenomas) and non-adenoma-like (sessile, irregular, ulcerated) lesions based solely on their endoscopic appearance. Some advocate treating adenoma-like DALMs with simple polypectomy and continued surveillance. The polyps must be discrete, completely removed and dysplasia must be absent elsewhere.[18] When dysplasia-associated lesions or masses are non-adenoma-like and cannot be entirely removed endoscopically, it is recommended to proceed with proctocolectomy because of the high probability of underlying neoplasia.

Flat low-grade dysplasia (LGD) detected during colonoscopic evaluation confers a reported ninefold increased risk of developing colorectal cancer and a 12-fold risk of developing an advanced lesion (high-grade dysplasia, or cancer).[19] Progression from colitis without dysplasia to colorectal cancer does not necessarily follow a sequence of low-grade dysplasia, high-grade dysplasia and ultimately carcinoma (inflammation–dysplasia–carcinoma sequence). Rather, LGD can progress directly to colorectal cancer.[20] Low-grade dysplasia can present as unifocal or multifocal and treatment is to some extent controversial, with some advocating prophylactic colectomy, while others recommend intensive colonoscopic surveillance.[20] Flat low-grade dysplasia has been shown to be a strong predictor of progression to advanced neoplasia (53% at 5 years) in surveillance colonoscopy, and in patients who underwent a colectomy an unexpected advanced neoplasia (high-grade dysplasia or cancer) was found in nearly 24%.[21] Other studies have shown the presence of LGD is as likely as high-grade dysplasia (54% vs 67%) to be associated with an already established cancer.[19] Repeated attempts to show low-grade dysplasia on endoscopic examinations should not be undertaken; rather, proctocolectomy is recommended to prevent progression to high-grade dysplasia or cancer.[22]

✓✓ A large meta-analysis of 20 surveillance studies showed the risk of developing cancer in patients with low-grade dysplasia is high. When LGD is detected on surveillance there is a ninefold risk of developing cancer and 12-fold risk of developing any advanced lesion.[19]

Flat high-grade dysplasia (HGD) has been shown to have a 42–45% rate of associated colorectal cancer at the time of colectomy, thus maintaining the recommendation that colectomy is mandatory in these patients, even with completely resected HGD or with HGD found on random biopsies.[23]

Several studies have suggested that surveillance colonoscopy in patients with UC significantly reduces the risk of developing neoplasia. To date, no randomised controlled trials have documented a reduced risk of colorectal cancer development or death by utilising surveillance colonoscopy.[24] The American Gastroenterological Association and British Society of Gastroenterology share international guidelines recommending surveillance colonoscopy every 1–2 years starting 8–10 years after a diagnosis of pancolitis, or 15 years after left-sided colitis. Recommendations are also advocated for random non-targeted biopsies performed every 10 cm in all four quadrants, equating to 20–40 biopsies per colon. Colitis-associated cancers have been shown frequently to arise from flat mucosa, be multifocal, broadly infiltrating, anaplastic and uniformly distributed throughout the colon. It is estimated that 33 non-targeted biopsies are required to detect dysplasia with 90% confidence, though studies show this is not often achieved.[25]

Patients with PSC and UC have an increased risk of colorectal cancer in comparison to those without PSC.[26] Cumulative colorectal cancer risk has been described as 33% at 20 years and 40% at 30 years after a diagnosis of UC. Surveillance colonoscopy is recommended at the time of diagnosis of PSC and yearly thereafter. In patients without a known diagnosis of UC, diagnostic colonoscopy with random biopsies is recommended to evaluate for subclinical evidence of disease.[23]

Flat and depressed colorectal lesions are often missed with conventional 'white light' colonoscopy and the utility of obtaining non-targeted random biopsies has been called into question.[27] Though highly specialised, time-consuming and not universally available, the use of high-magnification chromoscopic colonoscopy (dye spraying of the mucosal surface with indigo carmine or methylene blue) has been shown to have a significantly better correlation between endoscopic and histopathological findings than conventional colonoscopy, and also increased the number of neoplastic lesions identified. Chromoendoscopy (CE) has been repeatedly shown to increase the chance of detecting dysplasia compared to standard colonoscopic surveillance, allowing the endoscopist to take fewer, but rather higher yield, biopsies.[28]

Severity assessment

Disease severity is classified as mild, moderate or severe, and is based on the original descriptions provided by Truelove and Witts. Mild disease is characterised by less than four stools daily, with or without macroscopic blood, no signs of systemic toxicity (fever, tachycardia), mild to no anaemia and a normal ESR. Severe disease results in six or more bloody bowel movements daily, signs of systemic toxicity, anaemia (less than 75% of normal value) and an increased ESR.

Unlike the Crohn's Disease Activity Index, no gold standard index exists for evaluating the severity of UC. Rather, multiple indices have been developed to measure disease severity and activity in clinical trials, many with overlapping measured variables. Some assess the clinical and biochemical aspects of disease (Truelove and Witts Severity Index, Lichtiger Index, Powel–Tuck Index, Activity Index, Rachmilewitz Index, Physician Global Assessment, Ulcerative Colitis Clinical Score), others focus on endoscopy (Truelove and Witts Sigmoidoscopic Assessment, Baron Score, Powel–Tuck Sigmoidoscopic Assessment, Rachmilewitz Endoscopic Index), while further indices evaluate a combination of clinical and endoscopic criteria (Mayo Clinic Score, Sutherland Index). Common to all indices are numerical scoring systems. Scores at the elevated end of the spectrum indicate high disease activity, while lower scores signify milder or quiescent disease. Of the myriad scoring tools available to define disease activity, only two (Activity and Rachmilewitz Index) have been validated to date.[29]

Medical management

Inducing and maintaining clinical remission by promoting mucosal healing is the goal of medical treatment for UC. With several different medications to choose from (aminosalicylates, steroids, immunosuppressants, immunomodulators), therapy is modified in conjunction with the severity and extent of disease.

Clinical remission is characterised by symptom resolution of the inflammatory phase. This occurs with a decrease in diarrhoea, bleeding, urgency, tenesmus, the passage of mucopus and restoration of continence. Endoscopic remission will reveal regeneration of healthy mucosa, epithelial continuity, a return of a submucosal vascular pattern, and resolving ulceration, friability and granularity. Histological remission is achieved when an absence of neutrophils in the epithelial crypts is observed.

Just as there is no standard agreement amongst scoring systems measuring disease severity and activity, there are no universally validated means of defining disease remission. Prior to initiating maintenance therapy it is essential that clinical remission be achieved and verified. It has been demonstrated that high rates of relapse occur when endoscopic and histological remission has not been confirmed.[30]

✓✓ A prospective multicentre study revealed patients in clinical remission with less severe sigmoidoscopic scores (defined as normal-looking mucosa, with only mild redness and/or friability) after 6 weeks of acute treatment were less likely to relapse at 1 year than patients in clinical remission only (cumulative rate of relapse 23% vs 80%, respectively; P <0.0001).[30]

Proctitis

Disease limited to the rectum is best treated with topical therapy, including foams, enemas and suppositories. Mesalamine suppositories (1–1.5 g/day) administered nightly, or in daily divided doses, have shown superiority in comparison to oral 5-aminosalicylic acid (5-ASA) compounds. Maximal response is noted within 4–6 weeks and, if unresponsive, combination therapy with topical corticosteroids has been shown to be more effective than either therapy alone. In patients unwilling to make use of, or failing to respond to, topical therapy, oral mesalamine may be given as an alternative, though higher doses are typically required. Systemic steroids are only administered in individuals refractory to topical and oral therapy, or in cases of severe disease.

Mild to moderate distal colitis

Mild to moderate distal colitis (30–40 cm) is primarily treated with a regimen of oral aminosalicylates, topical mesalamine or topical steroids. Mesalamine enemas are the treatment of choice and achieve higher rates of remission than oral 5-ASA compounds or topical steroids. Nightly administered mesalamine enemas (4 g/60 mL) have documented remission rates of between 60% and 70%, with rates increasing as the duration of therapy increases. If symptoms persist, and no response is seen within 2–4 weeks, an additional mesalamine or hydrocortisone enema can be administered each morning. Combination therapy has been shown to be superior to either therapy alone.[31] The systemic side-effects from corticosteroid enemas occur as a result of a low first-pass hepatic metabolism, and can be significant in some patients. Budesonide, a newer corticosteroid formulation that has a high first-pass hepatic metabolism, reduces the systemic side-effect profile, and has been shown to be as effective as conventional corticosteroid enemas. Oral mesalamine can be added in combination with topical therapy for patients showing a poor response, and is superior to oral or topical therapies alone. For patients not responding to or refusing topical therapy, oral mesalamine can be administered and has been shown to be a valuable alternative, though it is not as effective. Oral and intravenous corticosteroids are only administered in patients refractory to topical steroids and 5-ASA compounds (oral and topical), or in cases of severe disease.

Mild to moderate extensive colitis

Extensive colitis involves the colon beyond the reach of topical therapy and necessitates oral pharmacotherapy. Oral sulfasalazine (2–6 g/day) is the treatment of choice, showing remission rates of up to 80%, though with a significant systemic sulphonamide side-effect profile and high rates of intolerability (30–40%).[22] Newer non-sulphonamide 5-ASA formulations have been shown to be as effective as sulfasalazine, though better tolerated without dose-limiting systemic side-effects. Distal colonic and rectal disease topical therapy can also be concomitantly administered and this combination has been shown to be more successful in inducing remission at 8 weeks than oral therapy alone. Enteral steroids are implemented in cases not responding to oral mesalamine, or when the side-effects of the 5-ASA compounds cannot be tolerated. Prednisone is typically administered, starting with doses of 40–60 mg/day until significant clinical improvement is observed. Once remission is achieved a taper of 5–10 mg/week is instituted until a daily dose of 20 mg is reached. A dose decrease of 2.5–5 mg/week is continued thereafter, while maintaining 5-ASA treatment, until completion.[22]

Thiopurines (6-mercaptopurine, azathioprine), with a primarily steroid-sparing benefit, are effective in patients who cannot be tapered off or tolerate corticosteroids. Their use is limited by a slow onset of action and prolonged duration is required to achieve optimal effectiveness (3–6 months).[22] Infliximab (Remicade) has shown effectiveness in inducing remission in patients failing corticosteroid and/or thiopurine, as well as aminosalicylate therapy. Infliximab is intravenously administered over a 2-hour period at a dose of 5 mg/kg at weeks 0, 2 and 6, and then at 8-week intervals. Those who fail to respond after the initial two doses are unlikely to respond to a third dose. Shortening the interval between doses or increasing the dose to 10 mg/kg can treat those who eventually lose responsiveness after an initial response. For those not responding to an escalated dose and decreased interval, treatment discontinuation is recommended.[32] Other biologic agents include adalimumab (Humira), certolizumab (Cimzia), golimumab (Simponi) and vedolizumab (Entyvio).

✅✅ Two randomised, double-blind, placebo-controlled studies – the Active Ulcerative Colitis Trials 1 and 2 (ACT 1 and ACT 2, respectively) – showed patients with moderate to severe active ulcerative colitis treated with infliximab at weeks 0, 2 and 6 and every 8 weeks thereafter were more likely to have a clinical response at weeks 8, 30 and 54 than were those receiving placebo.[32]

Severe colitis

The mainstay of therapy for patients with severe/fulminant colitis is intravenous corticosteroids with a daily dose equivalent of 300 mg for hydrocortisone or 60 mg for methylprednisolone. Higher doses have not been proven to be beneficial, and 20–40% will fail to respond to therapy. Studies have been unable to confirm any incremental advantage in administering or continuing oral 5-ASA compounds and topical regimens. The utilisation of empiric broad-spectrum antibiotics, although routinely administered, has not shown benefit when treating patients with severe colitis. Intravenous ciclosporin (2–4 mg/kg/day continuous infusion) has been shown to be an effective adjuvant (82% response) in those lacking improvement while being treated with maximal medical therapy over a period of 3–5 days. Infliximab has shown short-term efficacy in limited small trials, with approximately half of treated patients requiring a colectomy at 5 years. Patients failing to respond to maximal medical therapy or showing signs of deterioration are candidates for surgery.[22] Though published data are somewhat conflicting, several studies have shown that higher rates of anastomotic and infectious complications are seen in patients following ileal pouch–anal anastomosis when infliximab has been given within an 8-week period prior to surgery. Given these findings, a discussion with a surgeon to review surgical options is prudent before beginning infliximab therapy. Lightner and colleagues revealed that 37% of IBD patients who received vedolizumab within 30 days of a major abdominal operation experienced a 30-day postoperative surgical site infection, significantly higher than patients receiving TNFα inhibitors or no biologic therapy, and this remained the only predictor of 30-day postoperative surgical site infection on multivariate analysis.[33]

Surgical management

Surgery plays a pivotal role in the management of UC. Removal of the colon and rectum is essentially curative. Indications for removal include drug intolerability or unresponsiveness, intractability, life-threatening complications (perforation, bleeding, toxicity), dysplasia or malignancy, growth impediment in children, and for the attempted improvement of some extraintestinal manifestations refractory to medical treatment (pyoderma gangrenosum, erythema nodosum, peripheral arthritis, uveitis, iritis). The surgical approach depends on the presentation (emergency/urgent, elective) and can include: total abdominal colectomy with Brooke ileostomy, proctocolectomy with Brooke ileostomy, proctocolectomy with continent ileostomy, total abdominal colectomy with ileorectal anastomosis (IRA), and proctocolectomy with ileoanal reservoir/ileal pouch–anal anastomosis (IPAA). It is essential, when possible, to inform the patient, and have them site-marked preoperatively by an enterostomal therapist.

Emergency/urgent

Toxic fulminant colitis, toxic megacolon, haemorrhage and perforation are life-threatening complications necessitating emergency colectomy. Urgent typically refers to hospitalised patients who are failing maximal medical therapy.

Historically, the Turnbull 'blow-hole' procedure was used in severely debilitated (septic, malnourished) patients with megacolon who could not withstand a major abdominal operation. A loop ileostomy, a transverse colostomy and, if needed, a sigmoid colostomy was created (**Fig.11.1**). This allowed for faecal diversion, minimal handling of the bowel and patient convalescence for future

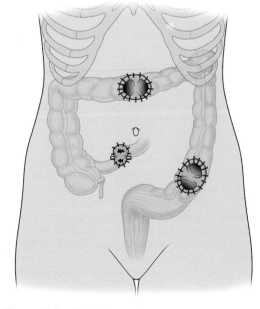

Figure 11.1 • Turnbull procedure.

colectomy, but did not eliminate the colitis nor the physiological impact of the inflammation on the patient. In rare circumstances (advanced pregnancy and toxic megacolon) the Turnbull approach could even now be considered.[34] Even so, recent experience in pregnant patients with fulminant disease suggests that total abdominal colectomy and Brooke ileostomy eliminates the systemic inflammatory consequences and can be done with low rates of maternal and fetal morbidity and mortality.[35]

✔ Subtotal colectomy and Brooke ileostomy for ulcerative colitis during pregnancy is safe. A multidisciplinary team that includes a gastroenterologist, high-risk obstetrician and experienced surgeon is necessary for an optimal outcome.[35]

For patients requiring urgent or emergency intervention, total abdominal colectomy with creation of a Brooke ileostomy and preservation of the rectum for a potential future restorative procedure is most commonly performed and recommended. It eliminates most of the disease and allows for restoration of health, as well as tapering of immunosuppressant medications.[36] When performing a total abdominal colectomy it is imperative to dissect as close to the ileocaecal valve as possible, thus preserving all of the ileocolonic branches for a possible restorative procedure. Deferring the proctectomy will simplify a restorative procedure by maintaining pelvic and presacral tissue planes. This not only reduces the potential complications (bleeding, infection, autonomic nerve damage) in an acutely ill patient, but also permits the opportunity pathologically to exclude Crohn's disease by examining the colonic specimen. Studies evaluating the outcome of a retained rectal stump have been conflicting. Some portend that leaving a diseased, thickened rectal stump is not associated with increased rates of postoperative pelvic sepsis or complications.[37] Others encourage exteriorisation (mucous fistula or subcutaneous placement) of long stumps, having found rates of pelvic sepsis as high as 12%, increased disease activity in the retained rectum and subsequent pelvic dissection for restorative procedures more difficult with a retained short stump. If a mucous fistula is not done, the rectum should be irrigated with a rigid proctoscope to remove bloody mucous and a transanally placed rectal tube left in place for 48 hours to decrease pressure on the closed rectal stump.

Elective

Indications for elective surgery consist of medical unresponsiveness, intolerability or intractability, dysplasia or malignancy, growth retardation in children, and for the attempted improvement of some extraintestinal manifestations. Depending on patient preference, continence, age, concerns of fertility and dysplastic changes, operative interventions include proctocolectomy with Brooke ileostomy, proctocolectomy with continent ileostomy, total abdominal colectomy with ileorectal anastamosis (IRA), and a restorative proctocolectomy with ileoanal reservoir/ileal pouch–anal anastamosis (IPAA).

Proctocolectomy with end ileostomy

A proctocolectomy with end Brooke ileostomy removes all disease and has a low rate of complications but leaves the patient with an incontinent stoma. Indications for this approach are patient preference, low rectal cancer and poor sphincter function.

The patient is placed in a modified lithotomy position. The colectomy portion of the procedure is carried out in a non-oncological approach unless neoplastic transformation has been identified. The rectal dissection and mobilisation may be done close to the perimuscular rectal wall in an attempt to minimise damage to the pelvic autonomic nerves. In the event of neoplastic changes both the colonic and rectal dissections are carried out in a standard oncological fashion. In the low anorectal region a perineal intersphincteric dissection is carried out (except in the presence of a low rectal cancer), preserving the external sphincter and levator ani muscles, which significantly improves wound healing. The perineum is closed in layers and the greater omentum, if present, is mobilised and placed in the pelvis. After closure of the abdomen the ileostomy is matured in a standard evaginated Brooke fashion, with an attempted ideal projection of 2.5 cm (**Fig. 11.2**).

Stoma complications including retraction, peristomal skin excoriation, stenosis, prolapse and herniation can occur, with up to 30% of patients requiring operative revision. When delayed healing

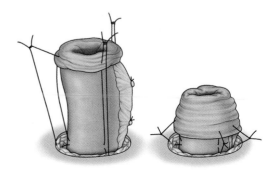

Figure 11.2 • Brooke ileostomy.

of the perineal wound occurs, evaluation for Crohn's disease and/or retained mucosa or foreign material (suture) should be carried out.

Proctocolectomy with continent ileostomy

Initially described by Nils Kock, the continent ileostomy still remains a viable alternative for motivated patients who are not candidates for an IPAA, but is only performed in a very few centres. Modifications and revisions to the original Kock continent ileostomy have been described and include the Barnett continent ileostomy reservoir (BCIR) and T-pouch, neither of which has supporting data to suggest they are better than the Kock pouch. Contraindications to construction of a continent ileostomy include Crohn's, obesity, marginal small bowel length, and anyone with a psychological or physical disability that would preclude understanding or being able to perform daily stomal intubation.

Surgical creation of a continent ileostomy is carried out by utilising 45–60 cm of terminal ileum and folding it into either a two-limb or S-pouch configuration. The pouch reservoir requires approximately 30 cm of ileum to construct, while a portion of the remaining distal outflow tract is intussuscepted to create a valve. As the pouch distends it causes an increase in pressure around the valve, thus occluding the outflow tract, preventing evacuation. The end of the ileum is brought out through the abdominal wall and matured flush with the skin. A wide-bore catheter is used to intubate the pouch by inserting it through the skin level stoma, which is placed to gravity drainage for approximately 10 days. The pouch is slowly distended over time by intermittently clamping the catheter. When the catheter can be clamped for 8 hours without discomfort it is removed and intermittent intubation is carried out three to four times per day.

Postoperative pouch complications requiring reoperation are common and include skin-level or valve strictures, volvulus, herniation, fistulisation and valve slippage. Subluxation of the nipple valve is suggested by the onset of incontinence of the stoma and difficulty in inserting the catheter. Valve slippage is the most common complication, with reported rates of nearly 30%. Contrast studies may show partial or complete prolapse of the valve. Fistulas occur in approximately 10% of patients and typically originate from the base of the nipple valve or the pouch itself.[39,40] Despite the high morbidity and need for reoperative intervention with a continent ileostomy, patient satisfaction and quality of life are extremely high. It has been documented that over 90% of patients would undergo the procedure again, as well as recommend it to friends and family.[41]

Ileorectal anastomosis

Colectomy with ileorectal anastomosis (IRA) should be considered only when the rectum is minimally inflamed, distensible and compliant, there is no rectal dysplasia, the patient has an intact sphincter mechanism and is willing to adhere to strict follow-up. Ileoproctostomy is an appealing alternative in younger patients of reproductive age in order to decrease the risk of impotence and reduced fecundity, as well as older patients with quiescent disease having colectomy for colonic dysplasia. Strict rectal surveillance must be adhered to due to the increased risk of future neoplastic changes. The risk of rectal carcinoma can reach up to 20% by 30 years.[42] Proctitis of the retained rectum can lead to bleeding, tenesmus, urgency, severe diarrhoea and pain. Topical, oral and systemic therapies can be utilised, but it has been documented that up to 45% of patients will not respond and eventually require a proctectomy.[43] In patients who require a completion proctectomy an end ileostomy, restorative IPAA or continent ileostomy are all options.

Restorative proctocolectomy/ileal pouch–anal anastomosis (IPAA)

Initially described in 1978 by Parks and Nicholls as an ileoanal ileal reservoir procedure, the restorative proctocolectomy has become the most common continence-preserving procedure performed for the management of UC in patients who are appropriate candidates. The restorative pouch can be fashioned in two-limb (J), three-limb (S), four-limb (W) or isoperistaltic (H) configurations (**Fig. 11.3**). The J-pouch, due to its ease of construction and excellent functional outcomes, has become the most common choice for most surgeons. The S-pouch provides additional length and can reduce anastomotic tension, though the 5-cm efferent limb of ileum projecting beyond the pouch can lead to evacuation difficulties and outlet obstruction. The isoperistaltic H-pouch, with its long outlet tract, can give rise to stasis,

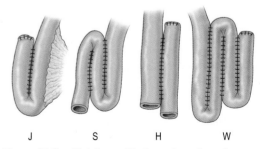

| J | S | H | W |

Figure 11.3 • Variations of ileal pouch configurations.

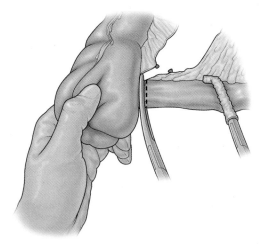

Figure 11.4 • Ileal transection adjacent to caecum.

distension and pouchitis. The W-pouch has been shown to have similar functional results when compared to the J-pouch, but it is more time-consuming and technically difficult to construct.

The patient is placed in a modified lithotomy position to allow access to the anus and abdominopelvic cavity. A total colectomy is performed and the ileum is transected flush with the caecum (**Fig. 11.4**). In order to provide adequate perfusion to the pouch it is imperative to preserve the ileal branches of the ileocolic and distal mesenteric arteries. At this point in the operation, if there is any doubt of the diagnosis, the colon should be removed and inspected with the pathologist. Once confident of the diagnosis of UC, evaluation for adequacy of reach of the small bowel to the deep pelvis should be undertaken. The proposed point of the pouch–anal anastomosis can be pulled down to the pubis, and if this point can be pulled 3–4 cm below the inferior edge of the pubis one can feel confident of successful reach for anastomosis. Strategies to decrease tension at the anastomosis include: complete mobilisation of the small-bowel mesentery to the root of the superior mesenteric artery cephalad to the head of the pancreas (**Fig. 11.5a**), proximal division of the ileocolic artery (**Fig. 11.5b**) and relaxing incisions of the mesentery over tension points along the superior mesenteric artery (**Fig. 11.5c**). Rectal dissection can be done in the total mesorectal excision (TME) plane or close to the rectal wall, depending on the concern for autonomic nerve damage and surgeon's experience with nerve-sparing proctectomy. Transection of the rectum should occur 2–3 cm above the dentate line in the anal transition zone, leaving a short rectal cuff (**Fig. 11.6**). After reach has been verified, a J configuration is fashioned, with each limb measuring between 12 and 15 cm

in length. The limbs are paired in an antimesenteric fashion and are held in position with interrupted stay sutures (**Fig. 11.7**).

Double-stapled technique

For a stapled technique an enterotomy is made in the antimesenteric portion of the apex of the pouch and a linear cutting stapler is used to divide the walls of the two limbs, creating a common channel (**Fig. 11.8**). A purse-string suture is then fashioned around the enterotomy and the anvil from a circular stapler is placed inside the pouch, where it is held in place by tightening the purse-string (**Fig. 11.9**). The circular stapler is then placed transanally (**Fig. 11.10**). After appropriate orientation, the trocar is advanced either above or below the transverse staple line and attached to the anvil. The stapler is then closed, approximating the pouch and anus (**Fig. 11.11**).

Hand-sewn technique

For a hand-sewn pouch–anal anastomosis, an anal canal mucosectomy is performed, starting at the dentate line (**Fig. 11.12**). Raising the mucosa with a submucosal injection of dilute saline and epinephrine (1:200 000) facilitates the dissection of the mucosa away from the internal sphincter muscle (**Fig. 11.13a,b**). After the circumferential mucosa and proximal rectum have been removed, the pouch is gently brought down to the level of the dentate line. An enterotomy is made in the apex of the pouch, if not already created, and it is anchored in position by placing a suture in each of the four quadrants incorporating a full-thickness bite of the pouch, internal sphincter muscle and mucosa. Sutures are placed between the anchoring stitches, in a clockface orientation, to complete a mucosally intact anastomosis (**Fig. 11.14**). An air insufflation leak test is performed and a protective loop ileostomy fashioned (**Fig. 11.15**). The operation can be carried out without the creation of a diverting loop ileostomy in highly selected cases, with good results. However, in a meta-analysis of nearly 1500 patients the rate of anastomotic leakage was significantly higher in patients not given a defunctioning ileostomy.[44]

✔✔ A review of 17 studies comprising 1486 patients revealed restorative proctocolectomy without a diverting ileostomy resulted in functional outcomes similar to those of surgery with proximal diversion, but was associated with an increased risk of anastomotic leak. Diverting ileostomy should be omitted in carefully selected patients only.[44]

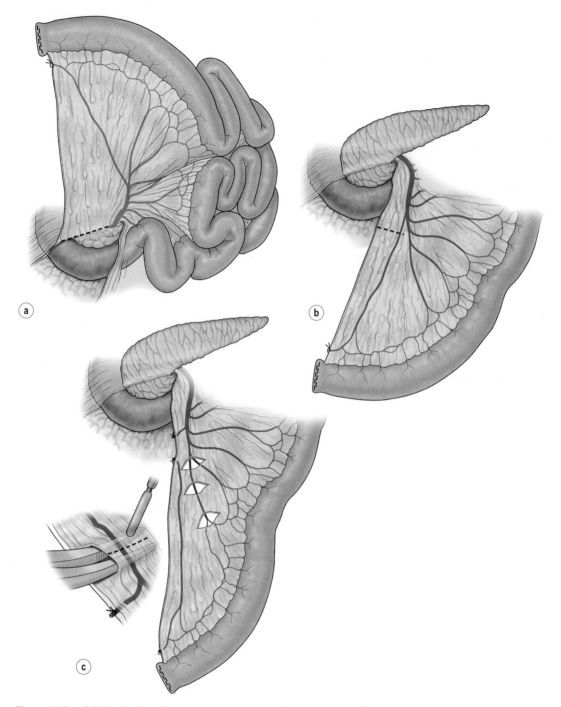

Figure 11.5 • (a) Mobilisation of the ileal mesentery around the duodenum. **(b)** Proximal division of the ileocolic artery. **(c)** Relaxing mesenteric incisions over the terminal portion of the superior mesenteric artery.

Outcomes in stapled versus hand-sewn anastomosis

Variations exist for the creation of a J-pouch, depending on the technique (hand-sewn versus double-stapled) chosen. A large meta-analysis demonstrated no significant differences between the two techniques. Nocturnal seepage and pad usage favoured the stapled anastomosis, in comparison to persisting symptoms due to inflammation or dysplasia in the cuff favouring the hand-sewn technique.[45] A single institution experience of over 3000 pouch procedures (474 hand-sewn and 2635

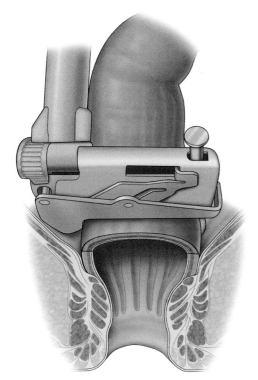

Figure 11.6 • Division of the rectum with stapler.

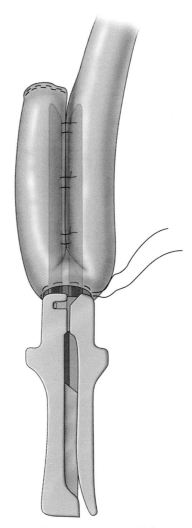

Figure 11.8 • Creation of reservoir with linear stapler.

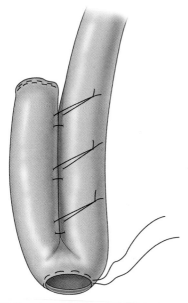

Figure 11.7 • J-pouch with orientation sutures.

✓✓ A large meta-analysis demonstrated no significant differences in postoperative complications between a mucosectomy and hand-sewn versus stapled anastomosis. Nocturnal seepage and pad usage favoured the stapled anastomosis, in comparison to persisting symptoms due to inflammation or dysplasia in the cuff favouring the hand-sewn technique.[45]

Neoplastic changes observed in the retained anal transition zone in patients undergoing double-stapled technique are rare. The majority of reports have been associated with pathological findings of dysplasia or cancer in the initial operative specimen. A hand-sewn technique, including a completion mucosectomy, nearly eliminates the possibility of leaving columnar rectal mucosa behind, though not completely. Studies have been able to demonstrate 14–21% of excised

stapled) revealed patients who underwent a stapled IPAA experienced better outcomes (incontinence, seepage, pad usage) and quality of life (dietary, social and work restrictions) in comparison to the hand-sewn group.[46]

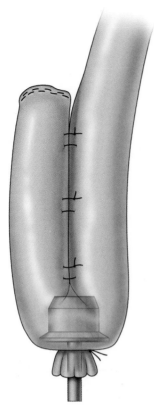

Figure 11.9 • Stapler anvil secured in J-pouch with purse-string suture.

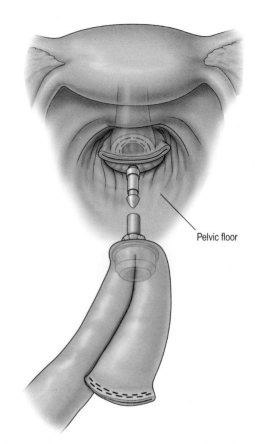

Figure 11.10 • Stapler placed transanally with spike posterior to transverse staple line.

pouches harbouring residual rectal mucosa.[47,48] A double-stapled technique, on the other hand, results in the retention of a small cuff of columnar mucosa. This can result in a 'cuffitis' or 'strip proctitis', and has been reported to occur in nearly 15% of stapled anastomoses, which can potentially progress to dysplasia.[49] Studies have demonstrated a 2.7–3.1% risk of developing low-grade dysplasia in the retained mucosa, although associated with a pre- or postoperative pathological diagnosis of concurrent dysplasia or cancer. In such patients a stapled technique may be less advisable and these authors recommend a mucosectomy and hand-sewn IPAA. For persistent or recurrent low-grade dysplasia, a completion mucosectomy, perineal pouch advancement and neo-ileal pouch–anal anastomosis is recommended.[50] Though studies recommending adequate pouch examination after an IPAA are lacking, long-term surveillance utilising annual endoscopy and biopsies is often recommended to monitor for dysplasia, although this is hard to achieve in practice.

Complications following pouch surgery

Major complications following pouch surgery include small-bowel obstruction, anastomotic stricture, pouch–vaginal fistula, pouchitis and pelvic sepsis. In

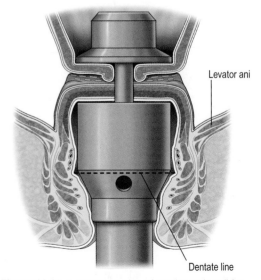

Figure 11.11 • Approximation of stapler and anvil for double-stapled anastomosis.

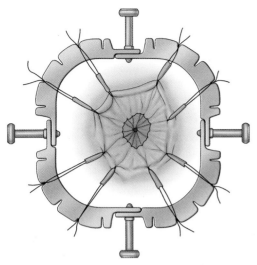

Figure 11.12 • Exposure for transanal mucosectomy using Lone Star retractor.

several series, morbidity after IPAA is a significant problem, with documented rates of over 60%.[51]

Small-bowel obstruction has been reported to occur in over 30% of patients, can present before or after loop ileostomy closure, and increases up to 10 years after operation. The cumulative risk has been shown to be 18% at 1 year, 27% at 5 years and 31% at 10 years. Adhesions are the most common cause of a small-bowel obstruction and surgical intervention is necessary in roughly 10% of patients by 10 years.[51,52]

Anastomotic strictures can cause pouch outlet obstruction with incomplete pouch evacuation and,

depending on how stricturing is defined, have been documented with rates as high as 38%. Stricturing can often be treated with finger or sequential dilator dilatation, depending on the degree of stenosis. If excessive fibrosis and stenosis are present, stricture excision and pouch advancement or removal may be necessary.[53]

Pouch–vaginal fistula is uncommon but is a devastating complication when it occurs. Obtaining a pouchogram prior to ileostomy closure, as well as a thorough vaginal and anal canal examination at the time of closure, can help exclude a fistula. Management depends on the level of the fistula (low versus high) and severity. Management includes placement of a seton, diversion, pharmacotherapy and transabdominal and perineal procedures.[54] A transanal or transvaginal approach for repairing low-lying fistulas has shown success in 50–70% of patients, though often requiring repeat procedures. Healing rates for higher fistulas after abdominal advancement of the pouch also show 50–70% documented success.[55] The presence of perianal abscess or fistula-in-ano preoperatively is associated with a 3.7- to 6-fold increase in the risk of developing pouch–vaginal fistula.[56]

The most common complication after IPAA is pouchitis, a non-specific inflammation of the pouch, which approaches 50% within 10 years. Symptoms include increased stool frequency, abdominal cramping, bleeding, urgency, tenesmus, incontinence and fevers. Diagnosis should be based on endoscopic and histological factors, rather than clinical symptoms alone. Hypothetically, pouchitis results from the overgrowth of anaerobic bacteria, local factors or ischaemia, though the exact aetiology

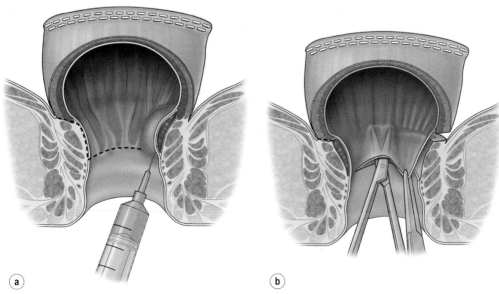

Figure 11.13 • (a) Submucosal injection. **(b)** Transanal mucosectomy.

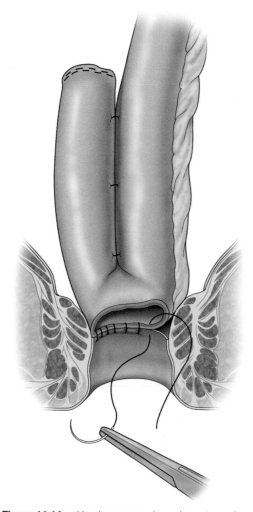

Figure 11.14 • Hand-sewn pouch–anal anastomosis.

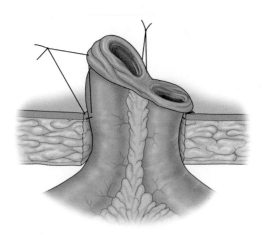

Figure 11.15 • Diverting loop ileostomy.

is unknown. Extraintestinal manifestations, specifically primary sclerosing cholangitis, and high serological levels of p-ANCA, have been shown to correlate with higher levels of pouchitis and chronic pouchitis.[57,58] Smoking, on the other hand, has been shown to decrease rates of pouchitis and probiotics (VSL#3) have shown promise in reducing episodes of acute pouchitis as well as maintaining remission.[59,60] Treatment depends primarily on the administration of antibiotics (metronidazole and ciprofloxacin), with response rates documented in over 80% of patients, though topical steroid or 5-aminosalicylate therapy is occasionally required.[61] Recurrent and refractory pouchitis is difficult to manage. Diversion with a loop ileostomy does not always affect the degree of inflammation and excision with construction of a new reservoir can be followed by recurrent pouchitis. Crohn's disease should always be suspected in patients with chronic pouchitis. Pouch excision is rarely necessary.

Pelvic sepsis has been documented to occur in as many as 20% of patients, and has the most clinically significant implications. Sepsis occurring in the early postoperative period confers a fivefold increased risk of subsequent failure, necessitating aggressive treatment with major or minor procedures in order to attempt to preserve the pouch. Pelvic sepsis can often be managed with CT-guided percutaneous drainage, but extreme cases will require operative intervention. Pouch failure and loss can occur immediately or several years following septic complication, with estimated cumulative 3-, 5- and 10-year failure rates of 20%, 31% and 39%, respectively.[62] If pouch salvage occurs in the setting of pelvic sepsis, pelvic fibrosis leads to compromised function of the pouch.

> ✅ The frequencies of permanent defunctioning and excision of a pouch in 131 patients with septic complications were 24% and 6%, respectively. The 5-year pouch failure rate increased in a subgroup of patients with septic complications at the pouch–anal anastomosis when the anal sphincter was involved (50% vs 29%). Surgery for septic complications is required in a high percentage of patients and repeated attempts are justified in order to decrease the risk of pouch loss.[62]

Female patients of reproductive age who undergo a proctocolectomy and creation of an IPAA have decreased postoperative fecundity, with reduced rates documented upwards of 50%.[63–66]

Studies have demonstrated no difference in fertility after a diagnosis of UC compared with before a diagnosis, but higher infertility rates (38%) in females who had pelvic pouch surgery in comparison to patients managed non-operatively (13%).[67]

The decreased fertility is hypothetically related to tubal occlusion secondary to adhesions and a large percentage (67%) of patients have demonstrated abnormal hysterosalpingography when evaluated postoperatively.[68] The ability to carry a fetus to term and successfully deliver vaginally has not been shown to be affected by an ileal pouch–anal anastomosis. Pregnancy has also not been shown to decrease pouch function or increase complications when followed long term.[66,69] Men report statistically improved sexual quality and function in relation to sexual desire, intercourse satisfaction, erectile function and overall satisfaction after IPAA when compared with prior to surgery.[70]

> ✓✓ A meta-analysis of eight studies revealed that an IPAA can increase the risk of infertility, defined as achieving pregnancy within 12 months of attempting conception, in women with ulcerative colitis by approximately threefold. Counselling female patients regarding decreased rates of fecundity following an IPAA is imperative.[65]

Risk factors found to be independent predictors of pouch survival include: patient diagnosis, prior anal pathology, abnormal anal manometry, patient comorbidity, pouch–perineal or pouch–vaginal fistulas, pelvic sepsis, anastomotic stricture and separation.[56] Pouch failure, defined as pouch excision or permanent diversion, is reported in several large series to range from 7% to 10% at 10 years and in one study, 8% at 20 years.[52,69,71]

Removal of the pouch has a significant early and late morbidity (62%), with readmissions and delayed healing of the perineal wound (persistent perineal sinus) in 40% of patients.[72] Thus, where failure is threatened by sepsis or poor function, it may be in the patient's interest to consider a salvage procedure that may be less traumatic and offers a chance of retaining satisfactory anal function. Recent success rates for salvage surgery following restorative proctocolectomy range from 75% to 94%.[73–75]

> ✓ The most common indications for pouch salvage are intra-abdominal sepsis, anastomotic stricture and retained rectal stump.[74] Surgical revision using a transanal or combined abdominoperineal approach has documented success rates of 74–94%.[73–75]

Functional outcomes

The frequency of bowel movements after an ileoanal–pouch anastomosis averages six in 24 hours, with minor incontinence of 11% during the day and 21% at night when followed for 20 years.[76] Nearly half will experience nocturnal leakage and minor spotting during the first 6 months, which improves over time, with rates of 20% noted at 1 year.[77] Studies comparing quality of life before and after an IPAA procedure document greater freedom in role function, improved body image and reduced negative effects caused by colitis or life with an ileostomy. Over 90% of patients report overall satisfaction with good or excellent adjustment following IPAA. The long-term functional and clinical outcomes of a restorative proctocolectomy are excellent, and patient satisfaction and quality of life are extremely high.[78,79]

Key points

- Ulcerative colitis is an idiopathic relapsing inflammatory bowel disease involving the mucosa and lamina propria of the rectum and variable segments of the proximal colon.
- The incidence is between 2 and 15 cases per 100 000 persons per year in more developed countries.
- The diagnosis is dependent on several factors, including the clinical presentation, radiological work-up, endoscopic evaluation and histopathological examination of tissue biopsies.
- Incidence rates for the development of cancer correspond to cumulative probabilities of 2% by 10 years, 8% by 20 years and 18% by 30 years.
- Toxic fulminant colitis, toxic megacolon, haemorrhage and perforation are life-threatening complications necessitating emergency surgical intervention, of which options are limited to the most expeditious and lowest risk procedures.
- Indications for elective surgery consist of medical unresponsiveness, intolerability or intractability, dysplasia or malignancy, growth retardation in children, and for the attempted improvement of some extraintestinal manifestations.
- Ileal pouch–anal anastomosis has become the most common continence-preserving procedure performed in patients who are appropriate candidates. Contraindications include incontinence, poor sphincter function and low rectal cancer.

- The foremost complication after completion of an IPAA is non-specific inflammation of the pouch (pouchitis), which approaches 50% within 10 years.
- Risk factors found to be independent predictors of pouch survival include: patient diagnosis, prior anal pathology, abnormal anal manometry, patient comorbidity, pouch–perineal or pouch–vaginal fistulas, pelvic sepsis, anastomotic stricture and separation.
- Pouch failure, defined as pouch excision or permanent diversion, is reported in several large series to range from 7% to 10% at 10 years and in one study, 8% at 20 years.
- Success rates for salvage surgery following IPAA range from 75% to 94%.

▶ Recommended videos:

- Restorative proctocolectomy with formation of ileoanal pouch – https://tinyurl.com/y6vuemcc
- Technical aspects of increasing length in ileoanal pouch surgery –https://tinyurl.com/ycrago33
- Stapled ileaoanal pouch construction – https://tinyurl.com/yavo6n2v

Key references

19. Thomas T, Abrams KA, Robinson RJ, et al. Meta-analysis: cancer risk of low-grade dysplasia in chronic ulcerative colitis. Aliment Pharmacol Ther 2007;25(6):657–68. PMID: 17311598.
   A large meta-analysis of 20 surveillance studies showed the risk of developing cancer in patients with LGD is high. When LGD is detected on surveillance there is a ninefold risk of developing cancer and 12-fold risk of developing any advanced lesion.

30. Meucci G, Fasoli R, Saibeni S, et al. Prognostic significance of endoscopic remission in patients with active ulcerative colitis treated with oral and topical mesalazine: a prospective, multicenter study. Inflamm Bowel Dis 2012;18(6):1006–10. PMID: 21830282.
   A prospective multicentre study revealed patients in clinical remission with less severe sigmoidoscopic scores (defined as normal-looking mucosa, with only mild redness and/or friability) after 6 weeks of acute treatment were less likely to relapse at 1 year than patients in clinical remission only (cumulative rate of relapse 23% vs 80%, respectively; P <0.0001).

32. Rutgeerts P, Sandborn WJ, Feagan BG, et al. Infliximab for induction and maintenance therapy for ulcerative colitis. N Engl J Med 2005;353(23):2462–76. PMID: 16339095.
   Two randomised, double-blind, placebo-controlled studies – the Active Ulcerative Colitis Trials 1 and 2 (ACT 1 and ACT 2. respectively) – showed patients with moderate to severe active ulcerative colitis treated with infliximab at weeks 0, 2, and 6 and every 8 weeks thereafter were more likely to have a clinical response at weeks 8, 30 and 54 than were those receiving placebo.

44. Weston-Petrides GK, Lovegrove RE, Tilney HS, et al. Comparison of outcomes after restorative proctocolectomy with or without defunctioning ileostomy. Arch Surg 2008;143:406–12. PMID: 18427030.
   A review of 17 studies comprising 1486 patients revealed that restorative proctocolectomy without a diverting ileostomy resulted in functional outcomes similar to those of surgery with proximal diversion but was associated with an increased risk of anastomotic leak. Diverting ileostomy should be omitted in carefully selected patients only.

45. Lovegrove RE, Constantinides VA, Heriot AG, et al. A comparison of hand-sewn versus stapled ileal pouch anal anastomosis (IPAA) following proctocolectomy: a meta-analysis of 4183 patients. Ann Surg 2006;244(1):18–26. PMID: 16794385.
   A large meta-analysis demonstrated no significant differences between a mucosectomy and hand-sewn versus a stapled anastomosis. Nocturnal seepage and pad usage favoured the stapled anastomosis in comparison to persisting symptoms due to inflammation or dysplasia favouring the hand-sewn technique.

65. Waljee A, Waljee J, Morris AM, et al. Threefold increased risk of infertility: a meta-analysis of infertility after ileal pouch anal anastomosis in ulcerative colitis. Gut 2006;55(11):1575–80. PMID: 16772310.
   A meta-analysis of eight studies revealed that an IPAA can increase the risk of infertility, defined as achieving pregnancy in 12 months of attempting conception, in women with ulcerative colitis by approximately threefold. Counselling female patients regarding decreased rates of fecundity following an IPAA is imperative.

Crohn's disease

Mark W. Thompson-Fawcett

Introduction

Crohn's disease is a chronic transmural inflammatory process that can affect the gastrointestinal tract anywhere from mouth to anus and which may be associated with extraintestinal manifestations. The disease is commonly confined to a region of the gut. Frequent disease patterns observed include ileal, ileocolic and colonic. Perianal disease may coexist with any of these. Often there are discontinuous segments of disease with areas of normal mucosa intervening. Inflammation may cause ulceration, fissures, fistulas and fibrosis with stricturing. Histology reveals a chronic inflammatory infiltrate that is typically patchy and transmural, and may reveal classic granulomas with giant cell formation. Clinically, patients have abdominal pain and diarrhoea, and they may develop bowel obstruction or intestinal fistulas. A combination of the clinical, macroscopic, radiological and pathological features is required to make the diagnosis. It is a chronic disease with varying lengths of remission interspersed with acute episodes.

Epidemiology

Crohn's disease has an incidence of 6–15/100 000 and a prevalence of 50–200/100 000 in the West, but much lower in other, particularly warmer regions. Peak age of onset is 20–30 years, with a higher incidence in females in many higher-incidence areas. There is no association with socioeconomic status or occupation, but an urban environment, cooler climate and increased standards of domestic hygiene may increase the risk. The incidence of Crohn's disease had steadily increased over recent decades but has now plateaued. Rates are lower but increasing in Southern and Eastern Europe, and Asia. Evidence of environmental effects is seen from studies of migrant populations. Current thinking is that environmental factors, rather than ethnicity, are a more important explanation for regional variation in incidence.[1] From genetic studies, there are some risk loci that are specific to ethnicity but many are shared.[2]

Aetiology

Crohn's disease involves interplay between environmental and genetic factors. The specific cause of the exaggerated inflammatory response at the mucosal level remains unclear. There are a number of areas where much investigation has been focused.

Smoking and oral contraception

Smoking increases the relative risk of Crohn's disease by two, in contrast with ulcerative colitis where smoking provides a protective effect. Oral contraception may be associated with a small increase in risk, but whether this is causal or by association is not clear. Evidence suggests that oral contraceptive use has no effect on disease activity.[1]

Infection

Mycobacterium paratuberculosis causes a granulomatous inflammatory disorder in the intestine of cattle (Johne's disease) and it has been hypothesised that Crohn's is the human form of this disease. Many remain sceptical as the evidence is conflicting; the issue requires resolution.[1,3]

It has been controversially proposed that measles virus infection or vaccination may cause the granulomatous vasculitis observed in Crohn's disease, but this has now been dismissed.[1]

Genes and the microbiome

Crohn's disease results from a genetic predisposition to an abnormal interaction between the immune system and environmental factors, especially the gut microbiota. It has been demonstrated that there is a dysbiosis in the microbiome of Crohn's patients at the time of diagnosis. Large-scale genetic studies have linked inflammatory bowel disease (IBD) to host–microbe pathways central to recognition and clearance, mucosal-initiated effector responses and mucosal barrier function.[4] Epigenetic factors have also been shown to play a role. Genetic research started with epidemiological studies that demonstrated familial aggregation. Of patients with Crohn's disease, 2–22% have a first-degree relative with IBD. There is greater concordance for IBD in monozygotic (20–50%) than dizygotic twins (0–7%). Early-onset disease has a higher familial prevalence rate, suggesting a greater genetic contribution compared with late-onset disease. Clinical patterns of IBD in affected parent–child and sibling pairs are concordant for each of disease type, extent and extraintestinal manifestations in the majority of cases. The relatives of patients with Crohn's disease also have an increased risk of developing ulcerative colitis. Crohn's disease and ulcerative colitis are polygenic disorders with some shared susceptibility genes.[5]

These familial patterns led to linkage studies between 1996 and 2004. The most significant finding of this era was the variants in the *NOD2* gene (initially *IBD1* and also *CARD15*). *NOD2* is associated with ileal disease, younger age at onset, ileocaecal resections and re-operation, and displays ethnic variation (less common in Northern Europe and Asia).[6] *NOD2* variants probably impair the innate immune system at mucosal level, limiting the ability to deal with some gut microbiota. Candidate gene studies followed linkage studies but were disappointing. It was proposed in the late 1990s that complex diseases like Crohn's were likely to be caused by numerous common variants of modest effect. Large numbers of cases are needed, to find both common variants of modest or small effect, and likely a large number of less common variants, that overall are still important contributors to susceptibility. Genome-wide association studies

(GWAS) enabled this to be explored. A 2012 meta-analysis of GWAS studies involving 75 000 individuals identified 140 susceptibility loci. Much of disease variability still remains unexplained. Next-generation sequencing with whole genome studies will identify the contribution of rare and low-frequency variants to disease risk. In the future, fine-mapping studies will lead to finding causal variants and thereby more understanding of biological mechanisms. The hope is this will lead to identification of therapeutic targets, and the ability to predict disease behaviour and response to medical therapy.[7]

Pathogenesis

Normally, the gut exists in a state of tolerance to the stream of microbial, dietary and other antigens in contact with the mucosa, but this tolerance and the ability to suppress an immune-mediated inflammatory response is lost in IBD. In Crohn's disease, defects in immunoregulation are coupled with an increased mucosal permeability due to leaky paracellular pathways.

Defects in immunoregulation may include disturbed innate immune mechanisms at the epithelial barrier, problems with antigen recognition and processing by dendritic cells, and effects of psychosocial stress via a neuroimmunological interaction. In Crohn's disease the cell-mediated response is predominant, with excessive activation of effector T cells (Th1) that predominate over the regulatory T cells (Th3, Tr) that turn off the process. Proinflammatory cytokines released by effector T cells stimulate macrophages to release tumour necrosis factor (TNF)-α, interleukin (IL)-1 and IL-6. In addition, abnormal dendritic cell function may further drive the inflammatory response. Leucocytes then enter from the local circulation releasing further chemokines, amplifying the inflammatory process. The result is a local and systemic response, including fever, an acute-phase response, hypoalbuminaemia, weight loss, increased mucosal epithelial permeability, endothelial damage and increased collagen synthesis. Due to immune dysregulation the inflammatory response in the intestinal mucosa proceeds unchecked, producing a chronic inflammatory state.[8]

Pathology

Distribution

The macroscopic appearance and distribution are the first important considerations that provide key information towards differentiating Crohn's disease from other forms of IBD, particularly ulcerative colitis. Frequencies of regions involved are:

1. small bowel alone, 30–35%;
2. colon alone, 25–35%;
3. small bowel and colon, 30–50% (usually ileocolic);
4. perianal lesions, over 50%;
5. stomach and duodenum, 5% (minor subclinical mucosal abnormalities in 50%).

Skip lesions (areas of disease separated by normal bowel) strongly suggest Crohn's disease, although occasionally a periappendiceal or caecal patch of overt colitis may be observed with distal ulcerative colitis.

Macroscopic appearance

The unmistakable appearance of Crohn's disease is of a stiff, thick-walled segment of bowel with fat wrapping. There is creeping extension of mesenteric fat around the serosal surface of the bowel wall towards the antimesenteric border. This is part of the connective tissue changes that affect all layers of the bowel wall. As inflammation is full thickness, there can be fibrinous exudate and adhesions on the serosal surface. Narrow linear ulcers with intervening islands of oedematous mucosa give the mucosal surface its classic cobblestone appearance. Ulceration is discrete, and serpiginous linear ulcers usually run along the mesenteric aspect of the lumen. Deep fissuring from linear ulceration may lead to formation of fistulas through the bowel wall. Closer inspection may reveal multiple aphthous ulcers that usually develop on the surface of submucosal lymphoid nodules. Aphthous ulcers are the earliest macroscopic lesions in Crohn's disease and are seen before the classic appearances of more established disease. Inflammatory polyps are often found in the involved colon but are unusual in the small bowel. Enlarged lymph nodes may be present in the resected mesentery but are not caseated or matted together. Strictures can vary from 1 to 30 cm in length. These may be stiff like a hosepipe, with turgid oedema, or tight fibrotic strictures from burnt-out inflammation. The narrowing of the lumen may be sufficient to produce obstruction and proximal dilatation, and there may be multiple dilated segments between multiple tight strictures. Fistulas, sinuses and abscesses are often present in the ileocaecal region but may arise from any segment of active disease and can communicate with other loops of bowel, stomach, bladder, vagina, skin or intra-abdominal abscess cavities.

Microscopy

Inflammation involves the full thickness of the bowel wall. Early mucosal changes show neutrophils attacking the base of crypts, causing injury and focal crypt abscesses. The formation of mucosal lymphoid aggregates followed by overlying ulceration produces aphthous ulcers. There is relative preservation of goblet cell mucin by comparison with ulcerative colitis, where there is usually mucin depletion. As the disease progresses, connective tissue changes occur in all layers of the bowel wall giving the stiff, thick-walled, macroscopic appearance. There is submucosal fibrosis and muscularisation. The muscularis mucosa and muscularis propria are thickened from increased amounts of connective tissue. Typically, the chronic inflammatory infiltrate and the architectural changes in the mucosa are patchy. Transmural inflammation is in the form of lymphoid aggregates seen throughout the bowel wall, leading to the formation of a Crohn's 'rosary' on the serosal surface. The following three features are diagnostic hallmarks of Crohn's disease:

1. deep non-caseating granulomas (excluding those that are mucosal or related to crypt rupture) are present in 60–70% of patients and are commonly located in the bowel wall but may be in the mesentery, regional lymph nodes, peritoneum, liver or contiguously involved tissue;
2. intralymphatic granulomas;
3. granulomatous vasculitis.

Pitfalls in differentiating Crohn's colitis from ulcerative colitis

Sometimes it is difficult even for an experienced gastrointestinal pathologist to differentiate between Crohn's colitis and ulcerative colitis on histology, and considerable interobserver variation is reported among pathologists. There can be overlap between the diseases and this can lead to the diagnosis of indeterminate colitis in 5–10% of patients with colonic involvement alone. During the course of the disease subsequent disease behaviour may change, leading to a change in diagnosis, usually towards Crohn's disease. For difficult cases, consideration of the macroscopic, microscopic, radiological and endoscopic features and the history and clinical picture is essential, for it is often the cumulative evidence that makes the diagnosis. A definitive diagnosis is more likely if the resected colon is available for assessment as opposed to mucosal biopsies. If only endoscopic biopsies are available, the endoscopic findings are important and must be discussed with, or shown to, the pathologist.

Rectal sparing may be seen in ulcerative colitis, especially if topical preparations have been used. Patchy inflammation is a feature of Crohn's disease, but treated ulcerative colitis can itself show patchy mucosal inflammation. Perianal disease is very suggestive of Crohn's, although patients with ulcerative colitis can develop cryptoglandular fistulas and abscesses. Lymphoid follicles may be seen in the base of the mucosa in severe ulcerative colitis, but they are a prominent feature of Crohn's disease, where they are transmural. In Crohn's disease there is relative preservation of goblet cell mucin, whereas mucin depletion is a feature of ulcerative colitis (with the exception of fulminant ulcerative colitis, where there may be surprisingly little mucin depletion). In established diversion proctitis or pouchitis it is difficult to exclude Crohn's disease as both these conditions may mimic Crohn's disease.

Clinical

Gastrointestinal symptoms

The clinical presentation varies depending on the site of disease. Acute first presentations of disease are uncommon, but ileal disease can mimic acute appendicitis and colonic disease may present as a fulminating colitis.

The majority of patients complain of diarrhoea (70–90%), abdominal pain (45–65%), rectal bleeding (30%) and perianal disease (10%). The symptom profile will reflect the disease location. Diarrhoea may result from mucosal inflammation, fistulation between loops of bowel, a short bowel from previous resections, bacterial overgrowth from obstructed segments, or bile salt malabsorption from terminal ileal disease. These latter two also produce steatorrhoea. Distal colitis and proctitis, and decreased rectal compliance, produce tenesmus and frequent bowel motions. Abdominal pain may be colicky from obstructing lesions or more continual from peritoneal irritation caused by acute inflammation. Terminal ileal disease is the most common site for obstructive lesions. Rectal bleeding is uncommon from terminal ileal disease, but does occur in 50% of patients with colonic disease. Massive bleeding occurs in 1–2%, though the site is often difficult to identify. When perianal disease is present, patients often complain of purulent discharge and minor leakage of faecal material with local discomfort. Fissures may be large, indolent and painless. Significant perianal pain suggests undrained sepsis. Fistulas extending to the bladder can produce pneumaturia and recurrent urinary tract infection, while those extending to the vagina may cause wind or faeces vaginally.

Systemic symptoms

Weight loss is reported by 65–75% of patients. This is usually of the order of 10–20% of body weight and is the result of anorexia, food fear, diarrhoea and, less often, malabsorption. The latter may be caused by inflammatory disease but more commonly is due to bacterial overgrowth as a result of coloenteric fistulas, blind loops or stasis from chronic obstruction. If there is extensive small-bowel disease, there may be poor absorption of fat-soluble vitamins leading to symptoms and signs of osteomalacia (vitamin D) or a bleeding tendency (vitamin K). Other deficiencies are uncommon; usually resulting from inadequate intake rather than increased losses, but may include deficiencies of magnesium, zinc, ascorbic acid and the B vitamins. Symptoms of anaemia are common and usually result from iron deficiency due to intestinal blood loss and, less commonly, from vitamin B_{12} or folate deficiency. After resection of more than 50 cm of terminal ileum, vitamin B_{12} absorption falls below normal. Malabsorption of bile salts and fats, which can cause diarrhoea, usually only follows an ileal resection of greater than 100 cm. The inflammatory process produces a low-grade fever in 30–49% of patients; where high and spiking, or the patient reports rigors, it is likely that there is a suppurative intra-abdominal complication.[9]

Extraintestinal manifestations

These are outlined in Box 12.1 and are more common in association with Crohn's colitis than isolated small-bowel disease. These manifestations are similar to those that occur in ulcerative colitis,

Box 12.1 • Extraintestinal manifestations of Crohn's disease

Related to disease activity
- Aphthous ulceration (10%)
- Erythema nodosum (5–10%)
- Pyoderma gangrenosum (0.5%)
- Acute arthropathy (6–12%)
- Eye complications (conjunctivitis, etc.) (3–10%)
- Amyloidosis (1%)

Unrelated to disease activity
- Sacroiliitis (often minimal symptoms) (10–15%)
- Ankylosing spondylitis (1–2%)
- Primary sclerosing cholangitis (rare)
- Chronic active hepatitis (2–3%)
- Cirrhosis (2–3%)
- Gallstones (15–30%)
- Renal calculi (5–10%)

and may precede, be independent of or accompany active IBD, and can cause significant morbidity. They may be experienced by up to 50% of patients and be present life-long in 25–30%. Gallstones are said to be common due to malabsorption of bile salts in the terminal ileum; however, symptomatic problems are not increased compared with the general population. Steatorrhoea promotes increased absorption of oxalate, thereby increasing the incidence of oxalate renal stones. Patients may have a fatty liver as a result of malnutrition or from receiving total parenteral nutrition. Mild abnormalities of liver function are common with active disease, and these do not imply significant liver disease.

Thromboembolic complications occur with IBD and are usually associated with severe active colonic disease. Common sites are the lower extremities and pelvic veins, but cerebrovascular accidents have also been reported. Metastatic Crohn's disease is an unusual complication in which nodular ulcerating skin lesions occur at distant sites including the vulva, submammary areas and extremities, and sometimes peristomal. Biopsies of these show non-caseating granulomas. Clubbing is seen in some cases of extensive small-bowel disease.

Amyloidosis is reported in 25% of patients with Crohn's disease at post-mortem but only 1% have clinical manifestations. It can occur in the bowel or within other organs, including the liver, spleen and kidneys. If renal function is affected, resection of the diseased bowel will result in regression of amyloid and improvement of renal function.[9]

Physical signs

Patients may appear well and have a normal physical examination. With more severe disease there may be evidence of weight loss, anaemia, iron deficiency, clubbing, cachexia, proximal myopathy, easy bruising, elevated temperature, tachycardia and peripheral oedema. Signs of extraintestinal manifestations may be present.

Abdominal examination can be normal but tenderness in the right iliac fossa is common. Thickened loops of bowel may be palpable and if matted together can produce an abdominal mass. A psoas or intra-abdominal abscess produces signs and occasionally there is free peritonitis. Enterocutaneous fistulas are most common when there has been previous surgery and usually present through a scar. Acute or chronic strictures or carcinoma may produce signs of obstruction. Compared to the general population, the relative risk of adenocarcinoma of the colon complicating Crohn's colitis is 1.4 to 1.9 and the relative risk of small-bowel carcinoma, 21 to 27.[10] Perianal disease varies from an asymptomatic fissure or inflamed skin tag to severe disease that may

look like a 'forest fire', with erythema, large fleshy skin tags, deep chronic fissures with bridges of skin and multiple fistulas creating the so-called 'watering-can perineum'. Fibrosis from chronic inflammation may have produced a woody, stiff anal canal or an anal or rectal stenosis.

Paediatric age group

In children and adolescents the gastrointestinal manifestations are similar but extraintestinal and systemic manifestations of disease become more important. About 15% have arthralgia and arthritis that often precedes bowel symptoms by months or years. Diagnosis may be delayed by a non-specific presentation with systemic symptoms of weight loss, growth failure and unexplained anaemia and fever. If active disease is dealt with promptly by medical or surgical treatment and adequate nutrition is maintained, retardation of growth and sexual development can usually be reversed.[9,10]

Pregnancy

This issue is often of concern as the disease frequently affects young adults. For the majority of patients with IBD fertility is normal but in some subgroups fertility rates are slightly reduced. Overall, patients with IBD do experience more adverse outcomes in pregnancy. In the absence of active disease, the outcome of pregnancy equals that of matched controls. With active disease at conception, there is an increase in spontaneous abortions and premature delivery, and a greater than 50% chance of relapsing disease during pregnancy. The risk of relapse is only 20–25% if disease is inactive at conception. It is therefore advisable to avoid conception during an acute phase of disease. Pregnancy probably does not affect the long-term course of the disease. Aminosalicylates, steroids and azathioprine are relatively safe in pregnancy. Azathioprine may be associated with a small increase in major congenital defects but this needs to be balanced against the importance of maintaining disease control. The use of methotrexate is contraindicated.[9,11]

Investigations

Laboratory

Anti-*Saccharomyces cervisiae* antibodies (ASCAs) and perinuclear antineutrophil cytoplasmic antibody (p-ANCA) can be useful to discriminate ulcerative colitis from Crohn's. ASCAs are positive in 35–50% of patients with Crohn's compared to less than 1% in ulcerative colitis. The specificity is around 90%. On the other hand, p-ANCA is often raised in ulcerative colitis with a sensitivity of 55% and specificity of about 90%. If p-ANCA is elevated in Crohn's, it is only with colitis. Faecal calprotectin and lactoferrin can play a role in diagnosis, monitoring disease activity and predicting relapse.[12,13]

In more severe or established disease, magnesium, zinc and selenium levels should be checked. Serum albumin is often low in active disease due to downregulation of albumin synthesis by cytokines (IL-1, IL-2, TNF). Mild episodic elevations of liver function tests are common but persistent abnormalities require further investigation. Evidence of anaemia should be sought, and investigated if present. A neutrophil leukocytosis usually indicates active disease or septic complications. Of the serum protein markers for inflammation, C-reactive protein and orosomucoid most closely match clinical disease activity. Erythrocyte sedimentation rate is useful in Crohn's colitis but not in small-bowel disease. Faecal fat excretion may be increased if malabsorption is present. Severe ileocaecal involvement can cause right hydronephrotic or sterile pyuria, and an enterovesical fistula will lead to bacteria in the urine.

Radiology

Small-bowel imaging is usually carried out as part of the diagnostic work-up or soon after diagnosis to determine the extent of the disease. A small-bowel barium study has traditionally been the key to confirming the presence of small-bowel disease. This has been superceeded by magnetic resonance imaging (MRI) and computed tomography (CT). Magnetic resonance enterography (MRE) (or enteroclysis, choice largely depending on local preference or radiologist), CT enterography and high-resolution ultrasound can all give good results. The clinical question, local expertise, desire to minimise radiation, availability and cost are factors taken into account when choosing a modality.

Although not commonly done now, small-bowel barium follow-through studies provide the best resolution, but this investigation only assesses the lumen and carries a radiation burden similar to CT. It is debated whether a barium study is best done by barium meal and follow-through techniques (better tolerated) or by a small-bowel enema with a nasoduodenal tube (enteroclysis); probably most important is a radiologist committed to producing good-quality images. More subtle features of small-bowel Crohn's include thickening of the valvulae coniventes, a granular mucosal pattern and aphthous ulcers. As disease progresses, features include wall thickening, cobblestoning and fissure-like ulcers, sinus tracts and fistulas. There may be stenosis

causing obstructive symptoms, commonly in the terminal ileum (**Fig. 12.1**). Multiple tight stenoses with intervening dilated segments produce a 'chain of lakes' appearance (**Fig. 12.2**).

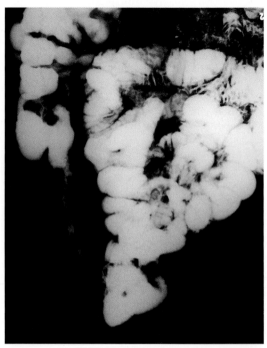

Figure 12.1 • Small-bowel enema with classic terminal ileal disease showing narrowing, cobblestone mucosa and fissures.

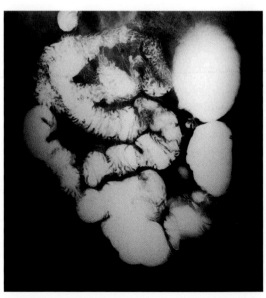

Figure 12.2 • Small-bowel enema showing multiple stenoses with intervening dilatation.

While CT enterography and MRE provide less luminal detail, they provide information on wall thickening (>3 mm), oedema in the bowel wall and mesenteric fat, any increase in fat adjacent to bowel, lymph node involvement, increased vascularity, fibrotic strictures, and sinuses and fistulas.

CT is frequently used to investigate acute abdominal pain. The diagnosis of Crohn's may be suggested in this context by seeing thickened small-bowel loops, especially in the terminal ileum (**Fig. 12.3**). CT is effective at detecting intra-abdominal abscesses and dilated segments of small bowel, and remains the most used modality for suspected acute complications including intra-abdominal sepsis and obstruction.

In addition to identifying stenosis (**Fig. 12.4**), MRI has the benefit of being able to demonstrate bowel wall oedema to assist in discriminating areas of inflammation from fibrosis. MRI is free of ionising radiation and not limited by poor renal function. Dynamic imaging also allows multiple sequences so

contractions can be delineated from true strictures more easily. However, respiratory movement and claustrophobia may be a problem and it is more costly. Its advantages, mainly less radiation, mean MRI has become preferred over CT for routine imaging and follow-up. If CT enterography is used, a low-dose protocol should be considered. MRI is also the investigation of choice for complicated perianal sepsis. High-resolution ultrasound is popular in Europe and effective at detecting inflamed bowel and demonstrating many of the features of Crohn's, although it is operator-dependent.[14]

A double-contrast barium enema of the colon is now rarely done and has been replaced by colonoscopy. In severe acute presentations of Crohn's disease, plain abdominal films should be done initially to look for evidence of obstruction, mucosal oedema or dilatation. Plain films can also be useful to identify constipation proximal to a segment of colonic disease.

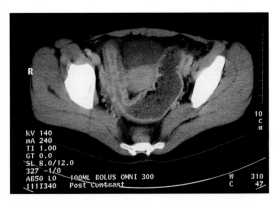

Figure 12.3 • CT scan showing thick-walled terminal ileum with proximal dilatation.

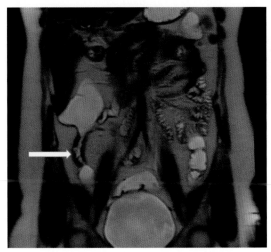

Figure 12.4 • MRI demonstrating strictured terminal ileum with thickened bowel wall (arrow).

Endoscopy

Colonoscopy provides a macroscopic view that can be recorded, allows biopsies to aid in the differential diagnosis, can assess and biopsy strictures, and can clarify the situation where significant symptoms are not backed up by clinical evidence of disease. Intubation of the ileocaecal valve allows examination and biopsy of the terminal ileum. Small aphthous ulcers are the early features of Crohn's disease, in contrast with the erythema and loss of vascular pattern in ulcerative colitis. In more severe disease the oedematous mucosa is penetrated by deep fissuring ulceration to give a cobblestone appearance. Multiple biopsies should be taken even if the mucosa appears normal, as granulomas may be present that can confirm the diagnosis. There is not usually a role for routine follow-up endoscopy and endoscopic findings correlate poorly with clinical remission. There is a cancer risk in long-standing Crohn's colitis and most apply the same colonoscopic surveillance as they do in cases of extensive ulcerative colitis, despite various objections and limitations.

Endoscopy of the oesophagus, stomach and duodenum is necessary if there are appropriate symptoms, or abnormalities on a barium meal. Findings may include rugal hypertrophy, deep longitudinal ulcers and a cobblestone mucosa, the latter being the main differentiating feature from peptic ulcer disease. Biopsies should be taken but granulomas are often absent.

The diagnosis of Crohn's disease may be made by capsule endoscopy; this may be in the context of investigating obscure chronic gastrointestinal bleeding when other investigations have been negative. Capsule endoscopy is more sensitive than MRE but only provides information from viewing the lumen. One of the technical problems is that the capsule may be held up by strictures and cause small-bowel obstruction. If there is any significant concern that this may happen, a dummy dissolvable capsule can be used first. Capsule endoscopy is considered a second-line investigation by most.

Disease activity assessment and quality of life

For clinical purposes, disease activity is best assessed by clinical features and the investigations outlined above. It is usually categorised as mild, moderate or severe. If patients are asymptomatic (and off steroids) and/or have no obvious residual disease they are considered in remission. A number of indices of disease activity have been developed for Crohn's disease, including the Crohn's Disease Activity Index (CDAI) and the Harvey–Bradshaw index. Their role has largely been confined to clinical trials for standardisation and comparison of patient groups. However, with the widespread use of expensive biological agents, in publicly funded health services a severity score over a certain threshold is often required to access these medications; usually this is the CDAI.

Health-related quality of life (HRQOL) is a quantitative measurement of the subjective perception a person has of their health state, including emotional and social aspects. If treatments are being compared, use of HRQOL instruments is essential for providing a valid and objective measure of a real change in health state.

Phenotyping

Different phenotypes of Crohn's disease are recognised and the clinical picture varies with the site of disease and the behaviour of the disease (i.e. stricturing or fistulating). To date it seems that the location of disease tends to be stable over time. However, the behaviour of Crohn's disease according to the location varies dramatically over the course of the disease. At 10 years, 46% of patients exhibit different disease behaviour than at diagnosis. Phenotype is important for genetic studies as differing phenotypes may correlate with particular genetic variations. Phenotype is also relevant for studying the outcome of therapy, medical or surgical. The Vienna classification was developed in 1998. This was modified to the current Montreal classification in 2005. At the time of diagnosis the following are recorded: age <16 years (A1), between 17 and 40 years (A2) or ≥40 years (A3); location of disease (ileal (L1), colonic (L2), ileocolonic (L3) and isolated upper gastrointestinal disease (L4) if present is added to the others); behaviour (non-stricturing/non-penetrating (B1), stricturing (B2), penetrating (B3), and perianal disease [P] is added if present).

Differential diagnosis

Small-bowel Crohn's disease

In most cases, after an appropriate work-up involving history and clinical, laboratory, radio-logical, endoscopic and pathological findings, the diagnosis will be fairly clear-cut. Box 12.2 shows the differential diagnoses of small-bowel Crohn's disease. Traditionally perhaps the two that cause most difficulty are *Yersinia* and tuberculosis. With

Box 12.2 • Differential diagnosis of small-bowel Crohn's disease

Differential diagnosis	Useful discriminating features
Appendicitis	History, CT scan
Appendix abscess	History, ultrasound/CT scan
Caecal diverticulitis	Older age, colonoscopy
Pelvic inflammatory disease	History
Ovarian cyst or tumour	Ultrasound
Caecal carcinoma	CT colonography/colonoscopy
Ileal carcinoid	Small-bowel enema
Behçet's disease	Painful ulceration of the mouth and genitalia
Systemic vasculitis affecting the small bowel	Underlying systemic connective tissue disorder
Radiation enteritis	History of radiotherapy
Ileocaecal tuberculosis	History of tuberculosis, circulating antibodies to *Mycobacterium*, stool cultures
Yersinia enterocolitica ileitis	Self-limiting, stool cultures, serology
Eosinophilic gastroenteritis	Gastric involvement, peripheral eosinophilia
Amyloidosis	Biopsy
Small-bowel lymphoma	Radiological appearance
Actinomycosis	Microscopy of fine-needle aspirate
Chronic non-granulomatous jejuno-ileitis	Clinical picture and histology

increased use of CT scanning for acute abdominal pain, thickened terminal ileum is a more common indication for a careful work-up.

Large-bowel Crohn's disease

When there is no small-bowel or perineal involvement, there are two areas where the diagnosis may be difficult. An isolated segment of disease, especially if it is a short segment, has to be differentiated from carcinoma, ischaemia, tuberculosis and lymphoma; occasionally, severe diverticular disease can appear as or disguise a segment of Crohn's disease. Inflamed diverticular disease can mimic Crohn's disease, with the presence of granulomas, transmural inflammation and fissuring ulceration. Isolated involvement of the sigmoid colon is not common in Crohn's disease, so care should be taken before making this diagnosis in the presence of diverticular disease. Differentiating Crohn's disease from ulcerative colitis has been discussed earlier.

Medical treatment

A summary of first-line medical treatment options for Crohn's disease is given in Box 12.3. The concept of treating Crohn's disease is to induce remission and then to maintain it. The most effective agent for inducing remission is a corticosteroid, and the second-line agents are the TNF inhibitors, infliximab or adalimumab. Budesonide has a role in ileocolic disease or right-sided colitis. It is not as effective for induction of remission as prednisone or methylprednisone but has fewer side-effects. For moderate to severe disease, steroids are commenced and at the same time as immunomodulators, usually with azathioprine. After some weeks or months, when the therapeutic benefit

Box 12.3 • Summary of medical treatment options for Crohn's disease

Induction of remission
Mild to moderate disease
- Prednisone 20–40 mg daily for 2–3 weeks then tapering
- Ileal and/or right colon: budesonide 9 mg per day
- Crohn's colitis: appropriate salicylate compound (oral and/or enema)
- Perianal disease: metronidazole 400 mg t.d.s. or ciprofloxacin 500 mg b.d.

Severe disease
- Intravenous prednisone 60–80 mg per day
- Infliximab, adalimumab or other biological (second-line)

Maintenance of remission
- Azathioprine, 6-mercaptopurine, methotrexate, budesonide 6 mg per day (ileal and/or right colon), infliximab or adalimumab

of immunosuppression commences, steroids can be removed. Aminosalicylates have modest efficacy for mild to moderate Crohn's colitis. As well as introducing treatment, with increased use of immunosuppression and associated risks, de-escalation of therapy is also important.[15] For more guidance on medical therapy readers are referred to the British Society of Gastroenterology guidelines[16] and the United Kingdom National Health Service, National Institute for Health and Care Excellence (NICE) guidelines (www.nice.org.uk/guidance/CG152).

Multidisciplinary care

✓ For the best outcomes, and for the safe and effective care of patients with IBD, multidisciplinary care is essential. With the introduction of expensive biological drugs, with at times limited efficacy, and more powerful immunosuppressive regimens, the surgeon must be involved in the complex decision-making for patients with moderate to severe Crohn's disease. Frequently patients do require surgery to achieve remission. Surgical input is needed to provide balanced decision-making, mindful that if the patient comes to surgery too late, the morbidity in a malnourished immunosuppressed patient is high. To contribute effectively to good decision-making the surgeon needs knowledge of the likely efficacy and outcome for the medical therapy options.

Aminosalicylates

Aminosalicylates have been used extensively in Crohn's but now have a limited role. Sulfasalazine and 5-aminosalicylic acid (5-ASA; also known as mesalazine or mesalamine) are used to treat disease of mild to moderate severity in the colon. Sulfasalazine consists of a sulfapyridine carrier linked to the active 5-ASA. In the colon bacteria cleave off the active 5-ASA, of which about 20% is absorbed. If 5-ASA is taken orally by itself, it is completely absorbed in the proximal small bowel. Although 5-ASA is the main active drug, the sulfapyridine produces most of the adverse effects, including nausea, vomiting, heartburn, headache, oligospermia and low-level haemolysis. These adverse effects are dose-related. There are also a number of hypersensitivity reactions unrelated to drug levels, including worsening colitis. Adverse effects occur in 30% of people taking 4 g daily of sulfasalazine. Other 5-ASA preparations use different carriers, or use pH- or time-dependent protective coatings that allow release to start in the jejunum, ileum or colon, thereby giving a much better adverse effect profile. If a 5-ASA preparation is used, one of the latter group is usually prescribed.

Aminosalicylates have historically had a significant place in the management of Crohn's disease, but their indications are now limited. Aminosalicylates may have a limited role for mild to moderate colonic disease but have marginal efficacy over placebo.[16] Mesalazine can be used for preventing recurrence after surgery, with a number needed to treat (NNT) of 13.[17]

Steroids

Systemically absorbed corticosteroids are the most effective and commonly used drugs for moderate to severe Crohn's disease and will induce remission in 70–80% of cases. Response should be seen within 2–4 weeks. They are less effective if only the colon is involved. Doses of prednisone range from 20–40 mg/day orally for moderate disease to 60–80 mg/day intravenously for severe disease. Steroids should be used in short courses and must be tapered when a clinical response is achieved. They can be useful in resolving the obstructive symptoms in early disease caused by narrowing due to inflammatory oedema. Steroids will not help with obstructive symptoms caused by established fibrotic stenosis. Steroids are useful for maintaining a steroid-induced remission in the short term, which implies steroid-dependent disease, but they do not have a role in maintenance beyond this. There is no advantage in combining salicylate therapy with steroids.

Rectal administration of steroid is effective for left-sided colonic disease, but steroid is still absorbed systemically, and prolonged therapy can cause adrenal suppression. 5-ASA foam enemas are equally effective and can be used in combination with oral steroids in an exacerbation of disease.

To avoid systemic adverse effects, topically active corticosteroids have been developed. Budesonide, formulated as a slow-release oral preparation, acts in the small bowel and colon or can be given as an enema. The systemic bioavailability of budesonide is only 10–15% because of rapid first-pass metabolism in the liver, but it can still produce some suppression of plasma cortisol levels. The response rates are slightly less than prednisone but with fewer side-effects.

✔✔ In active Crohn's disease, budesonide produced remission in 51–60% of patients compared with 60–73% on systemic steroids, but with a halving of reported adverse effects from 60% to 30%. When budesonide 9 mg daily was compared with mesalamine 4 g daily for ileal and/or ascending colon disease, remission in the budesonide group at 16 weeks was 62% vs 36% for mesalamine, and budesonide was better tolerated. Budesonide is not of value for maintenance therapy.[18,19] Budesonide was compared to placebo in a double-blind randomised controlled trial of endoscopic recurrence (at 3 and 12 months) after an ileal or ileocolic resection, with no overall benefit.[20]

Antibiotics

Metronidazole and ciprofloxacin are used to treat perianal disease. They both seem equally effective but ciprofloxacin may be better tolerated. They can reduce fistula discharge but probably have little impact on closure rates, and symptoms often return after cessation. Long-term use of metronidazole in doses >10 mg/kg is contraindicated because of the risk of peripheral neuropathy. There is evidence that metronidazole and ciprofloxacin have efficacy for ileal and colonic disease but are rarely used as alternative therapies are more effective.

Nutrition for therapy

The rationale for nutritional therapy is that intraluminal dietary antigens may drive the inflammatory response and that removal of these and bowel rest will bring remission.

✔✔ Total parenteral nutrition is effective in inducing remission in 60–80% of patients, which matches the effect of steroids, but combining both these therapies gives no added benefit over using only one. Relapse rates are high after cessation. Total enteral nutrition is equally as effective and has a similar relapse rate after cessation. Polymeric diets seem as effective as elemental and peptide-based diets, but polymeric diets are cheaper and more palatable and are therefore preferred.[21]

Polymeric or elemental intake as proportion of the diet is also effective at maintaining remission.[21] Enteral nutrition is frequently chosen as the first-line therapy for children with Crohn's disease.[22]

Immunomodulatory therapy

This is used to reduce and eliminate steroid requirements, particularly after a remission has been achieved, and in refractory disease. Azathioprine and 6-mercaptopurine are purine analogues, azathioprine being quickly metabolised to 6-mercaptopurine. They inhibit cell proliferation and suppress cell-mediated events by inhibiting the activity of cytotoxic T cells and natural killer cells. The onset of a therapeutic effect takes 3–6 months. Toxicity occurs in 20–30%, including 3–15% of patients who will develop pancreatitis. A significant proportion of toxicity, and possibly lack of efficacy, can be due to genetic variability in the metabolism of azathioprine that should be tested for and managed by measuring enzyme and drug levels.[23]

Fever, rash, arthralgias and hepatitis may occur and marrow suppression is dose-related. In trials to improve disease or to decrease steroid requirements, there is a success rate of about 70–80%, and this applies equally to all disease sites, including perianal disease. It is now thought thiopurines have a limited effect on inducing remission. They are effective in reducing steroids when in remission (64% vs 46% in placebo). Methotrexate is used occasionally for treating Crohn's disease. Limited data suggest it is as effective as azathioprine or 6-mercaptopurine and it can be prescribed for patients who do not tolerate or respond to the latter two drugs.[16,24,25]

'Biological agents'

'Biological agents' is the term used to refer to monoclonal antibodies targeted at mediators of the inflammatory response. The two agents in common clinical use are infliximab, introduced in the late 1990s, followed several years later by adalimumab. A number of other agents are under evaluation. Infliximab is a mouse–human chimeric monoclonal antibody to TNF-α delivered by intravenous infusion. Adalimumab is a fully human monoclonal antibody also directed at TNF-α, but has the added convenience of being delivered by subcutaneous injection. The RCTs evaluating these drugs are funded by the manufacturers, are complex in design with frequent crossovers, and require careful study to determine the real clinical efficacy. Occasional severe adverse reactions are reported and infectious diseases, especially tuberculosis, need to be excluded before treatment. There may be a possibility of an increase in the risk of malignancy in the long term. Unfortunately because of crossovers in RCTs there are few patients who remain purely in placebo arms to generate reliable long-term data on adverse outcomes. Perhaps the biggest drawback of these agents is their high cost. The initial landmark studies below build a fairly consistent pattern that about two-thirds of patients respond initially to biological agents but by a year this is probably a third (and probably half of these would have settled with placebo). If a first biological has failed and another is tried the response rates are about half those expected for the first treatment.

✔✔ The initial placebo-controlled trial with infliximab addressed induction of remission after a single dose. At 4 weeks after a single dose, an initial treatment response was seen in 65% (54 of 83) who received infliximab and 17% (4 of 24) in the placebo group; at 12 weeks this was 41% and 12%, respectively.[26] The ACCENT I study followed and

addressed the maintenance of remission with a year of treatment with infliximab; 573 patients were recruited. After an initial infusion, 58% responded. The responders were then randomised to placebo or infliximab at 2 and 6 weeks and then 8-weekly up to 54 weeks. At week 54, of initial responders, about 15% in the placebo group and 35% in the treatment group were in clinical remission.[27]

Similar results with initial moderate efficacy have been demonstrated using infliximab to treat fistulas. The ACCENT II study recruited patients with perianal (90%) and enterocutaneous draining fistulas. The primary endpoint of the study was a reduction in the number of fistulas by 50% or more. After three infusions at 0, 2 and 6 weeks, the study randomised responders at week 14 to placebo or infliximab infusions 8-weekly to week 54. The primary endpoint was loss of response, with fistulas reactivating or reappearing. Of 306 patients enrolled, 195 (64%) responders were randomised at week 14. At week 54, 23 of 98 patients receiving placebo maintained a response compared with 42 of 91 receiving infliximab. This means that of all 306 patients entered into the study, about 30% of patients treated with infliximab will maintain a response at 1 year, 22% having a complete response. In the placebo group after initial infliximab response, 19% (19 of 98) had a complete response.[28] The efficacy at 1 year judged by complete response is therefore modest.

Adalimumab (a human anti-TNF monoclonal antibody) has been evaluated in the CLASSIC I and II[29,30] and the CHARM studies[31] and has similar efficacy to infliximab. Adalimumab may be beneficial if infliximab therapy has not been successful and vice versa.

The CHARM study looked at maintenance therapy with adalimumab for 12 months using hospitalisation as an endpoint. After induction all patients were randomised to adalimumab or placebo. The Crohn's-related hospitalisation rate at 12 months was 8.4% on adalimumab and 15.5% on placebo. This means 14 patients are treated to prevent one admission. The study also looked at surgery rates. Three of 517 patients who had adalimumab and 10 of 261 who had placebo required major Crohn's-related surgery in the 12 months. Rates of surgery were higher but the follow-up is short.

Countries vary, but generally in publicly funded health systems conventional treatment with steroid and an immunosuppressant is first-line. If unsuccessful, biological agents are commenced and if response is achieved are continued for at least 12 months. At 12 months, if there is active disease treatment should continue. If in remission, there should be a discussion with the patient about the risks and benefits of stopping. It seems that up to 50% may relapse in the 12 months following stopping. Work on predictors of safe therapy withdrawal is ongoing.

Newer concepts in medical treatment include 'treat-to-target', 'step up versus top down' and biological drug and antibody level monitoring. A 'treat-to-target' target of 'deep remission' is symptom control and endoscopic mucosal healing. Adjusting treatment to meet these endpoints may produce better results. Another debate is 'step up' care versus 'top down'. The SONIC trial addressed this and for patients with predictors of more severe disease there is probably an advantage of a top down approach and introduction of a biological agent early with or without azathioprine. However, guidelines generally favour a 'step up' or 'accelerated step up' approach for most patients. Therapeutic drug concentration monitoring of biologicals to optimise dosing, including anti-drug antibody levels, is becoming part of management. Lower drug levels and higher antibody levels have been associated with less effective treatment. Immunomodulators may have a role in lowering antibody levels to biological drugs.[25]

While modern medical therapy is improving care for patients with Crohn's disease, population-based studies to date have not shown a clear drop in surgical intervention rates for Crohn's since the introduction of biologicals. Similarly, no alteration in surgical intervention rates was observed in the 1990s when the use of azathioprine and methotrexate became widespread.[32,33]

Surgery and immunosuppression

With increasing use of immunosuppressive therapies there is concern about the impact of these treatments on perioperative morbidity. Azathioprine does not cause problems in the perioperative period. Use of greater than 20 mg prednisone for more than 6 weeks probably has an impact and steroids should be reduced before surgery if possible. Reported outcomes when surgery is carried out within several months of infliximab infusions vary. From retrospective studies and meta-analysis of these it seems likely there is a small increase particularly in infective complications.[34]

✔ Biological drugs are effective so in the current era there will not be randomised studies to definitively answer the question about increased surgical morbidity. If possible, avoid an infusion within a week of surgery; otherwise it is reasonable to continue biologics if indicated. The focus for the surgeon should be on active involvement in multidisciplinary care to avoid the situation of a significantly malnourished immunosuppressed patient with active inflammatory disease presenting late for surgery. This is when there is a high risk of morbidity. In these sick patients care must be planned carefully and delivered to the highest standard.

Prophylaxis against recurrent disease after surgery

After surgery, medical treatment can be considered to prevent recurrence. Patients often prefer to be medication-free when these treatments have limited efficacy. The decision to commence prophylactic treatment requires weighing up the side-effects and burden of taking medication for several years, balanced against the modest benefit. For smokers it remains very important to stop, to halve their rate of recurrence. There is evidence that metronidazole, 5-ASA and azathioprine have a modest benefit (approximately 10% risk reduction) to prevent clinical recurrence after surgery.[35] Recently PREVENT RCT using infliximab was reported.[36] Although a difference in reduced endoscopic recurrence was seen (30 vs 60%), this did not carry over to a clinically significant difference (13 vs 20%). Some design issues and underpowering may have failed to disclose a real clinical benefit.

✔ Patients at higher risk of recurrence should have options for prophylaxis discussed with them. Benefits are limited. If it is available, patients at high risk of recurrence could have a colonoscopy at 6–12 months. If there is severe endoscopic recurrence, starting biological treatment could be considered if funding is available; however, there is not a strong association between endoscopic findings and clinical disease.

✔ The TOPPIC study has shown that for the subgroup who continue to smoke after resection, mercaptopurine taken postoperatively reduced the recurrence rate at 3 years from 46% on placebo to 10%. There was no benefit for non-smokers.[37]

Other drugs

Antidiarrhoeal medication and anticholinergic agents to relieve colicky pain are useful in mild to moderate disease but should be avoided in severe exacerbations. Non-steroidal anti-inflammatory drugs should also be avoided as they may make the disease worse, and opioids can increase bowel spasm. Cholestyramine is useful for treating bile salt diarrhoea.

Surgery

Development of surgery

Crohn and colleagues initially described radical resection of involved segments of bowel, but high recurrence rates led to an era of bypassing affected segments. Frequent complications with the bypassed segments caused a return to resectional surgery.

✅ Modern surgery for Crohn's disease involves resecting the least amount of bowel to re-establish satisfactory intestinal function. This is based on the concept that Crohn's is a gut-wide disease and that microscopic disease at the resection margin does not influence recurrence of disease.[38,39]

Furthermore, one small study has shown that asymptomatic endoscopic small-bowel lesions remaining after ileocolic resection did not correlate with clinical recurrence.[40] Although the term 'recurrence of disease' is widely used, a more accurate term is 'recrudescence', implying a new outbreak of already present disease.

It is important to avoid any unnecessary sacrifice of gut as these patients may need resection of further segments for future disease recrudescence. In the move to conservatism, however, it is important not to procrastinate when there is an indication for surgery. When patients were questioned on the timing of their surgery, most would have preferred to have had the procedure 12 months earlier because of the benefits it gave.[41] Low quality-of-life scores with active disease improve to normal when remission is obtained, whether by surgery or medical treatment.[42] When medical treatment does not induce remission or the adverse effects of therapy are unacceptable, in most cases the best course of action for the patient is to proceed to surgery.

Laparoscopic surgery is often feasible. Most surgeons favour an extracorporeal anastomosis. The mesentery is often thick and vascular in which case extracorporeal ligation of the mesentery may be better. Ileocolic resections can usually be accomplished with relative ease, giving the patient a small 3–5 cm midline incision through the umbilicus. Sometimes the incision will need to be lengthened to accommodate a large inflammatory mass. Two small RCTs showed no differences using an open versus laparoscopic approach. Case series and meta-analyses suggest 1–2 days shorter stay but 30 minutes more operating time for laparocopic surgery, but no other consistent differences.[43] Perioperative care for most bowel operations should follow enhanced recovery pathways.

Risk of operation and re-operation

Accurate population figures about patterns of disease and complications are not easy to obtain. Many of the data presented in this chapter are from specialist centres and these figures may not always apply to the Crohn's population at large. In one of the largest population-based cohorts reported of 1936 patients from Sweden, the cumulative rate of intestinal resection was 44%, 61% and 71% at 1, 5 and 10 years, respectively, after diagnosis; the subsequent risk of recurrence was 33%

and 44% at 5 and 10 years, respectively.[44] In another population-based study involving 210 patients with Crohn's disease at a mean of 11 years from disease onset, 56% required surgery; by life-table analysis the re-operation rate was 25% at 10 years and 56% at 20 years.[45]

In a tertiary referral centre experience of 592 patients with Crohn's disease, 74% required surgery at a median of 13 years' follow-up. The chance of surgery varied with the site of disease and was 65% in those with small-bowel involvement, 58% in those with colonic or anorectal disease and 91% in those with ileocolic disease.[46] Half of the patients in a tertiary referral centre who have had one operation will require re-operation for further disease with follow-up of more than 10 years.[47,48] Most studies report the annual rate of symptomatic recurrence to be 5–15% and the annual re-operation rate 2–10%. Recurrence is at the site of previous disease in the majority, but may be at a new site.[49] For patients presenting to a surgical service, the cumulative chance of a permanent stoma at 20 years is 14% and of a temporary stoma 40%.[50]

Risk factors for recurrence

Many studies have looked at risk factors for recurrence. Recurrence (or recrudescence) can be defined by radiological findings, endoscopic findings, the return of symptoms or the need for further surgery. Most studies have been retrospective, and although some claim to identify risk factors, others report no association for the same risk factor. There is no consistently robust evidence that age of onset of disease, gender, site of disease, number of resections, length of small-bowel resection, proximal margin length, microscopic disease at the resection margin, fistulising versus obstructive disease, number of sites of disease, presence of granulomas, blood transfusion or genetic markers have an important impact on recurrence.[51-53]

Although a recurrence frequently occurs immediately proximal to the previous anastomosis, there is no consistent or high-quality evidence to date that anastomotic technique (side-to-side, end-to-end, end-to-side, hand-sewn or stapled) affects recurrence.

✅✅ In an RCT it has been shown that there is no difference between a stapled side-to-side and a hand-sewn end-to-end anastomosis.[54]

✅ However, it is now clear that continuing to smoke after a surgical resection doubles the risk of recurrence and patients must be urged to stop smoking.[55-57] As above, prophylactic treatment should be discussed with patients, especially if still smoking.

Principles of surgery for Crohn's disease

Perioperative considerations

Excellent perioperative care is essential for a good outcome in patients with Crohn's disease. As there is always potential for colonic or rectal involvement with small-bowel disease, this should be borne in mind when planning surgery. Deep vein thrombosis prophylaxis using higher prophylactic doses of low-molecular-weight heparin, compression stockings and intermittent calf compression devices is important as patients with IBD are at higher risk of thrombotic complications.[58] Full postoperative anticoagulation may need to be considered if there is a history of thrombosis. Patients will often be at risk of adrenal suppression and the need for intravenous steroid cover should be considered every time. Before elective surgery, significant malnutrition should be restored by either enteral or parenteral nutrition, all potential electrolyte problems corrected and sepsis controlled. If these goals cannot be achieved, consideration should be given to a temporary stoma rather than an anastomosis. Joint management in a multidisciplinary team is an essential principle in the decision-making and hospital and post-discharge care. Psychological well-being always needs to be raised with the patient due to the chronic nature of the disease.

Technique

Patients with Crohn's disease can be among the most technically difficult cases a surgeon will face. Compromise of good technique can be unforgiving. Any part of the bowel can be affected or involved with Crohn's disease, so if there is any doubt, the patient should be placed in a modified lithotomy or Lloyd-Davies position. For open surgery a midline infraumbilical incision gives good access, is more easily reopened in the future and will not interfere with stomas that may be needed on either side of the abdomen. At each operation a full examination of the bowel should be carried out to stage the disease and the length of remaining and resected bowel measured. In the event of recurrence it is helpful to have marked anastomotic sites with a metal clip. At the first abdominal operation for Crohn's disease the appendix should be removed to prevent future diagnostic problems and confusion.

✅ Thick oedematous vascular mesenteric pedicles require special mention. A standard clamp and tie technique may allow a vessel to retract into the mesentery, resulting in a mesenteric haematoma with potential to compromise the blood supply to large segments of bowel. Thick pedicles should be dealt with very carefully and some recommend double-suture ligation. Spillage of gastrointestinal contents must be minimised and controlled, and meticulous haemostasis is important as there may be inevitable loss from oozing, inflamed, raw surfaces. Great care should be taken not to damage or perforate other loops of bowel or other organs in the presence of difficult adhesions and inflammation.

One of the benefits of laparoscopic surgery may be a decrease in adhesion formation, facilitating easier re-operation.

Surgery for small-bowel and ileocolic Crohn's disease

Indications

Surgery for small-bowel Crohn's disease is aimed at treating complications not amenable to medical therapy. Surgical interventions are required for:

1. stenosis causing obstructive symptoms;
2. enterocutaneous or intra-abdominal fistulas to other organs;
3. draining intra-abdominal or retroperitoneal abscesses;
4. controlling acute or chronic bleeding;
5. free perforation.

Of these, obstruction is the most frequent indication.

Gastroduodenal disease

Symptomatic gastroduodenal disease is present in 0.5–4% of patients and is usually associated with disease in other sites. The first and second parts of the duodenum are most commonly involved and the disease often extends into the gastric antrum. Most patients who require surgery require it for problems of stenosis or, occasionally, bleeding. Often it is difficult at endoscopy to differentiate Crohn's from peptic ulcer disease but a trial of medical ulcer therapy may help. Gastrojejunostomy is the standard procedure for duodenal or pyloric stenosis. Historically, vagotomy was often added to reduce stomal ulceration. Proton pump inhibitors can now be effective in this role and the potential side-effects of vagotomy avoided.

In selected cases pyloric or duodenal strictureplasty may be considered, and produce better function. Results of a duodenal strictureplasty are variable and complications can be significant.[59,60] Massive acute upper gastrointestinal bleeding is rare, but if endoscopic methods are unsuccessful, bleeding should be controlled by under-running the bleeding vessel with a suture. Balloon dilatation of benign upper gastrointestinal tract strictures is safe, but the limited experience in Crohn's disease suggests dilatation has little long-term benefit. Fistulas involving the duodenum occur in 0.5% of patients with Crohn's disease and generally arise from other diseased segments fistulating into the duodenum. Surgical therapy for these is usually successful and prognosis relates to the severity of disease in the primary segment. Closure of secondary duodenal defects with a jejunal serosal patch or Roux-en-Y limb may be preferable to primary suture.

Ileocolic disease

The cumulative operation rate for patients with distal ileal disease at 5 years from the time of diagnosis is up to 80%. Ileocaecal disease is treated with a limited ileocaecal resection, including a few centimetres of macroscopically normal bowel at each end, and either a side-to-side or end-to-end anastomosis is satisfactory.[54]

After a first operation the re-operation rate at 5 years is 20–25% and at 10 years 35–40%. Re-operation rates for second and subsequent operations are the same. Further disease is usually on the ileal side of the anastomosis and it is important to stress that this is new disease and does not relate to an inadequate resection margin. Although recurrent disease rates are high and on average a patient will need an operation every 10 years, surgery is highly successful at relieving symptoms and restoring health when disease is refractory to medical treatment.

Balloon dilatation of selected symptomatic ileocolic strictures, usually short anastomotic strictures, is a treatment option with at least short-term benefit in 60–80% (with a risk of perforation of 2–11%) and with longer-term benefit in 40–60%.[61] Suitable strictures are less than 4 cm long, without active disease and without angulation. As it is not possible to get the scope through the stricture before dilatation, cross-sectional imaging is important to document the length of the stricture and plan treatment.[62]

Ileal and jejunal multisite disease

If there is isolated small-bowel disease, it is most commonly in the terminal ileum and is usually suited to a limited resection. More extensive disease can produce obstructive strictures throughout the small bowel. In the past, these patients requiring surgery had multiple resections, with a risk of short-bowel syndrome. In an endeavour to maximise conservation of bowel length the concept of strictureplasty was introduced, and this technique is now preferred for all suitable lesions. It is ideally suited to short fibrotic strictures but it may be used for strictures up to 25 cm long. Long strictures with active inflammation are usually better managed with resection unless there is concern about bowel length because of previous resections. In most series half the patients having a strictureplasty will also have a segmental resection.

The Heineke–Mikulicz technique is usually used for strictures <10 cm. In a small number of cases with longer strictures (10–25 cm) where bowel conservation is required, a Finney or a Jaboulay strictureplasty may be used. For even longer narrowed segments (>25 cm) a side-to-side isoperistaltic technique described by Michelassi et al. may be used.[63] For this, the diseased bowel is divided at its midpoint, the diseased portion opened on the antimesenteric border, the ends spatulated, the proximal and distal ends advanced so that the diseased segments lie side by side, where they are anastomosed to each other, trying to ensure stenotic segments are complemented with dilated segments. Despite often long suture lines, results are similar to other strictureplasty techniques. Most candidates for strictureplasty have three or four strictureplasties but in some cases there may be 10–15. To ensure no significant strictures have been missed a Foley catheter or ball should be passed along the small bowel through an enterotomy. Using a catheter the balloon is inflated with a measured amount of saline to a diameter of 25 mm and pulled back through the bowel, and strictures not easily seen externally will be identified. Alternatively, a marble or stainless steel ball with a diameter of 25 mm can be traced through the bowel to identify strictures. The ball technique perhaps enables better control of spillage of bowel content but a stricture cannot be passed until it has been corrected, whereas a balloon can be deflated.

Results of strictureplasty have proved it to be a safe and effective technique. Overall morbidity is 10–20%. Postoperative abdominal septic complications occur in 5–10%, and overall 98–99% have symptomatic relief. Postoperative bleeding from a strictureplasty site occurs in about 3% of patients, but this usually resolves with conservative measures. Recurrence requiring re-operation is about 30% at 5 years. Re-operation rates after a strictureplasty are similar whether or not a limited resection is included in the operation. The re-operation rates are similar after first, second and third recurrences requiring surgery. Less than 10% of the strictureplasties themselves re-stricture, so most of the recurrent disease occurs at new sites.[62,64–68]

Fistulas and abscesses

Enteric fistulas may affect up to 30% of patients with Crohn's disease and in a referral centre about 40% are internal, 40% external and 20% mixed. Internal fistulas are usually spontaneous and external ones postoperative. Fistula tracts have an associated abscess, at least initially, in most cases. In expert hands surgical repair is successful in closing the fistula in more than 95% of cases, but failure after an attempt at definitive surgery can result in life-threatening morbidity.

Enterocutaneous fistulas and intra-abdominal abscess

Enterocutaneous fistulas in Crohn's disease are a common cause of intestinal failure and patients who develop intestinal failure are best managed in a specialised unit with a multidisciplinary team. Intra-abdominal abscesses that are drained externally will often result in a fistula. When abscesses complicate existing fistulas it is necessary to convert these fistula/abscess complexes into a well-draining fistula. Fistulas, whether postoperative or spontaneous, will drain along the line of least resistance, which is often previous scar tissue from incisions or drain sites.

Management principles

Although spontaneous and postoperative fistulas behave differently, the same management principles apply. The steps are outlined below.

1. Resuscitate the patient, correcting electrolytes and restoring haemoglobin levels. Control sepsis by open or percutaneous drainage and antibiotics; occasionally, exteriorisation of the bowel ends will be required. Attempts at repair and anastomosis should never be made in a patient with significant nutritional compromise or sepsis. Protect the skin from the fistula output by expert application of stoma appliances.

✔✔ There has been a vogue for using somatostatin analogues to decrease fistula output but it has shown no benefit.[69] Some may still argue to use it for very high volume proximal fistulas, which were not part of this trial.

---

2. Establish nutrition by either enteral feeding or total parenteral nutrition.
3. Support morale as these patients are often emotionally very fragile. They are upset and angry about what has happened to them and often demoralised and frightened as well. The surgeon should at all times recognise this and regard addressing these concerns with the patient as a priority.
4. Mobilise the patient to restore health. If it is reasonable to anticipate closure with conservative measures, or if the fistula is postoperative, wait for at least 6 weeks. If a fistula has not closed by 12 weeks, it probably never will. However, a fistula will generally close spontaneously by 6 weeks unless it:

(a) originates from a diseased segment of bowel;
(b) arises from an anastomotic breakdown greater than 50% of the circumference of the bowel;
(c) has a very short tract or communication between skin and mucosa;
(d) has bowel obstruction distal to it.

5. Plan a definitive operation with:
(a) complete adhesiolysis;
(b) en bloc resection of the diseased or damaged bowel and the fistula tract with primary anastomosis.

The work-up includes radiological imaging to (i) define the extent of intestinal disease, (ii) exclude any obstructing lesions and (iii) delineate the fistula tracts. Avoid the temptation to carry out earlier and repetitive imaging unless the results will alter management. There are reports of vacuum-assisted dressings and gelfoam embolisation of the fistula tract achieving closure; whether the closure is simply accelerated or whether surgery can be avoided is unknown.

Spontaneous enterocutaneous fistulas

In Crohn's disease this implies that there is a segment of diseased bowel that will require resection. This group generally benefits from earlier surgery for the following reasons:

1. The fistula will not heal spontaneously.
2. There is no concern about a more recent laparotomy making surgery difficult.
3. The bowel perforation occurs slowly and abdominal sepsis is usually localised, lessening the initial systemic insult.
4. Although the aim is to optimise the patient's general and nutritional state before surgery, active Crohn's disease will limit what is achievable.

Postoperative fistulas

In contrast to spontaneous fistulas, these will usually close with conservative measures if there is no downstream obstruction because the previously diseased bowel has been removed. However, the patient is often very ill and can have extensive abdominal contamination, which will usually drain by the incision or a drain site but may require added open or percutaneous drainage. On occasions the abdominal wound may be better left open initially and managed with a vacuum-assisted dressing, although there are some concerns that enterocutaneous fistulas can be induced in this way.

Intra-abdominal fistulas

These fistulas are usually spontaneous. The origin of the fistula, or primary defect, may arise from any segment of diseased bowel but is most commonly from the ileocaecal region. Similar management principles apply to these fistulas as to those described above, but the patients are generally in better health and less symptomatic. About half of the fistulas are diagnosed clinically, the remainder being asymptomatic and discovered at surgery. A fistula should always be suspected between two loops of adherent bowel. The secondary defect can occur in the stomach, duodenum, vagina, fallopian tube, ureter or urethra, but the sigmoid colon, small bowel and bladder are the most common sites. Most high vaginal fistulas are from the rectum but some are from the ileum.

Surgery involves en bloc resection of the primary defect and fistula with primary anastomosis and often only simple closure of the secondary defect, but with the exception of the duodenum.

Spontaneous free perforation in the small bowel or colon

Free perforation occurs in about 1% of patients with Crohn's disease and involves the small bowel and colon with similar frequency. Best results are from operation within 24 hours, with resection of the diseased segment and exteriorisation of the bowel ends.

Surgery for colonic and rectal Crohn's disease

Indications

The most common indication for colonic surgery is intractable disease that is not well controlled with medical therapy. The need for surgery and the choice of operation will depend on the extent of the disease. About one-third of patients will have segmental disease, a third left-sided disease and a third total colitis. Overall a third will have associated perianal disease. After 10 years about half will have had surgery and a quarter will have an ileostomy.[70] Many of those with severe colitis will settle with medical treatment. However, half of these patients will require colectomy within 1–2 years.[71]

Emergency colectomy and colectomy and ileostomy

Acute colectomy for Crohn's disease constitutes a small portion of operations for acute Crohn's disease. The indications for this include toxic dilatation, haemorrhage, perforation and severe colitis not responding to medical therapy. If medical treatment for acute severe colitis brings a response in 48–72 hours and urgent surgery is avoided, early elective colectomy should be considered as the chance of recurrent toxic colitis in the following years is significant and symptomatic control is often poor. Severe haemorrhage and perforation both occur in about 1% of patients with colitis. Urgent surgery is usually a total colectomy and ileostomy.

Completion proctectomy, if possible, is usually left until the patient is in good health, but severe haemorrhage can be a problem. The rectal stump, if left initially, will usually need to be removed to control residual symptoms. If the rectum is retained long term there is a risk of cancer and surveillance is required. In selected cases a loop ileostomy can be used to defunction moderately severe colitis. This will allow clinical improvement in over 80%. Half will be able to have the stoma closed initially, but only 20% continue without relapse after medium-term follow-up.[72]

In some cases a colectomy and ileostomy may be chosen over a proctocolectomy in the first instance if there is severe anorectal disease and concern about perineal wound healing. After colectomy with a period of maximal medical therapy the perianal disease may settle, facilitating better results with proctectomy, but doubt remains as to whether this is effective.

Segmental colectomy

Segmental colectomy is appropriate for a symptomatic stricture. In some cases it may be required to exclude cancer. The pattern of recurrence is similar to that seen with segmental small-bowel disease (Table 12.1). A meta-analysis of case series has compared segmental colectomy to colectomy and ileorectal anastomosis. If there were multiple colonic segments involved, recurrence was earlier with segmental resections, but there was no difference in permanent stoma rates. Treatment choices should be guided by the extent of colonic disease.[77]

Total colectomy and ileorectal anastomosis

In patients needing a colectomy for Crohn's colitis, 25% have rectal sparing, with a normally functioning rectum and sphincter mechanism. These patients are suitable for an ileorectal anastomosis. Some patients with a mild proctitis and/or mild perianal disease may even achieve reasonable function. With more severe disease, colectomy and ileorectal anastomosis may be done in two stages.

Clinical recurrence is reported in 50% at 10 years. Of those who lose their ileorectal anastomosis, many will still have obtained 4–5 years of useful function, and this can be particularly important if a stoma is deferred for teenage and young adult years. At 10 years, over half will retain their rectum. The development of perianal disease usually leads to proctectomy.

Table 12.1 • Long-term outcome of patients with segmental colonic Crohn's disease who have a segmental resection

Reference	n	Mean follow-up (yr)	Clinical recurrence (%)	Re-operation rate at 10 years (%)	Permanent stoma avoided (%)
Allan et al.[73]	36	–	–	66	–
Makoweic et al.[74]	142	12	60	32	88
Prabhakar et al.[75]	48	14	77	33	86
Polle et al.[76]	91	8.3	–	33 (at mean 8.3 years)	56*

The series by Prabhakar et al.[75] includes 10 patients who had the majority of their colon removed.

*Some patients had a stoma formed after segmental resection.

Panproctocolectomy

This operation is clearly the most definitive for colorectal disease and is associated with the lowest recurrence rate, albeit at the price of a stoma. Recurrence usually involves small-bowel disease, but it can be from perineal Crohn's after removal of the anorectum. Recurrence rates after panproctocolectomy are of the order of 15–25% at 10 years. Patients report a good quality of life after colectomy and ileostomy for disease confined to the colon.[47] In addition, a portion will need revisional surgery for ileostomy complications.[50]

Removal of the rectum requires particular care not to damage the pelvic nerves, and a technique of intersphincteric and perimuscular dissection (close to the rectal wall) of the rectum has been used. As there is no natural anatomical plane, perimuscular dissection is more vascular and time-consuming than dissection in the mesorectal plane. It is probably safe for the specialist to carry out most of the dissection in the mesorectal plane, perhaps coming inside the mesorectal plane at the critical points, anteriorly and laterally in relation to the parasympathetic nerves. Whichever technique is preferred, the surgeon has to be prepared to modify this to take account of severe perineal or perirectal disease that can make the dissection very difficult. The perineal wound is best treated with primary closure and suction drainage (if desired) from above. Delayed wound healing is frequently a problem, although 60–80% will have uncomplicated healing. Up to 30% have traditionally taken 4–6 months to heal completely, but vacuum-assisted closure systems may now reduce this in many cases. About 10% will have longer-term problems with perineal sinuses, most of which settle with further surgical procedures. These may include several attempts at scraping the sinus tract to remove necrotic tissue and freshen the walls, and excluding an enteroperineal fistula (**Fig. 12.5**) and cutaneous Crohn's disease. Some cases eventually need local excision of the sinus. In troublesome cases of active perineal disease after proctectomy, there is a role for wide excision and a vertical rectus abdominis transpelvic musculocutaneous flap reconstruction. Disappointingly, in a small

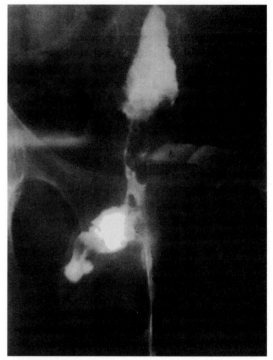

Figure 12.5 • Sinogram examination demonstrating an enteroperineal fistula.

number the flap of normal skin can also develop granulomatous cutaneous Crohn's disease.

Restorative proctocolectomy

Crohn's disease has traditionally been regarded as a contraindication for an ileal pouch because of the risk of developing small-bowel or perianal disease that will lead to pouch excision. Now some surgeons are prepared to offer an ileal pouch to a well-informed patient who has isolated colonic Crohn's and requires a proctocolectomy. Other surgeons still regard Crohn's as an absolute contraindication.[78] The risk of pouch failure (and excision) is in the range of 10–45%, and is higher than for ulcerative colitis. However, for Crohn's disease at other sites re-operation rates of 50% at 10 years are acceptable, and small-bowel recurrence probably involves a similar sacrifice of bowel to that of excising a pouch.[79,80] The group in Paris who controversially promoted pouches in selected patients with colorectal Crohn's disease have reported 10-year follow-up documenting Crohn's-related events in 35%, with 10% requiring pouch excision.[81]

Crohn's colitis and cancer

With extensive Crohn's colitis it is now accepted that there is an increased risk of colorectal cancer similar to ulcerative colitis.[82–84] Field change in the colonic mucosa with areas of dysplasia is observed, as in ulcerative colitis.[85] Surveillance colonoscopy should be offered to patients with Crohn's colitis and this is probably best done with dye spray and targeted biopsies. Particular care is needed in the presence of colonic strictures, which should always be regarded as malignant until proven otherwise; this may entail a resection to make the diagnosis.

Perianal disease

Perianal disease should be considered as a separate entity or phenotype of Crohn's disease. It is associated with more severe luminal disease and earlier age of onset. Some 30–70% of patients with Crohn's disease will have a degree of involvement of the anal canal, ranging from minor skin tags to severe disease. However, only a much smaller proportion will need surgical intervention for anal disease.[86] In different cohorts perianal disease has been reported either as more frequent in association with colonic disease or rectal disease or ileal disease.[87,88] A small percentage of patients have their initial presentation with anal disease, but over time half of these will develop disease at other intestinal sites. The activity of anal disease is unrelated to more proximal disease activity.

Generally, the prognosis is good, with only 5–10% of patients with perianal Crohn's requiring a proctectomy. If rectal disease is also present, proctectomy will be needed in up to twice this proportion. Fissures or fistulas may be asymptomatic, and after some years about half will have healed spontaneously and a further 20–30% will heal after a surgical procedure. Carcinoma is a rare but recognised complication, and hidradenitis suppurativa may coexist. The benign course of most perianal lesions caused by an incurable disease has led many (but not all) surgeons to a general policy of conservative treatment, but with active attention to draining sepsis. Carefully selected cases without active disease can benefit from active surgical management. Preserving a functioning sphincter must remain a paramount concern in these patients. Box 12.4 outlines a classification of lesions described by Hughes and Taylor.[89] This

Box 12.4 • Hughes' classification of perianal lesions in Crohn's disease

Primary lesions
- Anal fissure
- Ulcerated oedematous pile
- Cavitating ulcer
- Aggressive ulceration

Secondary lesions
- Skin tags
- Anal/rectal stricture
- Perianal abscess/fistula
- Anovaginal/rectovaginal fistula
- Carcinoma

Incidental lesions
- Piles
- Perianal abscess or fistula
- Skin tags
- Cryptitis
- Hidradenitis suppurativa

From Hughes LE, Taylor BA. Perianal lesions in Crohn's disease. In: Allan R, Keighley M, Alexander-Williams J, et al., editors. Inflammatory bowel disease, 2nd ed. Edinburgh: Churchill Livingstone; 1990. p. 351–61. With permission from Churchill Livingstone.

classification is useful to help understand aetiology and development of anal lesions. In practice, lesions are usually described as they are observed. Surgery is most frequently indicated for secondary and incidental lesions.

Investigation

Careful examination, often under anaesthesia, is the most useful investigation and often an essential part of the work-up. MRI and/or endoanal ultrasound in combination with examination under anaesthesia allow accurate identification of obscure tracts and collections.[90]

Medical treatment

Ciprofloxacin, metronidazole, azathioprine, infliximab and adalimumab are probably effective at controlling or improving perianal disease (see above), but most of the claims in the literature are small case series and the impact of medical therapy on reducing complications or the need for surgery is not known. Case series suggest that while the initial response rate is reasonable, the long-term closure rate is little improved by adding infliximab to established medical and surgical treatment. In those with active disease, however, it seems reasonable to employ any measure that is likely to help the symptomatic patient and avert proctectomy. Treatment decisions are case by case. Currently, it is common to insert setons to achieve drainage and to commence a biological agent. If there is a good response, setons are usually removed some months later. Ciprofloxacin or metronidazole are used for septic problems and can be used as first-line medical treatment. Ciprofloxacin is better tolerated. With the above approach in the biological era, case series with medium-term follow-up report two-thirds respond or close, and then a third recur.[91,92] The length of time biological agents are continued depends on response and disease at other sites, and similar factors are considered for stopping as discussed above. The overall benefit of biologicals to improve long-term fistula closure is modest.[93]

Anal fissure

Most fissures are in the midline posteriorly, one-third are multiple and two-thirds are asymptomatic. Anal canal pressures are similar to those in controls and 50–70% heal with conservative or concurrent medical therapy.[94] Initially a conservative approach should be adopted for chronic fissures. Treatment options include topical glyceryl trinitrate or diltiazem, and botulinum toxin injection. All efforts should be made to conserve the internal anal sphincter in Crohn's disease. However, if all else fails and the patient has significant symptoms, the fissure will usually heal after a lateral anal sphincterotomy without compromising continence. This should probably not be done in the presence of active proctitis. Healing the fissure may prevent future abscesses and fistulas arising from its base.[95]

Abscesses

Abscesses may arise from deep cavitating ulcers or distorted anal glands (**Fig. 12.6**). The first sign of an abscess is often increasing perianal pain. An MRI can confirm clinical suspicion if little is obvious on initial examination. Occasionally, abscesses may be above the levator muscles. Examination under anaesthesia will identify the problem, in combination with MRI for difficult cases. Collections should be drained by removing a small area of overlying skin to allow drainage. In larger cavities it may be useful to insert a mushroom catheter to facilitate drainage and irrigation. It is usually inadvisable to lay open a primary tract at this stage.

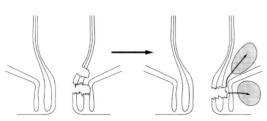

Figure 12.6 • Pathogenesis of anal suppurative disease. Deep cavitating ulcers give rise to extrasphincteric and supralevator abscesses.

Anal fistulas

Fistulous disease may range from an incidental fistula to a 'watering-can' perineum. If a fistula has been judged incidental or there is no active inflammation in the perianal region or rectum it is reasonable to progress to a standard surgical procedure. If there is active disease no more than drainage and seton insertion should be considered until the disease is in remission. This lessens the risk of poor healing and allows time for medical therapy to be implemented. Once acute inflammatory disease is controlled or absent, options to eliminate the fistula may be considered. Sphincter preservation is particularly important. A lay open or fistulotomy may be done if the tract is superficial. If the fistula is higher and trans-sphincteric a rectal advancement flap, or ligation of intersphincteric tract (LIFT) procedure are options giving a success rate as high as 50–70% at 2–3 years.[86,96] Later recurrence after initial success is not uncommon. Bovine collagen fistula plugs are likely to be more successful with single tracts than complex fistulas and seem to work in about 50% of cases where applied.[97] The newest promising treatment is stem cell injection into fistula tracks, but more data are needed. A covering stoma is probably not of benefit for the majority of cases. In complicated fistulas or in the presence of active inflammation, the aim is to establish adequate drainage and this is best done with a loose seton, which may be left long term with a good functional result. Supralevator fistulas are a difficult problem and usually involve perforating disease from the rectum or even more proximal bowel. Again, the primary aim is drainage and identification of the internal origin, but these cases are more likely to need a proctectomy. Fistulas arising from deep cavitating ulcers are difficult to manage and proctectomy is often unavoidable in the long term.

Rectovaginal fistulas

The distressing problem of passing faeces or wind through the vagina means that these fistulas usually require surgical therapy. They occur in 10% of women presenting to specialist centres with Crohn's disease. In one series 37% had a proctectomy, but only one-third of these were primarily for the rectovaginal fistula.[98] They are more frequently associated with colon rather than small-bowel disease. The fistula, if low, will usually be identified on examination that may need to be done under anaesthesia with initial insertion of a seton to control sepsis. An MRI will give information about surrounding sepsis and may identify the fistula. For difficult high fistulas a vaginogram may be used.

Medical therapy should be optimised. It is doubtful whether biologicals are helpful to close the fistula. If the disease is quiescent a variety of surgical approaches can be employed. Depending on the condition of local tissues, options include a rectal advancement flap, a rectal sleeve advancement flap, an anocutaneous advancement flap, a vaginal advancement flap, a Martius graft, a gracillis interposition or sphincteroplasty.[99,100] With persistence and possibly more than one procedure, closure rates of over 50% may be a reasonable expectation. A temporary stoma may be considered for complex repairs.

Defunctioning ileostomy for perianal disease

A temporary ileostomy has a role in providing symptomatic relief to the desperate patient while more definitive treatment options are discussed or tried. In this situation, the majority will experience symptomatic improvement but with longer follow-up only a small number have intestinal continuity restored and following this an even smaller number remain in clinical remission.[72]

Long-term complications of perianal disease

Longer-term complications of perianal Crohn's disease may include rectal or anal strictures and incontinence due to fibrosis and sphincter damage. Symptomatic strictures should be gently dilated to not more than 20mm, remembering that with an impaired sphincter there is a risk of precipitating or worsening incontinence. About half the patients who develop an anal or rectal stricture will require proctectomy.[101]

Prognosis

Standardised mortality rates are higher for patients with Crohn's disease, with a ratio of 1.4. This particularly relates to patients who have the onset of their disease before the age of 20 years, and the risk is particularly high early in the course of the disease, although the absolute numbers dying remain small. Causes of death include sepsis, perioperative complications, electrolyte disturbances and gastrointestinal tract cancers.[10]

Quality-of-life issues are important to these patients and they express concerns over energy levels, fear of surgery and body image. Often, loss of energy and malaise contribute more to functional disability than specific gastrointestinal symptoms. In terms of academic success and advancement, patients are not hampered by the disease, and employment rates are the same as for matched healthy controls. However, patients frequently express impairment of employment, recreation, and interpersonal and sexual relationships. Most patients continue to function optimistically and adapt successfully. However, Crohn's patients are twice as likely to suffer anxiety and depression disorders and are more likely to require treatment with psychotropic drugs. Disease relapses produce considerable stress, and psychological support from counsellors, psychiatrists, non-medical and patient support groups should be utilised.[102]

Key points

- Patients with Crohn's disease usually enjoy reasonable health punctuated by periods of increased disease activity, initially managed medically.
- Many patients will require surgery at some stage.
- Multidisciplinary management is essential now that biological treatments are well established. Surgical input into medical treatment decisions is important so that all options are considered.
- Surgery is restricted to dealing with troublesome segments that cannot be managed medically.
- Surgery for small-bowel disease is usually necessary because of complications of disease such as strictures and fistulas.
- Surgery for large-bowel disease is usually necessary because of inability of medical treatment to control symptoms.
- Severe disease in young people can be life-threatening and expert surgical care is required.

🌐 Full references available at **http://expertconsult. inkling.com**

Key references

16. Mowat C, Cole A, Windsor A, et al. Guidelines for the management of inflammatory bowel disease in adults. Gut 2011;60(5):571–607. PMID: 21464096.
   IBD Section of the British Society of Gastroenterology UK guidelines.

18. Benchimol EI, Seow CH, Otley AR, et al. Budesonide for maintenance of remission in Crohn's disease. Cochrane Database Syst Rev 2009;(1): CD002913. PMID: 19160212.
   A Cochrane Database review.

19. Thomsen O, Cortot A, Jewell D, et al. A comparison of budesonide and mesalamine for active Crohn's disease. N Engl J Med 1998;339:370–4. PMID: 9691103.
   Budesonide is twice as effective as mesalamine in treating active Crohn's with the benefit of fewer side-effects than systemic steroids.

20. Hellers G, Cortot A, Jewell D, et al. Oral budesonide for prevention of postsurgical recurrence in Crohn's disease. Gastroenterology 1999;116:294–300. PMID: 9922309.

    Budesonide does not have a role in prophylaxis after surgery.

21. Akobeng AK, Thomas AG. Enteral nutrition for maintenance of remission in Crohn's disease. Cochrane Database Syst Rev 2007; 3:CD005984. PMID: 17636816.

26. Targan SR, Hanauer SB, van Deventer SJ, et al. A short-term study of chimeric monoclonal antibody cA2 to tumor necrosis factor alpha for Crohn's disease. Crohn's Disease cA2 Study Group. N Engl J Med 1997;337:1029–35. PMID: 9321530.

    The first RCT of biological agents in Crohn's disease demonstrating moderate efficacy in inducing remisson.

27. Hanauer SB, Feagan BG, Lichtenstein GR, et al. Maintenance infliximab for Crohn's disease: the ACCENT I randomised trial. Lancet 2002; 359(9317):1541–9. PMID: 12047962.

    Many centres took part with small numbers each. There is drug company representation on the writing committee. Infliximab is moderately effective at inducing remission but at 12 months is only a little better than placebo. The data need to be interpreted carefully, infliximab is very expensive, has a poor cost–benefit ratio and there are concerns about serious long-term side-effects. On the other hand, there are many anecdotes of dramatic clinical responses when other measure have failed. It has a role to induce remission in refractory cases.

28. Sands BE, Anderson FH, Bernstein CN, et al. Infliximab maintenance therapy for fistulizing Crohn's disease. N Engl J Med 2004;350(9):876–85. PMID: 14985485.

    This study looks at the role of infliximab for fistulating Crohn's disease and is a similar design to ACCENT 1. Similar comments apply as for ACCENT 1 above.

29. Hanauer SB, Sandborn WJ, Rutgeerts P, Fedorak RN, Lukas M, MacIntosh D, et al. Human anti-tumor necrosis factor monoclonal antibody (adalimumab) in Crohn's disease: the CLASSIC-I trial. Gastroenterology 2006;130(2):323–33. PMID: 16472588.

    First RCT to establish the efficacy of induction therapy with adalimumab.

30. Sandborn WJ, Hanauer SB, Rutgeerts P, et al. Adalimumab for maintenance treatment of Crohn's disease: results of the CLASSIC II trial. Gut 2007; 56(9):1232–9. PMID: 17299059.

    First RCT to demonstrate the efficacy of adalimumab for maintenance of remission out to 56 weeks after successful induction therapy with adalimumab in CLASSIC I.

31. Colombel JF, Sandborn WJ, Rutgeerts P, et al. Adalimumab for maintenance of clinical response and remission in patients with Crohn's disease: the CHARM trial. Gastroenterology 2007;132(1):52–65. PMID: 17241859.

    This RCT looked at the frequency of dosing for maintenance of remission, every other week (40%) versus every week (47%) versus placebo (17%) at 56 weeks.

54. McLeod RS, Wolff BG, Ross S, et al. Investigators of the CT. Recurrence of Crohn's disease after ileocolic resection is not affected by anastomotic type: results of a multicenter, randomized, controlled trial. Dis Colon Rectum 2009;52(5):919–27. PMID: 19502857.

    Good quality RCT to finally address the question about technique for ileocolic anastomosis.

69. Scott NA, Finnegan S, Irving MH. Octreotide and postoperative enterocutaneous fistulae: a controlled prospective study. Acta Gastroenterol Belg 1993;56(3–4):266–70. PMID: 8266769.

    Octreotide is not helpful in closing enterocutaneous fistula. There still may be a role though to help manage high-output fistulas. This subgroup is not specifically addressed by the study.

74. Travis SP, Stange EF, Lemann M, et al. European evidence based consensus on the diagnosis and management of Crohn's disease: current management. Gut 2006;55(Suppl 1):i16–35. PMID: 16481629.

    European Crohn's and Colitis Organisation Consensus Development Conference series. Evidence based consensus statements that includes opinions of experts both for and against the various recommendations.

13

Intestinal failure

Carolynne Vaizey
Janindra Warusavitarne

Introduction

The term intestinal failure (IF) encompasses a spectrum of conditions that manifest as an inability to maintain adequate nutritional, fluid and electrolyte homeostasis without supportive therapy.[1] The vast majority of cases are transient, without significant gut pathology, and are routinely managed in general surgical units. They frequently occur secondary to postoperative ileus. However, there are a group of cases distinguished by loss of functional gut that results in prolonged intestinal failure lasting months to years, some patients requiring permanent parenteral nutrition (PN). These cases may be due to massive gut loss following surgery, or loss of functioning intestine available for absorption, as can occur after enterocutaneous fistula formation.

Management of these cases may be complex, prolonged and expensive, in terms of financial cost and clinical input. The care of these patients should therefore be in a specialist IF unit. Such a unit should include a nutrition support team with the capacity to facilitate transition of the patient's care from a hospital environment to a home environment. The care of patients with IF is prolonged and involves specialist gastroenterological, surgical and nursing input. Surgical treatment is generally the last of many steps in the management but accounts for an important part of the workload of specialised IF units.[1]

The nursing staff on the ward and in clinic, specialist nutrition nurses and the home PN team are the backbone of delivery of care to these patients and their families. The different functions of each of these groups and their separate locations make it imperative that all are coordinated in their approach to each patient. Failure to achieve this results in confusion and demoralisation of this psychologically vulnerable group of patients, who are faced with prolonged hospital admission, debilitating illness, the prospect of no longer being able to eat normally (or at all) and the likelihood of incomplete functional recovery. Those who do survive find it difficult to accept the major limitations to their opportunities in life, especially in the case of young adults who constitute a significant proportion of these patients. A high level of technical training of the carers is required, which necessitates a specialist centre to maintain the technical base to these skills.

Guidelines on surgical management have been published by the Association of Surgeons of Great Britain and Ireland and the European Society of Coloproctology.[2,3] The National Health Service has set up and funded two national units in England through the National Specialist Commissioning Advisory Body. One is at St Mark's Hospital in London, the other is at Hope Hospital in Salford.

Intestinal failure: criteria for referral

The following criteria[4] are an indication of the type of cases that warrant referral to a nationally designated intestinal failure unit:

1. Persistence of intestinal failure beyond 6 weeks, without any evidence of resolution and/or complicated by venous access problems.
2. Multiple intestinal fistulation in a totally dehisced abdominal wound.

3. An intestinal fistula outside the expertise of the referring unit (e.g. recurrent in a non-specialist unit) or second and third recurrences in a colorectal centre.
4. Total or near-total small-bowel enterectomy, resulting in less than 30 cm of residual small bowel.
5. Recurrent venous access problems in patients needing sustained parenteral nutrition. This definition includes recurrent severe infections and recurrent venous thrombosis, where all upper limb and cervical venous access routes have become obliterated.
6. Persistent intra-abdominal sepsis, complicated by severe metabolic derangement (characterised by hypoalbuminaemia), that is not responding to radiological/surgical drainage of sepsis and provision of nutritional support.
7. Metabolic complications relating to high-output fistulas and stomas and to prolonged intravenous feeding, not responsive to medication and adjustment of the feeding regimen. Disorders of hepatic and renal function associated with intravenous nutrition that are resistant to metabolic and nutritional supplementation.
8. Chronic intestinal failure (from whatever cause) in a hospital without adequate experience/expertise to manage the medical/surgical and nutritional requirements of such patients.

Epidemiology

The prevalence of IF is unknown, but estimates can be made by considering those who require home PN. The incidence of home PN in Europe is estimated to be 3 per million population and the prevalence at 4 per million population, of whom 35% have short-bowel syndrome (SBS).[5] In the USA the use of home PN is estimated to be 120 per million population, of whom approximately 25% have SBS.[6] Such data do not include the patients who have not required home PN or those who have been successfully weaned off home PN. In the UK the estimated incidence of IF requiring treatment at a specialised unit is 5.5 per million population.[1]

As SBS is an uncommon condition, specialised centres with expertise in SBS have been created.[1,7,8] A recent study showed an overall survival rate of 86% in patients undergoing autologous surgical reconstruction at a median follow-up period of 2 years in a specialised unit.[9] Similar results have been achieved in other units and highlight the importance of multidisciplinary care.[1,10]

Causes

The causes of IF are multifactorial but can be categorised into four broad areas:

1. loss of intestinal length;
2. loss of functional intestinal length;
3. loss of intestinal absorptive capacity;
4. loss of intestinal function.

Loss of intestinal length

In the adult population, IF is most commonly related to a loss of intestinal length as a result of multiple or one massive intestinal resection.[11,12] Multiple resections are most common in recurrent Crohn's disease; an isolated massive enterectomy usually follows a vascular catastrophe, such as mesenteric arterial thrombosis or embolism or a venous thrombosis. Massive resection can also be necessary in cases of volvulus, trauma or, in the case of children, necrotising enterocolitis or gastroschisis.

The relation between the amount of bowel removed and the degree of IF is variable, influenced by the age of the patient, the site of resection and the presence or absence of colon. The normal small bowel is around 600 cm in length but may range between 300 and 800 cm. The important figure is not how much small bowel is removed but how much remains. An approximate figure of less than 100 cm in the presence of an ileostomy or less than 50 cm with colon present is likely to result in dependence on PN at 3 months. Children may function with shorter bowel as small-bowel adaptation (see below) can be very dramatic. The function of the remaining bowel may also be influenced by the presence of active Crohn's disease as well as the presence or absence of colon, as this may have a significant absorptive function.

Loss of functional absorptive capacity

Enterocutaneous fistula (ECF) is the commonest cause of IF where the mechanism is loss of functional absorptive capacity. Fistulous disease commonly bypasses otherwise normal functional small intestine. This is usually the result of an ECF, but hidden internal fistulas may also be responsible.

At a specialised IF unit, 42% of patients had Crohn's disease and the commonest complication necessitating admission was formation of ECFs.[1] The second most common cause of fistulas is abdominal surgery. The majority of fistulas occurring in postoperative patients[13,14] are the consequence of anastomotic breakdown. Risk factors for this include the age of the patient, the state of the bowel undergoing anastomosis, preoperative nutritional status and the site of anastomosis.[14] When associated with malignancy, factors including tumour fixity, presence of obstruction, previous radiotherapy, associated abscess and surgical technique all affect the risk. Non-absorbable mesh can erode into the bowel and cause fistula, particularly where there is fragile postoperative or diseased bowel. The use of vacuum-assisted closure (VAC) systems in the open abdomen can result in fistula when applied next to the bowel wall. In patients with intestinal or peritoneal inflammation and/or multi-organ failure there is a 20% rate of intestinal fistulisation associated with the use of a VAC system.[15] Newer VAC systems designed to prevent the sponge from making direct contact with the bowel have yet to be evaluated.

Other causes of fistulas include colorectal cancer, diverticular disease and radiation. Fistulas resulting from radiation damage are usually complex and carry a high mortality. Rarer conditions include trauma and congenital fistulas, such as a patent vitellointestinal tract. Tuberculosis may fistulate as a complication of an ileal mass, and actinomycosis is an alternative possibility. Ulcerative colitis may fistulate, but this is more commonly postoperatively, and occasionally the diagnosis needs reviewing with regard to the possibility of Crohn's disease.

Loss of intestinal absorptive capacity

Inflammatory conditions of the small bowel can result in non-functioning enterocytes that reduce absorptive capacity. Such conditions include inflammatory bowel disease, scleroderma, amyloid, coeliac disease and radiation enteritis.

Loss of intestinal function

In the acute setting, postoperative ileus is the commonest reason for a loss of intestinal function, but this is usually self-limiting and does not require more than short-term supportive treatment. More chronic conditions, such as pseudo-obstruction, gastroparesis, visceral myopathy or autonomic neuropathy, can result in functional disability and present a significant challenge for management.

Pathophysiology

The three stages of intestinal failure

Following the initiating event, intestinal 'recovery' results in three recognisable phases that have implications for management.

Stage I: hypersecretory phase

Of the 7 litre's secreted daily by the duodenum, stomach, small intestine, pancreas and liver, about 6 litres are reabsorbed proximal to the ileocaecal valve and a further 800 mL are reabsorbed in the colon, leaving just 200 mL of water in the farces.

Lack of absorption results in large volume losses. This phase can last 1–2 months and is characterised by copious diarrhoea and/or high stoma or fistula outputs. The main focus of treatment is on fluid and electrolyte replacement while PN may be required to maintain nutrition.

Stage II: adaptation phase

The process of intestinal adaptation involves a series of histological changes in the intestinal mucosa that permit enhanced mucosal absorption within the residual intestine. The triggers for adaptation are the maintenance of fluid and electrolyte balance and the gradual introduction of enteral feeding. The process of adaptation takes 3–12 months and the degree of adaptation varies with age (more adaptation occurs in the paediatric population), underlying disease extent, and the site of resection (ileum has better capacity for adaptation than jejunum).

Stage III: stabilisation phase

Maximum intestinal adaptation may take up to 1–2 years and the extent and route of nutritional support will vary. The overall goal for the patient is to achieve as normal a lifestyle as possible, which means achieving stability at home.

Normal physiological functioning of the intestine involves complex fluid, electrolyte and nutrient exchanges to maintain homeostasis. Interruption of this can result in gross imbalances that require supplementation enterally or parenterally. The normal physiology of the intestine is discussed below.

Fluid and electrolytes

Sodium absorption in the small bowel is actively linked to the absorption of glucose and certain amino acids. Water absorption is passive and follows the sodium. The jejunum is freely permeable to water, so the contents remain isotonic.

✅✅ Movement of sodium into the lumen occurs if luminal sodium concentration is low, and absorption of sodium, and hence water, occurs only when the concentration is greater than 100 mmol/L.[16]

Sodium absorption normally occurs in the ileum and colon. In the absence of the absorptive capacity of the ileum and colon the net sodium losses are expectedly high. This occurs in the presence of a high fistula or jejunostomy; the daily net loss of sodium and net loss of water from the body will be approximately 300–400 mmol and 3–4 L, respectively. This highlights the importance of sodium replacement when there is a high jejunostomy or fistula. Oral fluid concentrated in sodium will help reduce enteric fluid losses. The minimum required daily oral sodium replacement is 100 mmol. The sodium concentration that is absorbable is limited by palatability.[17]

The colon has a significant absorptive capacity, amounting to 6–7 L of water, up to 700 mmol of sodium and 40 mmol of potassium per day. Connection of colon in continuity with the residual small bowel will significantly reduce water and sodium losses.

Potassium absorption is usually adequate unless there is less than 60 cm of small bowel. In this scenario, standard daily intravenous requirements of potassium are 60–100 mmol. Magnesium is usually absorbed in the distal jejunum and ileum. Loss of these will result in significant magnesium loss and deficiency. Magnesium deficiency may precipitate calcium deficiency because hypomagnesaemia impairs the release of parathyroid hormone.

Nutrients

Carbohydrates, proteins and water-soluble vitamins

The upper 200 cm of jejunum absorbs most carbohydrates, protein and water-soluble vitamins. Nitrogen is the macronutrient least affected by a decrease in the absorptive surface and utilisation of peptide-based diets rather than protein-based ones has demonstrated no benefit.[17] Water-soluble vitamin deficiencies are rare in patients with SBS, although thiamine deficiency has been reported.[18]

Fat, bile salts and fat-soluble vitamins

Fat and the fat-soluble vitamins (A, D, E and K) are absorbed over the length of the small intestine,[19] hence loss of ileum will impair absorption. Bile salts are also reabsorbed in the ileum and bile salt deficiency will contribute to reduced fat absorption. However, bile salt supplements such as cholestyramine have shown no benefit and may worsen steatorrhoea due to binding of dietary lipid[20] and may also worsen fat-soluble vitamin deficiency. In view of multifactorial metabolic bone disease, vitamin D_2 supplements are often given empirically along with calcium supplements. Vitamin A and E deficiencies have been reported, but usually an awareness that visual or neurological symptoms may indicate deficiency, combined with infrequent monitoring of serum levels, are all that is necessary. If the patient is wholly dependent on PN, then replacement along with vitamin K injections is required. Most patients have lost their terminal ileum and so require vitamin B_{12} replacement. Trace elements appear not to be a problem, with normal levels being found in patients on long-term PN.

Loss of bowel results not only in decreased absorptive capacity but also rapid transit. Reduced time for absorption will exacerbate nutritional deficiencies.

Adaptation

Following massive small-bowel resection there are changes in the mucosal surface of the remaining small intestine. Most experimental work has been in small animals such as rats. It appears that adaptation will occur only if there is enteral feeding. Patients who are wholly dependent on PN have mucosal atrophy, which is reversed on re-feeding enterally. The mechanism for this is at present unknown, but various trophic factors have been proposed. Current theory is that increased crypt cell proliferation leads to lengthening of villi and deepening of crypts, so resulting in increased surface area. Because the ileum has shorter villi it is able to adapt further, but is unfortunately more frequently resected. The stimulation to adapt appears to be threefold: (i) direct absorption of enteral nutrients leading to local mucosal hyperplasia; (ii) enteral nutrition resulting in the release of trophic hormones and a paracrine effect; and (iii) increased fluid and protein secretion with subsequent resorption, leading to increased enterocyte workload and adaptation.[19]

Another form of adaptation occurs in neonates, infants and young children, where continued developmental growth of the small intestine may make the difference between dependence on PN and managing with an enteral diet.[20]

Role of the colon in short-bowel syndrome

The colon has significant absorptive capacity, not only for fluid and electrolytes as described above, but also for short-chain fatty acids.[21,22] These are an energy substrate and in the region of 500 kcal may be derived in this way. It is estimated that having a colon is the equivalent of approximately 50 cm of small bowel for energy purposes.[23] The colon will also slow intestinal transit, particularly if the ileocaecal valve is present, which will improve absorption.

Having overcome the immediate problems of fluid balance and nutritional replacement, a frequent problem for those patients who still have their large bowel in continuity is diarrhoea. Excessive carbohydrate entry into the colon may result in osmotic diarrhoea.[24,25] Alternatively, choleric diarrhoea may be brought on by failure to reabsorb bile salts completely. Colonic bacteria deconjugate and dehydroxylate these into bile acids, which stimulate water and electrolyte secretion. In more extreme cases of SBS, bile salt depletion may occur that will give rise to steatorrhoea from incompletely digested long-chain fatty acids. Bile salts increase colonic permeability to oxalate. As the undigested fatty acids bind calcium in preference to oxalate, there is a resultant increase in enteric oxalate uptake and hence increased renal stone formation.[24]

> ✅✅ There is an increased frequency of mixed gallstones, possibly because of interruption of the enterohepatic circulation.[26]

Lastly, D-lactate acidosis[27] is a rare syndrome that comprises headache, drowsiness, stupor, confusion, behavioural disturbance, ataxia, blurred vision, ophthalmoplegia and/or nystagmus. The exact mechanism is unknown. It may be provoked by a carbohydrate load and is relieved by antibiotics. Whether it is a direct result of D-lactate or whether this is a marker for some other substance is unclear. There is anecdotal evidence that neomycin or vancomycin has led to improvements. Polymyxin E (Colistin), an antibiotic that has been shown to eradicate certain resistant strains, may also be useful in reducing the risk but specific evidence is lacking as the condition itself is uncommon.[28]

Surgical catastrophe and management

The management of IF and ECF can present a paradigm of multidisciplinary care. In patients who do not heal spontaneously, surgical treatment is generally one of the last of many steps in treatment. Owing to the heterogeneity of this condition, randomised controlled trials have not been performed and most recommendations are based on expert opinion. The multidisciplinary approach to management involves initial 'damage control' and medical management followed by definitive surgical management. It is vitally important to initiate wound and psychological management early in order to prevent and reduce effluent-associated excoriation and prepare the patient mentally for what may be at least a few months of therapy.

Resuscitation

The scenarios in which patients usually develop IF are often acute catastrophes, and the very nature of IF is such that patients are often severely fluid- and electrolyte-depleted. In the light of this, urgent fluid and electrolyte replacement is vital. This will often have been undertaken when the patient was first admitted to hospital, before transfer to a specialist intestinal failure centre.

Restitution

The key components of restitution may be summarised by the acronym SNAPP, representing sepsis, nutrition, anatomy, protection of skin and planned surgery.

Sepsis

Sepsis is often present in patients who have developed IF and adversely influences outcome.

> ✅ In a study of patients with enterocutaneous fistulas, Reber et al.[14] reported an overall mortality of 11%, with 65% of these associated with sepsis. In patients who had their sepsis controlled within 1 month the mortality was 8%, with spontaneous closure of the fistula in 48%. In those where sepsis remained uncontrolled the mortality was 85%, with a spontaneous closure rate of 6%.

Awareness of the high probability of associated sepsis is vital, and if the suspicion arises patients should be thoroughly investigated. Currently the optimum tool to identify collections is computed tomography (CT). Management includes appropriate antibiotics and drainage of sepsis. This is usually possible and successful radiologically, which is the preferred option. Surgical drainage carries a high risk of further bowel damage.

Nutrition

Sepsis and inflammatory bowel disease can add to patients' state of malnutrition. Replacement of fluid, electrolytes and nutrients, including carbohydrate, protein, fat and vitamins, is vital. Monitoring fluid and electrolyte replacement is a key part of nutritional support and involves serum electrolyte measurements and regular weight measurements. Hiram Studley in 1936 commented that 'weight loss is a basic indicator of surgical risk' and this still remains true today.

Fluid and electrolytes

Following resuscitation, fluid and electrolyte requirements will depend on the patient's losses. As described above, the first stage of IF is a hypersecretory phase, with high outputs and gastric hypersecretion. Fluid and electrolyte replacement should be by the intravenous route, with the following daily requirements:

- Water: losses + 1 L
- Na^+: losses (100 mmol/L effluent) + 80 mmol
- K^+: 80 mmol
- Mg^{2+}: 10 mmol

Nutritional support

Early return to enteral nutrition should be the aim as soon as the patient is haemodynamically stable and fluid and electrolyte replacement complete. Parenteral nutrition should be regarded as a support mechanism rather than the main source of calories. Overall energy requirements depend on the size and weight of the patient, activity levels and metabolic status, with sepsis increasing demand. Generally males require 25–30 kcal/kg/day and females 20–25 kcal/kg/day of non-protein energy. For research purposes, more exact estimates can be made using the Harris–Benedict equation:

$$\text{Male energy expenditure} = [66 + (13.7 + W) + (5 + H) \\ - (6.8 + A)] + SF$$
$$\text{Female energy expenditure} = [665 + (9.6 + W) + (1.7 + H) \\ - (4.7 + A)] + SF$$

where W represents weight (kg), H height (cm), A age (years) and SF stress factor.

However, the Harris–Benedict equation is inconvenient for daily use. Replacement should also include 1.0–1.5 kg/day of protein.

Daily requirements from the American Gastroenterological Association[29] for patients with SBS are recorded in Table 13.1.

Parenteral nutrition will provide calories (carbohydrate and fat), protein (amino acids), vitamins and trace elements. The volume should also be considered as part of the daily fluid requirement, with additional fluid given as normal saline.

Reduction of output

Losses from stomas, fistulas or the anus may be very substantial, making replacement and simple management difficult. A number of strategies should be introduced to reduce these losses. Although they should be allowed to eat solids, patients should be restricted to around 500 mL of water orally per day, as hypotonic drinks will increase output in patients with SBS. They should be cautioned against consumption of plain water and be given electrolyte solution, which will reduce intestinal fluid and electrolyte losses. There are several commercially available formulas. The St Mark's electrolyte solution is made from 1 L of water to which is added 20 g of glucose (six tablespoons), 3.5 g of sodium chloride (one level 5-mL teaspoon) and 2.5 g of sodium bicarbonate (one heaped 2.5-mL half teaspoon). This provides 100 mmol of sodium per litre. The problem is palatability, although this may be improved by the addition of orange squash or similar flavourings. Patients at home can make up this solution themselves. The World Health Organisation recommendations are similar but also contain 20 mmol of potassium chloride.[30]

Medication is given to reduce gastric hypersecretion. H_2-receptor blockers can reduce gastric hypersecretion,[31] as can proton pump inhibitors, but not always enough to obviate the need for parenteral fluid supplements.[32,33]

Patients are routinely started on high-dose omeprazole to reduce gastric output. Octreotide produces a similar action but is more expensive and has been shown to be of little benefit.

A review of all controlled studies evaluating the effects of somatostatin or octeotride showed that none demonstrated a significant increase in the rate of fistula closure.[34] Medication to slow intestinal transit or gastric emptying should in theory improve absorption,[31] so both codeine phosphate and loperamide[35,36] are used on an empirical basis. They are given before meals and often at higher doses than normal, frequently crushed. However, codeine runs the risk of addiction and clinical trials are equivocal as to the benefit of both,[37] so monitoring the effluent and weighing patients daily are essential for individual assessment. Bulking agents have shown no benefit in reducing stomal effluent. Cholestyramine may be used to treat hyperoxaluria, but it has no

Table 13.1 • Dietary macronutrient recommendations for short-bowel syndrome

	Colon present	Colon absent
Carbohydrate	Complex carbohydrate, 30–35 kcal/kg daily soluble fibre	Variable, 30–35 kcal/kg daily
Fat	MCT/LCT, 20–30% of caloric intake, with or without low fat/high fat	LCT, 20–30% of caloric intake, with or without low fat/high fat
Protein	Intact protein, 1.0–1.5 g/kg daily, with or without peptide-based formula	Intact protein, 1.0–1.5 g/kg daily, with or without peptide-based formula

LCT, long-chain triglyceride; MCT, medium-chain triglyceride.
Reproduced from Buchman AL, Scolapio J, Fryer J. AGA technical review on short bowel syndrome and intestinal transplantation. Gastroenterology 2003;124:1111–34. With permission from Elsevier.

place in those with a jejunostomy, and in those with a colon in continuity it may reduce jejunal bile salt concentration to a level below the minimal micellar concentration for absorption of fat, resulting in steatorrhoea. A review of long-term medication is always useful, paying particular heed to site of uptake. Enteric-coated tablets are unlikely to be useful.

Dietary modification

Oral feeding should be introduced gradually with additions made one at a time and assessed. Patients should remain fluid-restricted and continue on oral rehydration solution, gastric antisecretory drugs and antidiarrhoeal medication, the latter taken 30–60 minutes before meals. Drinking should be avoided during meals as this increases losses. It is important to continue intravenous maintenance therapy during this time as this will reduce the pressure on the patient to drink. In the early part of the second clinical stage it may be necessary to feed the patient wholly using PN, as gastric hypersecretion in response to even the smallest volume of enteral feeding can prejudice newly stabilised fluid balance.

A change of eating pattern to one of 'grazing' or 'little and often' increases the absorption window for the small intestine. Alternatively, overnight nasogastric tube or percutaneous endoscopic gastrostomy feeding can utilise otherwise unproductive absorption time.[38]

Oral magnesium oxide capsules, 12–16 mmol daily, are started and intravenous therapy is gradually withdrawn. Magnesium replacement may need to remain intravenous, albeit intermittent.

The precise balance between oral and parenteral requirements will vary between patients. Generally, daily stoma/fistula losses below 1500 mL may be managed with oral replacement alone; losses between 1500 and 2000 mL require sodium and water replacement, usually as subcutaneous or intravenous fluids, but no PN; and losses of more than 2000 mL per day require PN. Requirements will change over time as adaptation occurs; this can continue for up to 2 years and in the case of children can be very dramatic.

Outcome aims and monitoring

Clinically, the aim is for the patient to have no thirst or signs of dehydration, with acceptable strength, energy and appearance. Biochemical targets should include the following:
Gut loss: <2 L/day

- Urine: >1 L/day
- Urine Na^+: >20 mmol/L
- Serum Mg^{2+}: >0.7 mmol/L
- Body weight within 10% of normal.

The mainstays of monitoring in the first stage are those used in the normal postoperative patient (temperature, pulse, lying and standing blood pressure, urine output, and daily urea and electrolytes), combined with random estimations of urinary sodium osmolality. If urinary sodium content falls below 20 mmol/L, then deficiency is likely. As the patient stabilises, fluid balance is monitored with daily weight measurement and the observations are reduced in frequency. A meticulous watch is kept on the input/output volumes, with specifically designed charts for ease and clarity of recording. With the fluid balance under control and the eradication of any associated sepsis, reassessment of the underlying trend in the patient's nutritional status is performed. This is done by calculating body mass indices, skinfold thickness and serum albumin, and by making an estimate of likely return to normal activities. As the patient moves into the third stage of maximum adaptation, the common nutrient deficiencies are assessed (Table 13.2) and the rarer complications are clinically looked for (Box 13.1).

Parenteral nutrition

PN is used either as a temporary measure to maintain fluid and energy intake while the remaining small bowel undergoes adaptation or as definitive treatment in itself. The advantages of maintaining some enteral nutrition, even if not totally sufficient in terms of energy needs, include maintenance of normal gut flora, increased gastrointestinal adaptation and prevention of biliary sludge accumulation. With better understanding has come a willingness to maintain patients at home on PN. This is a great advantage for those who are dependent on PN and who have not otherwise responded to medical therapy. The benefits of the home environment cannot be overestimated in terms of morale and psychological well-being in an otherwise chronically hospitalised patient.[39] Home PN depends upon a stable physiological condition, a suitable social set-up and good patient education, coupled with a dedicated PN team providing technical support and advice. Even then, it is not without complications, the chief among them being catheter sepsis.[40,41] Meticulous aseptic technique on the part of the team and patient is essential if this is to be avoided. It takes about 3 weeks as an inpatient for the nursing staff to teach sufficiently rigorous self-care of the feeding line. Other complications, such as catheter occlusion, hepatic dysfunction, gallstones and bone disease, may occur.[42] Guidelines to its use are well established.[43]

Fistuloclysis

Fistuloclysis or distal enteral feeding involves cannulating the distal limb of a fistula and providing feeding to the distal non-functioning part of the bowel. Before fistuloclysis is carried out it is

Table 13.2 • Supplementation required in patients with intestinal failure depending on whether the patient needs partly enteral or wholly parenteral feeding

Nutrient	Parenteral	Partly enteral	Route
Potassium	Yes	If <60 cm and a jejunostomy	In PN or oral supplement
Magnesium	Common with a jejunostomy Uncommon with a colon		Magnesium oxide 12–24 mmol daily
Calcium	Uncertain	Vitamin D_2 400–900 IU daily	
Vitamin D	Uncertain		
Vitamin A	Uncommon		Watch for visual and neurological symptoms and monitor levels 3-yearly
Vitamin E	Uncommon		
Vitamin K	Yes	Normal	Monthly injections
Vitamin B complex	Yes	Normal	In PN
Vitamin C	Yes	Normal	In PN
Vitamin B_{12}	If terminal ileum lost (most patients)	Bimonthly hydroxycobalamin 1000 μg	
Iron	Yes	Normal	In PN
Zinc	Yes	Normal	In PN
Copper	Yes	Normal	In PN

PN, parenteral nutrition.

Box 13.1 • Complications of intestinal failure

Early
- Dehydration
- Hyponatraemia
- Shock
- Hypokalaemia

Intermediate
- Morale
- Weight loss
- Immune compromise
- Peptic ulcers
- Gastro-oesophageal reflux disease
- Proximal small-bowel inflammation
- Diarrhoea
- Bacterial overgrowth
- Peristomal excoriation

Late
- Vitamin deficiency syndromes
- Growth retardation in children
- Depression
- PN-induced liver disease
- Recurrent sepsis
- Intravenous line-related complications
- Cholelithiasis
- D-Lactate acidosis
- Urolithiasis

essential to ensure that there is no obstruction in the distal bowel and the efferent limb of the fistula can be cannulated easily. As shown in **Fig 13.1** the catheters can often be left in the bowel and covered by the stoma appliance. The fistula output can be re-fed into the distal bowel or a commercially available enteral feeding solution can be administered. In a specialised centre using fistula output has been shown to reduce the need for PN.[44] Patients may find the process cumbersome and as such it has not become common practice.[45]

Anatomy (mapping)

Defining the anatomy is important in terms of both planned management and prediction of long-term outcome. This may vary from determining how much small bowel remains, which may give an indication as to the likely necessity for permanent PN, to defining the anatomy of ECFs that will enable planned surgery later. The key facts to identify therefore are small-bowel anatomy, site of origin of a fistula (if present) and the anatomy of fistulous tracts.

Radiological contrast studies are the investigations of choice for assessing remaining bowel length and may include small-bowel follow-through or enema, and fistulograms. CT enteroclysis and MR[33] enteroclysis can also be very useful in examining pathological bowel and areas of other pathology, such as areas of ongoing obstruction or septic

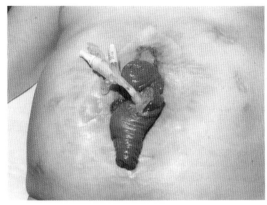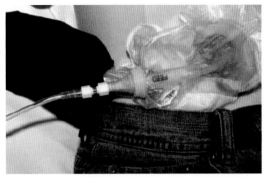

Figure 13.1 • The distal feeding catheter placed in the distal limb and subsequently covered by a stoma appliance.

collections.[46–48] CT scanning can also provide valuable information, such as safe sites of entry into the abdominal cavity. Active discussion between the IF team and the radiologists is essential as each case is unique and poses different questions.

Protection of skin

Protection of the skin is an essential component of management of patients with intestinal failure. Small-bowel output is caustic and excoriation of skin around a stoma or fistula is a painful, demoralising and highly visible immediate complication. The extent of the problem will vary, ranging from a standard end ileostomy, through patients with an ECF, to those with a laparostomy and multiple open loops of small bowel visible in the wound. This requires specialist stoma care from highly skilled nurses who use a wide variety of shaped appliances, wide-necked bags and protective dressings and pastes to protect the skin and contain the small-bowel contents. In exceptional situations, emergency surgery is indicated to either refashion a stoma or construct a controlled proximal stoma in the presence of a more distal fistula. An example of the need for this may be an enterovaginal fistula, where a proximal stoma is the only means of control possible.

The resolution of wounds over time may be very significant. This is usually a result of time, nutrition and skin protection. In the case of patients with laparostomy, there is usually significant reduction in the diameter of the wound and bowel loops become indistinguishable following growth of granulation tissue over them.

Planned surgery

Surgical intervention should be planned and is usually delayed. In the case of IF associated with ECF, early operative intervention to close the fistula is contraindicated by the associated high mortality due to re-fistulisation, sepsis, malnutrition and difficulties with fluid balance.[49] Delaying surgery for 6–12 months after the last operation has been shown to reduce both the mortality and fistula recurrence rates at subsequent definitive surgery (Table 13.3).[50–54]

Early surgery should be avoided if at all possible. Rarely the surgeon is forced to intervene for:[55]

1. excision of ischaemic bowel;
2. laying open of abscess cavities or removal of abdominal wall mesh;
3. construction of a controlled proximal stoma, for example in high output enterovaginal fistula.

These are usually the most septic patients and there is an associated high mortality with these procedures. Only in life-threatening situations should surgery be undertaken early in these patients and the decision should not be taken lightly as early surgery can result directly in multiple complications.

Patients managed with an open abdomen have a higher mortality and ECF rate when compared with historical case-matched controls with a closed abdomen,[56] patients with an open abdomen having a mortality rate of 25% and fistula formation rate of 14.8%.

Table 13.3 • The risk of mortality and ECF recurrence after surgery

Timing of Surgery	Early	3–12 weeks	6–12 months
Mortality	30–100%	7–20%	3–9%
ECF recurrence	40–60%	17–31%	10–14%

Reconstruction

When considering reconstructive surgery, the aim is to have a well patient, with no signs of dehydration or evidence of sepsis and with good nutritional status. The aim of the management described above is to produce this scenario, such that surgery can be undertaken as safely as possible. The decisions then concern when to operate and what to do.

The decision about when to operate is vital. In the 1960s, Edmunds et al. proposed that early intervention using a conservative approach was associated with 80% mortality compared with 6% mortality for an operative approach. Supportive care has changed significantly since that time, however, particularly the use of PN. In 1978, Reber et al.[14] proposed planned intervention following eradication of sepsis. In the case of ECF, they reported a proportion of spontaneous closures, of which 90% occurred within 1 month, 10% within the next 2 months and none thereafter.

As discussed above, early surgery is made extremely difficult by the severity of adhesions. It is important to delay surgery until these adhesions have softened, thereby reducing the risk of iatrogenic complications. This will often necessitate a delay of 5–6 months following the patient's previous surgical intervention. Clinically, this may be indicated by the identification of prolapse of stomas or fistulas, and by the impression, on examination, that the abdominal wall is moving separately from the underlying bowel (**Fig. 13.2**).

The second decision is what definitive reconstruction to undertake and this must be individualised. It may range from connecting an end ileostomy to the remaining colon, with the aim of bringing the colon into continuity, to closure of multiple complex fistulas in a hostile abdomen full of severe adhesions.

Surgery to increase nutrient and fluid absorption by either slowing intestinal transit or increasing intestinal surface area is not commonly undertaken in the adult population. The operations include reversed small-bowel segments,[57–59] colonic interposition and tapering with small-bowel lengthening.[60–62] The first two attempt to slow the transit of luminal contents by antiperistaltic activity or interposition of colonic tissue. They have achieved some clinical success but run the risk of further sacrifice of small bowel, obstruction or anastomotic leakage. Tapering with small-bowel lengthening (the Bianchi technique) has been applied in children with some success.[63] It involves dividing the dilated adapted bowel in two longitudinally, while maintaining mesenteric blood supply via careful dissection in the axis of the mesentery, allocating vessels to either segment. The bowel is then tubularised and joined sequentially.[64–66] However, no new mucosa is formed and there are risks of multiple adhesions and leakage or stenosis from the long anastomotic line.

The serial transverse enteroplasty (STEP) procedure involves serially stapling the dilated short bowel, leaving a lumen of 1–2 cm. The staple direction is alternated between the mesenteric and antimesenteric borders and the bowel length (but not overall surface area) is increased. Sudan et al. describe their experience with both the Bianchi and STEP procedures. In a combined analysis incorporating both children and adults, 69% of patients were off PN after intestinal lengthening. The exact benefit of intestinal lengthening procedures in the adult population is unclear in this analysis.[67]

Artificial valves, recirculation loops, electrical pacing,[68–70] tapering and plication, growth of neomucosa and mechanical tissue expansion[71] are all experimental techniques that are either untried in clinical practice or limited to case reports only.

Enterocutaneous fistula

High-output proximal small-bowel fistulas are associated with IF by producing functionally short bowel, and are often associated with significant problems with sepsis, malnutrition and difficulties with fluid balance.[49] Initial management is as described above.

Natural resolution of the fistula depends on the underlying pathology. Postoperative fistulas heal in around 70% of cases,[72] usually within the first 6 weeks of starting PN. Factors preventing healing may be specific to the fistula itself, as indicated in Table 13.4, or general, including ongoing sepsis, nutritional deficiency, or infiltration of the tract by underlying disease such as malignancy, Crohn's or tuberculosis.

Surgical intervention tends to be somewhat 'freestyle' as, despite detailed investigations, findings at surgery may be unexpected. General principles are well described.[73] The abdominal cavity is

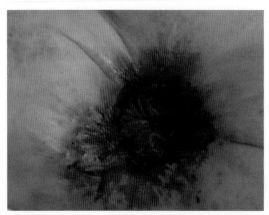

Figure 13.2 • Intestinal fistula with prolapsing bowel indicating correct time for surgery.

Table 13.4 • Factors influencing spontaneous fistula closure

	Unfavourable	Favourable
Anatomy	Jejunum	Ileum
	Short and wide fistula	Long and narrow fistula
	Mucocutaneous continuity	Mucocutaneous discontinuity
	Discontinuity of the bowel	Continuity of the bowel
Small bowel	Active disease	No active disease
	Distal obstruction	No distal obstruction

entered and the small bowel mobilised carefully as the adhesions are usually considerable. The fistula-bearing segment(s) of bowel is resected en bloc and the remaining ends of bowel re-anastomosed. This includes resection of any cutaneous abdominal wall component of the fistulous tract. If an anastomosis is likely to be in an area of residual sepsis, a stoma is usually advisable.

Abdominal wall closure may be problematic and may necessitate a component separation abdominoplasty in order to obtain fascial closure due to tissue loss from the abdominal wall, or the use of a biological mesh. In some circumstances where the loss of domain is quite significant tissue flaps may be required to treat the abdominal wall defects. The risk of refistulisation is particularly high if abdominal wall reconstruction is carried out with cross-linked porcine collagen mesh or synthetic mesh.[74]

Rehabilitation

The goal of therapy is for the patient to resume work and a normal lifestyle, or as normal a one as possible. This can be a considerable undertaking as the patient will generally have spent a prolonged period of time in hospital. Sending patients home on PN whilst they await surgery reduces the time to long-term rehabilitation.

Rehabilitation must be multidisciplinary, involving stoma care, physiotherapy, dietetics and occupational health. There needs to be detailed stoma care for patients with high-output stomas and referral to a community continence service for patients with intestinal continuity and incontinence due to liquid stools. Referral to a medical social worker for assistance with social security benefits is important. A proportion of patients will need to remain on intravenous therapy, either saline or PN. Patients must be taught how to manage their tunnelled feeding lines appropriately in order to allow them to move from a hospital environment to home.

Considerable psychological support may be required and patients should be put in contact with supporting organisations. Long-term sequelae must also be considered. This may involve long-term home PN or recurrence of the underlying disease. Long-term care will include regular monitoring and review of therapy, vitamin B_{12} replacement if more than 1 m of terminal ileum has been resected, and review of other nutrients such as zinc, iron, folic acid and fat-soluble vitamins.

Transplantation

Around two patients per million commence home PN and 50% are suitable for consideration of small-bowel transplantation. In the UK this results in a possible 50 cases per year (50% children). A study of 124 consecutive adult SBS patients with non-malignant disease at two centres in France reported survival of 86% at 2 years and 75% at 5 years.[75] Dependence on PN was 49% at 2 years and 45% at 5 years. Small-bowel transplantation remains an experimental procedure.

The latest update of the international intestinal transplant registry showed that 2887 transplants were carried out in 2699 patients since 1985. These procedures were carried out in 82 centres and individual centre volumes were low. It was difficult to determine specific reasons for graft failure from the registry data. Actuarial survival rates of 76%, 56% and 43% at 1, 5 and 10 years have been described. When a segment of colon was involved the function was better. Patients with a transplanted liver component, those with induction immune suppression and those who were not hospitalised in the period prior to transplantation were more likely to have better graft survival.[76]

A recent review of the adults in the Scientific Registry of Transplant Recipients showed that the risk of rejection is approximately 40% and prior to the year 2000 Crohn's disease was associated with a higher risk of rejection but after 2000 there has been no difference based on aetiology.[77] Five-year survival rates for intestine-only transplants of 100% and multivisceral transplants of up to 70% have been reported in individual centres in recent years, indicating the potential benefits of experience and potentially more effective immunosuppressive medications.[78]

The most recent evaluation has reported 1-year patient and graft survival of 79% and 64%, respectively, for intestine-only transplants, and 50% and 49%, respectively, for intestine/liver transplants. Long-term patient and graft survival for intestine-only transplants is 62% and 49%, respectively, at 3 years, and 50% and 38% at 5 years.[66]

Because survival is poorer than that of patients on home PN, the indication for transplantation is SBS not maintainable on dietary supplements, and in whom PN is no longer possible due to severe complications. These usually include lack of access sites because of central venous occlusion, or cholestatic liver disease progressing to fibrosis and cirrhosis. The possibility of gut-lengthening operations must be considered first. The portal vein must be patent and should be checked by Doppler studies, as should the other great veins, in a search for vascular access for the perioperative period.

Complications are chiefly due to graft rejection and immunosuppression. Rejection leads to bacterial translocation and sepsis in an immunosuppressed patient who is often already malnourished. Current immunosuppressives such as tacrolimus have been paramount in reducing graft sepsis but have adverse effects of neurotoxicity, nephrotoxicity and glucose intolerance. The antiproliferative agents may cause bone marrow suppression. The consequences of chronic steroid use are osteoporosis, cataracts and diabetes, and growth retardation in children. Opportunistic infections are a major problem, particularly cytomegalovirus.[79]

Supporting organisations

Like most chronic conditions, a supporting structure has evolved to assist in overall management. The patient support group is Patients on Intravenous and Nasogastric Nutrition Therapy (PINNT). The paediatric version is called half-PINNT. Apart from the functions of providing advice and understanding from patients in a similar condition, the association also enables the borrowing of portable equipment to allow holidays away from home.

The professional supporting body is the British Association of Parenteral and Enteral Nutrition (BAPEN). Keeping an overall view of intestinal failure is the British Artificial Nutritional Survey (BANS), which maintains a census of patients on long-term nutritional support. Most importantly, the pharmaceutical firms that supply the various nutritional preparations are also involved in providing and delivering the bags to patients at home; this includes maintenance contracts that ensure continued functioning of the necessary fridges and emergency back-up in case of failure.

Summary

Recent developments in IF, including home PN and a greater understanding of the pathophysiology of massive intestinal resection, have allowed clinicians to treat and maintain such patients, resulting in long-term survival. The complex medical and surgical management is prolonged and multidisciplinary. It is summarised in Box 13.2.

Box 13.2 • St Mark's intestinal failure protocol

Stage 1: Establish stability
Restrict oral fluids to 500 mL daily

Achieve and maintain reliable venous access
Administer intravenous sodium chloride 0.9% until the concentration of sodium in the urine is greater than 20 mmol/L

Maintain equilibrium by infusing:
1. Fluid: calculated from the previous day's losses and daily body weight records
2. Sodium: 100 mmol/L for every litre of previous day's intestinal loss plus 80 mmol (more if the intestinal loss is excessive)
3. Potassium: 60–80 mmol daily
4. Magnesium: 8–14 mmol daily
5. Calories, protein, vitamins, trace elements: only if enteral absorption is inadequate

Stage 2: Transfer to oral intake
1. Continue intravenous maintenance therapy
2. Start low-fibre meals
3. Start antidiarrhoeal medication 30–60 minutes before meals
4. Start gastric antisecretory drugs
5. Start oral rehydration solution. Discourage drinking around meal times
6. Restrict the intake of non-electrolyte drinks to 1 L daily
7. Encourage snacks and supplementary nourishing drinks, within above limits

Consider the need for enteral tube feeding
1. Start oral magnesium oxide capsules 12–16 mmol daily
2. If intestinal losses remain high, start octreotide 50–100 mg s.c. t.d.s.
3. Gradually withdraw intravenous therapy

Stage 3: Rehabilitation

1. The patient and family should by now understand the physiological changes that have occurred and the rationale for treatment
2. There needs to be detailed stoma care for patients with high-output stomas
3. Referral to community continence service for patients with intestinal continuity and incontinence due to liquid stools
4. Referral to medical social worker for assistance with social security benefits
5. If intravenous therapy cannot be withdrawn because of continuing intestinal losses (>2 L/day), teach the patient/family to perform intravenous therapy at home

Stage 4: Long-term care

1. Regular monitoring and review of therapy
2. Vitamin B_{12} replacement if more than 1 m of terminal ileum resected
3. Review other nutrients such as zinc, iron and folic acid and also fat-soluble vitamins

Key points

- Intestinal failure is a multifactorial entity with improved long-term outcome with developments in nutritional and specialised care.
- A clear understanding of normal intestinal physiology is required to understand the pathophysiology of IF.
- Prevention of IF is important and involves meticulous attention to anastomotic technique and techniques to preserve intestinal length in conditions such as Crohn's disease. The use of non-absorbable mesh and VAC dressings should be avoided in the setting of intestinal inflammation.
- Nutritional requirements will vary according to phase of IF. In the hypersecretory phase the aim is to maintain fluid balance and reduce stoma output, and PN may be required. In the adaptation and stabilisation phases enteral nutrition is encouraged and TPN requirements may be reduced or weaned.
- A staged approach to management will ensure good long-term outcome. Nutritional management, defining the anatomy by radiological means and skin protection should be the initial steps in management. Any definitive surgery should be deferred until nutritional optimisation has been achieved, all sepsis is eradicated and maturation of adhesions has occurred.
- The multidisciplinary team approach to management of IF is the standard of care and consideration should be given to referring these patients to a centre dedicated to the management of IF.
- Intestinal transplantation is a valuable addition to the armamentarium of treatments available for IF.

Full references available at **http://expertconsult.inkling.com**

Key references

16. Spiller RC, Jones BJ, Silk DB. Jejunal water and electrolyte absorption from two proprietary enteral feeds in man: importance of sodium content. Gut 1987;28:681–7. PMID: 3114056.

Highlights the importance of sodium concentration in water reabsorption in the intestinal lumen.

26. Nightingale JM, Lennard-Jones JE, Gertner DJ, et al. Colonic preservation reduces need for parenteral therapy, increases incidence of renal stones, but does not change high prevalence of gall stones in patients with a short bowel. Gut 1992;33:1493–7. PMID: 1452074.

Seminal paper on the role of the colon in reducing extraintestinal manifestations of intestinal failure.

14

Incontinence

Paul-Antoine Lehur
Gregory P. Thomas

Introduction

Faecal incontinence (FI), the involuntary loss of solid or liquid stool, is a debilitating condition with potentially devastating consequences for both physical and psychosocial well-being. Although surveys of the adult population have estimated the prevalence of FI to be between 1% and 19%,[1] the majority of sufferers do not seek medical help due to embarrassment and social stigmatisation.[2] As a result, the condition remains largely undiagnosed.

It is estimated that FI affects over half a million adults in the UK. This symptom/functional disorder has very profound negative consequences for the patient. Fear of embarrassment or public humiliation can impose major restrictions on individuals and their families.

> ✅ Faecal incontinence (FI) occurs when a person loses the ability to control their anal sphincter and bowel movements, resulting in leakage of faeces.

Aetiology

The ability to maintain continence to stool relies on a coordinated interplay of several factors, including stool consistency, rectal capacity and compliance, intact neural pathways, normal anal sphincter and pelvic floor function, and normal anorectal sensation. Deficiencies or failures in any component can lead to incontinence. In many cases, the aetiology of FI is multifactorial and it is impossible to ascertain the relative contribution of each factor, adding to the complexity of managing this condition.[3]

FI is most commonly an acquired disorder, so finding a cause is the first step to manage the disorder adequately (**Fig. 14.1**). Faecal loading or impaction is a major contributor to FI in an elderly, frail population. A rectum impacted with faeces can result in 'overflow incontinence'. It is easily diagnosed on digital examination. A rectally administered treatment is required to clear the bowel, followed by regular checks to avoid recurrence. When 'empty' on digital examination or when there is no relief from incontinence after evacuation of the rectum, the three main mechanisms (sometimes acting in combination) contributing to FI are: diarrhoea or loose stool, rectal volume/compliance reduction, and anatomical and/or functional injuries to the anal sphincter complex (Fig. 14.1).

Sphincter injury

In adult females, the most common cause of sphincter injury is obstetric trauma. After vaginal delivery, up to 10% of primiparous women have a clinically recognised sphincter disruption (**Fig. 14.2a**), and the incidence of occult injuries diagnosed sonographically can be as high as 30% after normal delivery.[4,5] More complicated deliveries, such as those involving instrumental delivery (forceps/vacuum-assisted), a large birth weight or a prolonged second stage of labour increase the risk of FI, and an episiotomy has not been shown consistently to protect against sphincter injury.[4-8]

Anorectal surgical procedures responsible for direct trauma to the anal sphincters with resultant incontinence include haemorrhoidectomy and

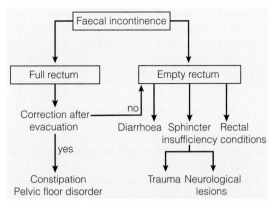

Figure 14.1 • The various mechanisms responsible for faecal incontinence: a guide to identifying a cause.

fistulotomy.[9-11] With the former, some patients report minor degrees of incontinence to flatus and/or faecal soiling due to loss of the normal anal cushions allied to sensory impairment in the anal canal. Risk factors for incontinence following fistula-in-ano surgery include high or complex fistulas or repeated procedures for recurrence or persistence (Fig. 14.2b). Manual anal dilatation for anal fissures has been associated with incontinence rates of up to 20% (in contrast, the use of lateral internal sphincterotomy has resulted in much lower rates). Incontinence may also arise following major colorectal resections, such as low anterior resection with colorectal or colo-anal anastomosis, due to the reduction in or loss of the rectal reservoir capacity and also to the disruption of intramural

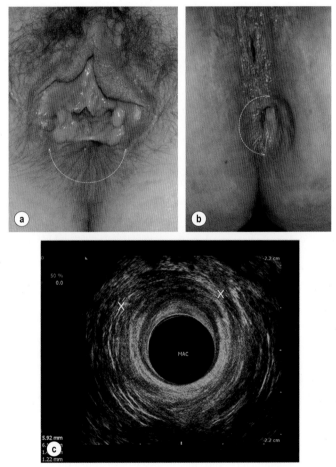

Figure 14.2 • **(a)** Examination in lithotomy (gynaecological) position: anterior anal sphincter defect, a sequela of fourth-degree tear following vaginal delivery. Obstetric injury of the perineum is classified as a first-degree tear if confined to vaginal mucosa and perineal skin, second-degree if the perineal muscles are torn, third-degree if the anal sphincter is torn, and fourth-degree if both sphincter and anorectal mucosa are torn. In the illustrated situation, the anal sphincter muscles and perineal body have separated, leaving a large anterior hemi-circumferential defect splaying open the anal sphincters in a horseshoe-type configuration (*arrows*). Here the defect was such that the anal and vaginal mucosa have healed to form a cloacal defect. **(b)** Examination in lithotomy (gynaecological) position: left lateral anal sphincter defect, sequela of an extensive fistulotomy for complex anal fistula, resulting in a gaping anus (*arrows*). **(c)** Endoanal ultrasonography (EAUS). Anterior defect of internal and external sphincters (*between marks*) visualised on two-dimensional image of the anal canal.

nerve pathways. Function can be further adversely affected by chemotherapy and/or radiation. This forms part of what is referred to today as low anterior resection syndrome (LARS).

Trauma to the perineum or pelvis, such as pelvic fractures or impalement injuries, can be associated with significant damage to both the anal sphincter and its nerve supply,[6,10] along with collateral damage to other pelvic floor structures, such as the bladder and urethra. Occasionally, injuries associated with a sexual assault may result in faecal incontinence.

Neurological diseases, such as multiple sclerosis, muscular dystrophies or congenital myelomeningocoele (spina bifida), can cause incontinence, frequently coupled with constipation and evacuation problems.

The sequelae of congenital abnormalities, like anal agenesis or Hirschsprung's disease treated in childhood, can also be responsible for later faecal incontinence, with their own specific management.

Rectal compliance

The rectum can become stiff and uncompliant, so that it will not adapt to filling, due to conditions such as inflammatory bowel disease (Crohn's disease, ulcerative colitis), radiation proctopathy and irritable bowel syndrome.[11]

'Idiopathic' faecal incontinence

Often, the precise aetiology is unclear and the incontinence is termed 'idiopathic'. Pudendal neuropathy, conceptually demonstrated by delayed pudendal nerve terminal motor latency and an increase in mean nerve fibre density (which can be hard to show in practice), is considered to be present in the majority of these patients.[12] Low squeeze pressures and decreased anal canal sensation are usually found. Idiopathic faecal incontinence may result from chronic straining during defecation and perineal descent, as first described by Parks.[13] Perineal descent also appears to be related to the number of vaginal deliveries, thereby leading to another way in which the pudendal nerves can be damaged. Indeed, a majority of cases of FI secondary to obstetric damage is due to a combination of traumatic injury to the anal sphincters and the associated trauma to the pelvic floor nerve supply, the latter only becoming evident many years later at the onset of menopause. To make matters worse, these patients present frequently with associated urinary incontinence (double incontinence), which should be identified and managed accordingly.

This multifactorial aetiology results in a wide variation in clinical presentation and much overlap between the above groups. Clinically, patients may present with either a pattern of 'urge incontinence', where they are unable to actively defer a bowel movement, 'passive incontinence', with the patient unaware of stool leakage, or a 'mixed pattern'. While a patient presenting with urge incontinence may suggest external anal sphincter pathology, this may also be a feature of rectal pathology, such as proctitis or carcinoma. Conversely, passive soiling is more suggestive of a deficient internal anal sphincter or an anatomical deformity from a fistula-in-ano or post-surgical scarring.

Added to the complexity is the frequent coexistence of other pelvic floor pathologies, such as rectal intussusception, which can itself result in patients presenting with varying combinations and severity of urge and passive incontinence or post-defecatory leakage. Indeed, up to 75% of patients with rectal intussusception have incontinence, with some presenting only with this symptom.[14] Although the exact mechanism remains unclear, it is postulated that rectal intussusception stretches the internal anal sphincter and inappropriately triggers the rectoanal inhibitory reflex, leading to temporary reversal of the pressure gradient in the anal canal and soiling. The accompanying incomplete rectal emptying of this defecatory disorder can also contribute to post-defecatory leakage.

> ✅ Faecal incontinence is a symptom, not a diagnosis. This symptom should not be ignored as something can be done. It is important to identify the underlying causes for each individual and this is often multifactorial.

Presentation

History

Clinical assessment starts with a detailed history. The frequency and severity of incontinence episodes are best quantified using a 3-week stool diary completed by the patient. It is an essential and simple tool to ascertain a baseline of incontinence episodes. It will serve as a useful comparator when referred back to during treatment. Standardised scoring systems are a useful complement and provide an objective assessment tool (Table 14.1).[15] It is also important to assess stool consistency using the Bristol stool chart, which rates it on a seven-point scale from hard to liquid. Finally, a quality of life assessment is provided by the Faecal Incontinence Quality of Life (FIQoL) instrument that attempts to measure any impairment in quality of life 'due to accidental bowel leakage' in four different domains: lifestyle, coping and behaviour, depression, and embarrassment.[16]

Table 14.1 • St Mark's Incontinence Score[15]

	Never	Rarely	Sometimes	Weekly	Daily
Incontinence for solid stool	0	1	2	3	4
Incontinence for liquid stool	0	1	2	3	4
Incontinence for gas	0	1	2	3	4
Alteration in lifestyle	0	1	2	3	4
			No	Yes	
Need to wear a pad or plug			0	2	
Taking constipating medicines			0	2	
Lack of ability to defer defecation for 15 minutes			0	4	

Definitions: *Never*: no episodes in the past 4 weeks. *Rarely*: one episode in the past 4 weeks. *Sometimes*: more than one episode in the past 4 weeks but less than one a week. *Weekly*: one or more episodes a week but less than one per day. *Daily*: one or more episodes a day.
Add one score from each row: minimum score = 0 (perfect continence); maximum score = 24 (totally incontinent).

The history offers clues to the possible aetiology of incontinence. In women, an obstetric history is mandatory, including number of pregnancies, mode of delivery, birth weight and type of presentation. The hormonal status is recorded, as well as the presence of any concomitant urinary incontinence, which could suggest a more global pelvic floor deficiency. A history of anal surgery is important, particularly in men, because up to 25% of male patients with faecal incontinence have an iatrogenic sphincter injury.

It is too simplistic to attribute all patients with urge incontinence and all patients with passive incontinence as having external and internal sphincter weakness, respectively. The scenario is often more complex, with patients presenting with an overlap of symptoms. Some may even present with mixed symptoms of faecal incontinence and obstructed defecation, which should make the clinician consider a possible rectal intussusception.[17]

Examination

A general examination (abdomen and neurological examination of the back and lower limbs) should be performed. Next, the perianal skin should be inspected for any scars of trauma or surgery (Fig. 14.2), as well as skin excoriation that might suggest long-term seepage of stool. The pelvic floor should be examined for evidence of a descended perineum. A gaping anal orifice when pulling apart the buttocks suggests decreased resting tone, absent or weak voluntary contraction and pudendal neuropathy. The patient should be asked to strain to accentuate a descending perineum or exteriorise any rectal prolapse or rectocele. An external prolapse may become more evident if the patient is examined on the lavatory. In addition, when examining the patient in the gynaecological position any mid- or anterior compartment deficiencies should be visible, including utero-vaginal prolapse and cystocoele respectively.

Sensory perception at the anal margin must be checked and a digital rectal examination performed to assess resting and squeeze anal pressures and contraction of the puborectalis muscle, as well as to confirm the presence of a rectocele. With an educated finger, defects in the sphincter muscles can be felt, and straining can also reveal subtle cases of rectal intussusception and enterocele. Finding impacted stool suggests overflow as a possible mechanism for incontinence.

Investigations

The indications for and extent of diagnostic work-up are guided by duration and severity of symptoms, response to initial conservative management, and ultimately fitness for surgery (see Box 14.1). It is also imperative to exclude any coexisting organic pathology that could lead to symptoms of faecal incontinence and warrant urgent attention.

Anorectal physiology studies are essential in providing an objective assessment of anal sphincter pressures, rectal sensation, rectoanal reflexes and rectal compliance, all of which guide management.[6] Manometry is a simple method for measuring internal (resting) and external anal sphincter (squeeze) tone, which are usually low in patients with faecal incontinence. Although the findings of anorectal physiology studies do not consistently correlate with symptom severity, they may influence the treatment options and guide biofeedback training modalities.[3]

Box 14.1 • Work-up for faecal incontinence: a summary

A. Symptom assessment
- Careful history-taking
- Three-week stool diary
- Faecal Incontinence Score[15]
- Bristol stool chart[18]
- Faecal Incontinence Quality of Life instrument[16]
- Urinary incontinence
- Constipation

B. Clinical assessment
- General examination (including neurological)
- Anorectal examination
- Assessment of the anterior compartment
- Cognitive assessment (if needed)

C. Investigations
- Exclude organic pathology
- Colonoscopy – or flexible sigmoidoscopy
- Pelvic ultrasound – cervical smears
- Anorectal physiology tests
- Endoanal ultrasonography
- Standard or MRI dynamic defecography

✅ Baseline assessment in faecal incontinence relies on a structured evaluation, including patient reporting of symptoms, careful and sensible clinical examination, and investigations that arise from this focused history-taking and examination.

Management of faecal incontinence in adults

The treatment of faecal incontinence is mainly guided by the severity of symptoms, the aetiology and the structural integrity of the sphincter muscles. Despite a number of publications on the topic, it has to be borne in mind that current recommendations are based more on expert opinion than high-quality evidence. Indeed, most of the published literature in this field reports single series studies. Very few are large randomised comparative studies. Given this absence of truly strong objective evidence, the patient's own views are all the more important. It is also worth remembering that this is a 'benign' problem. Although it will affect quality of life significantly, it is not life-threatening. Many of the surgical interventions described below carry the risk of complications, of varying degrees of severity. The risk of these must be balanced against the patient's individual condition. A proposed treatment algorithm is shown in **Fig. 14.3.**

✅ Management of faecal incontinence is multi- and trans-disciplinary, often involving several specialists working to provide holistic care to help the patient cope with the broad range of needs, including consideration of the psychological impact of this potentially stigmatising handicap. With a few exceptions, conservative measures should be used first before more invasive treatments.

Endoanal ultrasonography (EAUS) provides a dynamic assessment of the thickness and structural integrity of the external and internal sphincter muscle using an intra-anal probe. It is the procedure of choice to diagnose sphincter defects in patients with suspected sphincter injury. When performed by an experienced clinician, EAUS approaches 100% sensitivity and specificity in identifying internal and external sphincter defects.[19] However, the presence of a sphincter defect does not necessarily correlate with incontinence. In a study of 335 patients with incontinence, 115 patients who were continent and 18 asymptomatic female volunteers, EAUS detected sphincter defects in 65%, 43% and 22%, respectively.[20]

Dynamic standard or magnetic resonance imaging (MRI) defaecography is not a routine test in incontinent patients as it relies on the patient's ability to retain paste. However, it is useful in selected cases when there are mixed symptoms, including obstructed defecation, where an occult prolapse may be responsible for the incontinence, particularly when other tests have failed to identify a clear cause (e.g. normal or near-normal anal pressures and intact anal sphincters).

At first glance, pelvic floor electrophysiological assessment, including pudendal nerve terminal motor latency, might be considered useful, but lack of a direct impact on treatment strategy, the operator-dependent nature of the test and patient discomfort have significantly limited its use in many centres.

Conservative measures

First-line treatment of faecal incontinence is conservative. These measures can also be used as adjuncts to subsequent surgical procedures.

Dietary modification and medications

Liquid stools exacerbate faecal incontinence. An increase in dietary fibre may improve stool consistency. Stool bulking agents (e.g. psyllium) also improve stool consistency and decrease symptoms of incontinence. The recommended dose is 25–30 g/day. A gradual increase in fibre intake will minimise the associated abdominal

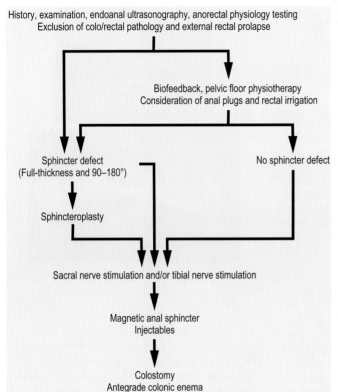

Figure 14.3 • Proposed treatment algorithm for faecal incontinence.

History, examination, endoanal ultrasonography, anorectal physiology testing
Exclusion of colo/rectal pathology and external rectal prolapse

Biofeedback, pelvic floor physiotherapy
Consideration of anal plugs and rectal irrigation

Sphincter defect
(Full-thickness and 90–180°)

No sphincter defect

Sphincteroplasty

Sacral nerve stimulation and/or tibial nerve stimulation

Magnetic anal sphincter
Injectables

Colostomy
Antegrade colonic enema

bloating and discomfort. Dairy products should be avoided in patients with lactose intolerance. Antidiarrhoeal agents are also useful and the first drug of choice should be loperamide (0.5–16 mg/day as required). This should be started with low doses (less than 2 mg) to avoid constipation, and loperamide hydrochloride syrup should be considered if fractions of a conventional dose are required. People unable to tolerate loperamide hydrochloride should be offered codeine phosphate or co-phenotrope. Cholestyramine chelates bile salts, the latter being occasionally responsible for diarrhoea, and may be worth a try.

Small retrograde enemas and suppositories can promote more complete bowel emptying and as a consequence reduce soiling. In more intractable cases, such as spinal cord-injured patients with overflow incontinence from severe faecal impaction, a regular enema programme using specially designed apparatus has proved to be highly effective[21] (**Fig. 14.4**). Rectal irrigation may also be helpful in those with non-neurogenic incontinence.[22] It may also be useful in situations where the patients have cognitive impairment or in the elderly infirm, in order to prevent skin excoriation and infections from frequent soiling.

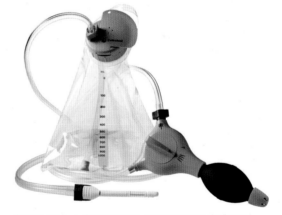

Figure 14.4 • Conservative management: dedicated material for transanal retrograde colonic enemas/irrigation.

Biofeedback and pelvic floor muscle retraining

Biofeedback (BFB) – also known as 'behavioural therapy' – uses visual, auditory or verbal feedback techniques, with three main goals: strength training, sensory training and coordination training.

The treatment protocol should be customised for each patient based upon the supposed underlying pathophysiological mechanism. A set of 10–15 sessions (two per week) is recommended to assess the efficacy of the biofeedback, with regular 'recall' sessions every 6 months for surveillance of progress. Supportive counselling and practical advice regarding diet and skin care play an important role in the success of biofeedback. More recently, some units offer group sessions rather than individual consultations. Anecdotal reports suggest that this may be an efficient and effective approach. This may, in part, be due to the reassurance that patients gain from seeing others in the same predicament.

The benefit of BFB varies, with a wide range of improvement reported (64–89%).[6] Exact assessment of its effect is difficult due to the different definitions of success, differing therapeutic regimens, varied selection criteria, fluctuating individual motivations and therapist enthusiasm. Improved rectal sensation after biofeedback is one of the most consistent predictors for improved continence.

The most recent Cochrane review concluded that the poor quality of published evidence does not allow a definitive assessment of the role of pelvic floor exercises and biofeedback in the management of faecal incontinence. Nevertheless, the authors suggested that biofeedback with electrical stimulation is likely to be more beneficial than exercises or electrical stimulation alone. In general, some elements of biofeedback and sphincter exercises are likely to be beneficial.[23] The current consensus is that BFB as a treatment for faecal incontinence is possibly effective and is recommended because it is painless and risk-free, after other behavioural and medical management has been tried and inadequate symptom relief has been obtained. Pelvic floor muscle exercises are recommended as an early intervention based upon low cost, no morbidity and some weak evidence suggesting efficacy.

Anal plug

The Peristeen anal plugs (Coloplast Ltd, UK) are disposable devices that expand when soaked with rectal mucus and control continence by blocking the passage of stool. Unfortunately, they can become uncomfortable and are poorly tolerated by many. They may be helpful in preventing faecal incontinence in selected groups, such as patients with neurological impairment (spina bifida) who have less anal sensation and thus greater toleration.[24] A newer anal plug, called the Renew device (Renew Medical Inc. Ca, USA) (**Fig. 14.5**) has had encouraging reports. Lukacz and colleagues[25] reported the outcome of a single group study. Eighty per cent persisted with this device, with 77% of those who completed the course of treatment reporting a

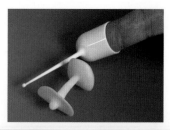
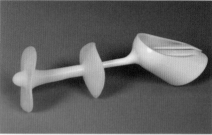

Figure 14.5 • Renew anal plug, with and without applicator.

greater than 50% reduction in incontinent episodes. More work is needed to further evaluate this device.

> ✅ A patient is referred for surgical consideration after conservative treatment has failed. The surgeon should ensure that these measures of conservative management have been correctly and adequately administered before embarking on surgery.

Surgery

Surgical treatment for faecal incontinence is reserved for patients who in whom conservative therapy has failed. The available techniques range from direct repair of damaged sphincters (e.g. sphincteroplasty) to techniques that augment the function of (e.g. injectables, sacral nerve and tibial nerve stimulation) or replace the native anal sphincter complex (e.g. artificial bowel sphincter, dynamic graciloplasty or magnetic anal sphincter). The relatively lower morbidity of the neuromodulatory treatments such as sacral and tibial nerve stimulation, means that these are often considered first before more invasive treatments. A stoma should not be perceived as a failure of management and when appropriately chosen can significantly improve nursing care and provide a better quality of life for affected patients.

Sphincteroplasty

'Anal sphincteroplasty' describes a secondary (delayed) repair of the anal sphincter muscles. It is distinct from an 'anal sphincter repair', a term used to describe primary (immediate) repair of the anal sphincters following direct trauma, in the UK often being performed by the attending obstetrician.

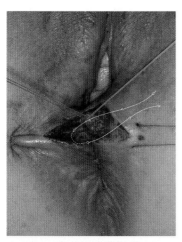

Figure 14.6 • Sphincteroplasty for anterior sphincter defect following obstetric injury. Overlapping anal sphincter repair: two edges of detached sphincter muscles dissected free and mobilised with the scar tissue; The U-shaped suturing (*arrows*) uses either non-absorbable or absorbable sutures to bring both muscle ends together.

Anterior sphincteroplasty following an obstetric injury is the most common type of reconstruction performed. Overlapping sphincteroplasty is the standard of care (**Fig. 14.6**). Normally, both the external and internal sphincters are included together in the repair; separation and individual repair of these is not thought to confer any benefit. It is performed under general anaesthesia with the patient either in the prone jack-knife or lithotomy position.[26] An incision is made transversely between the anus and the vaginal introitus. The scar tissue and muscle ends are dissected from the anal canal posteriorly and the vagina anteriorly without separate identification and repair of the internal anal sphincter. Adequate mobilisation is necessary to ensure a tension-free wrap. The scar tissue is then divided and the two ends are overlapped over the midline and stitched with 2/0 mattress sutures. A levatorplasty can be added, taking great care not to narrow the vagina excessively, which can cause dyspareunia. A 'T'-closure of the skin with interrupted absorbable sutures is often feasible. A small opening can be left in the centre of the wound or a Penrose drain inserted. A small study of 10 patients suggested that reinforcement of the repair with a small collagen porcine mesh may be beneficial.[27] However, this has not been investigated in larger studies.

✔ Preoperative counselling should highlight postoperative wound infection and delayed healing as the most common complications.[26]

Sphincteroplasty confers substantial benefits in patients with localised (from 90 to 180 degrees of circumference) full-thickness sphincter defects. There are no established factors that predict outcome, but it is thought that those with poor function of the residual sphincter muscle preoperatively are probably unlikely to have a good result. The young patient who attends with a cloaca type defect should be considered for a sphincteroplasty and perineal reconstruction, irrespective of residual function. There may or may not be a gain in function, but the restoration of anatomy will be of significant benefit to this particular patient group.

The presence of a persistent sphincter defect after repair may be associated with early failure.[28] These may be amenable to a repeat repair. Short-term outcomes suggest good-to-excellent results in a majority of patients. There is, however, increasing evidence that continence deteriorates over 5–10 years.[29] A systematic review analysed the outcome of over 900 reported repairs. Marked heterogeneity of symptom reporting was found. However, there appeared to be good results initially, which tailed off. There was poor correlation between symptoms and quality of life, and all articles reported high satisfaction scores despite decline in continence.[30] Adjuvant biofeedback therapy after surgery may improve quality of life and help sustain symptomatic improvement with time. Previous sphincter repair does not seem to affect the clinical outcome of a subsequent repair. In a comparative study, the outcome was similar between patients with or without a previous sphincter repair, with good results obtained in 50% and 58% of patients, respectively.[31] Indeed, the long-term benefit of a repeat sphincter repair was similar to an initial repair.[32]

Pelvic floor repair (postanal, preanal or total)

Different types of pelvic floor repair have been described in the past.[33] These are rarely practised today, and are of historical interest only. The aim of postanal repair[34] was to increase the length of the anal canal, restore the anorectal angle and recreate the flap valve mechanism, which at the time was thought essential for maintaining faecal continence. Despite initial improvement, the long-term results of postanal repair or total pelvic floor repair for neurogenic faecal incontinence have been disappointing. Postanal repair or total pelvic floor repair now have no place in the treatment of neuropathic faecal incontinence, as better options are available.

Sphincter reconstruction – muscle transposition

Non-stimulated[35] and stimulated muscle transpositions[36] have been devised to replace the anal sphincter (*neosphincter*) when local repair is not possible or has failed. Transposition of one or both gluteal muscles from the buttock (*gluteoplasty*) has been used, as well as transposition of the gracilis muscle from the leg, which is wrapped around the anus to form a new sphincter (*graciloplasty*). Improved results were noted when an implantable electrical stimulator was applied to the transposed gracilis muscle.[36] However, this was not maintained in the medium to longer terms. Considerable postoperative morbidity was noted in many of these patients. For these reasons, muscle transposition procedures are rarely performed these days.

Artificial sphincters

Artificial sphincters can be defined as any kind of implanted device intended to replace or reinforce the native sphincteric mechanism. They aim to be a substitute for normal sphincters. As such, it is necessary that they are efficient for both terminal bowel functions, of continence and evacuation; their implantation is safe and reproducible, with a limited need for patient/medical intervention and follow-up after implantation; finally, they should be cost-effective.

Artificial bowel sphincter

Artificial sphincters initially used in humans were silicone, pressure-regulated devices restoring continence through an inflatable cuff placed around the lower rectum or upper anal canal. The majority of the published literature concerns the Acticon Neopshincter ™ (American Medical Systems (AMS), Minnetonka, MN, USA) artificial bowel sphincter (ABS). It comprises a fluid-filled cuff that encircles and compresses the anal canal. A pressure-regulating balloon is implanted in the retropubic space of Retzius. A pump placed in the labia majora or scrotum, which is accessible to the patient, controls the system. To initiate defecation, squeezing the pump empties the cuff by transferring fluid into the balloon, permitting passage of stool. The cuff then refills automatically from pressure built up in the balloon.

Few of these, if any, are implanted currently since the device is no longer commercially available. Concerns about the high complication rate, late mechanical failure due to perforation of the cuff, and the availability of less invasive treatments, are likely to be responsible for this. Much of the recent data have described long-term outcome of these devices in expert centres that have mastered the technique; they report rather satisfactory results.[37] The ABS in its present state has no role in severe faecal incontinence as it has been superseded by less invasive treatments.

Magnetic anal sphincter

Studied in small trials, the magnetic anal sphincter (MAS; FENIX®, Torax Medical Inc., Shoreview, MN, USA) is a novel device designed to augment the native anal sphincter (**Fig. 14.7**). It consists of a series of titanium beads with magnetic cores hermetically sealed inside. The beads are interlinked with independent titanium wires to form a flexible ring that rests around the external anal sphincter in a circular fashion. The device is manufactured in different lengths determined by the number of beads (14–20) necessary to accommodate the variation in anal canal circumference.

One of the advantages of this still investigational device over the previous artificial sphincters is that it begins working immediately, without the need for subsequent manipulation by either the patient or surgeon. The procedure for implantation is also substantially simpler than the ABS because access to the perineum alone is required.

A multicentre feasibility study demonstrated good short-term restoration of continence with limited morbidity.[38] Subsequent non-randomised comparative cohort studies compared the results of MAS with the ABS[39] and SNS.[40] Both showed that the MAS was similarly effective in restoring continence and quality of life without any difference in morbidity. Further studies have demonstrated its efficacy.[41] It is uncertain where the MAS should lie in the treatment algorithm of faecal incontinence. The SaFaRI study is a large multicentre study, currently underway in the UK.[42] This aims to compare the MAS with SNS. The results of this trial are keenly awaited. In carefully selected patients, MAS appears to be a promising innovation as it offers a less invasive and simpler alternative of anal reinforcement than the ABS. However, with only short-term follow-up available, it remains to be seen if the promise of the MAS can withstand the test of time.

Sacral nerve stimulation

Sacral nerve stimulation (SNS) was first described for use in urological disorders and was adapted for use in faecal incontinence in 1995.[43] The mechanism of action of SNS is unclear. There are no consistent anal or pelvic floor motor responses evident in the literature.[44] It is believed to work by alteration, or modulation, of ascending spinal sensory pathways. This may have an effect on local colonic and rectal reflexes and also on the sensory cortex.[45] Because of this, it is often referred to as sacral neuromodulation rather than stimulation. Its effect appears to be genuine. A crossover study in 34 patients comparing active with deactivated devices demonstrated a significant improvement in incontinent symptoms during the active stage.[46]

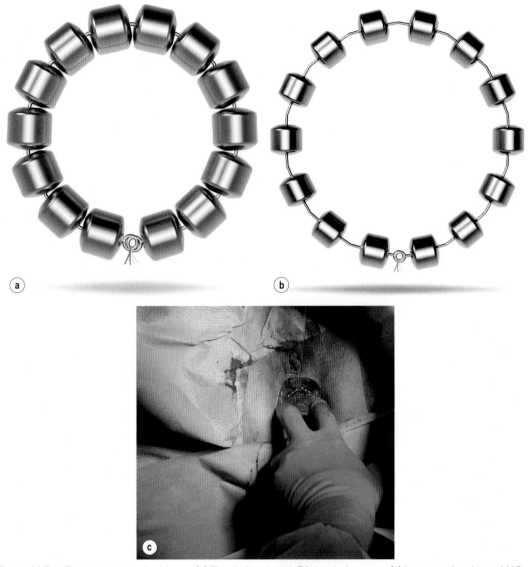

Figure 14.7 • The magnetic anal sphincter. **(a)** The device closed; **(b)** the device open; **(c)** intraoperative view at MAS implantation.

SNS consists of a *screening phase* of peripheral nerve evaluation (PNE), followed by a second *therapeutic phase* of permanent neurostimulator implantation (**Figs 14.8** and **14.9**). In the initial diagnostic phase of PNE, which can be performed under local or general anaesthesia with the patient in the prone position, the S3 foramen is preferentially cannulated under fluoroscopic guidance with an electrode through which stimulation is performed, looking for an appropriate 'bellows response' of the pelvic floor and plantar flexion of the ipsilateral great toe. This is sometimes repeated on the contralateral side to select the best response, with some surgeons routinely screening the S2 and S4 positions as well.

Once a location is decided upon, the electrode is secured in place and connected to a portable external stimulator. The patient then undergoes a 3-week trial of stimulation while filling out a bowel-habit diary. Only patients with significant clinical improvement, demonstrated by a reduction in frequency of episodes or days of faecal incontinence of at least 50%, are then selected for the *therapeutic phase*, of permanent stimulator implantation. The permanent stimulator is placed subcutaneously in the gluteal area under local anaesthesia. The pulse generator is activated and stimulation parameters are set by telemetry. The patient can deactivate it with a small, hand-held device, the 'patient programmer'.

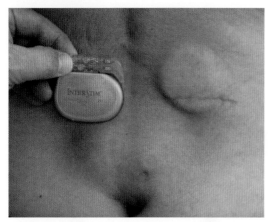

Figure 14.8 • Sacral nerve stimulation: Interstim™ pulse generator (left) and the implanted generator in a thin patient (right).

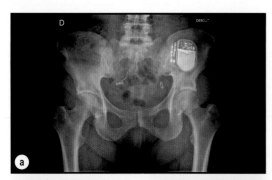

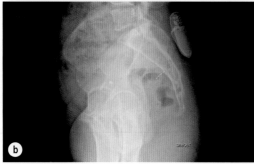

Figure 14.9 • Sacral nerve stimulator on plain X-ray: **(a)** AP and **(b)** lateral views.

> ✓ SNS is a minimally invasive technique with low morbidity. The decision to implant a permanent neurostimulator is made on the basis of clinical improvement during test stimulation.

Sacral nerve stimulation is an attractive treatment option for several reasons. It is minimally invasive, a trial phase allows one to decide on the suitability for permanent implantation, and it has minimal morbidity. Studies have shown that SNS is feasible,

with sustainable long-term results. In a series of 228 patients long-term improvement was seen in 71% at a median follow-up of 84 (70–113) months. The frequency of incontinent episodes per week fell from 7 to 0.5, and the St Mark's incontinence score improved from a median of 19 to 6 (both $P < 0.001$). Fifty per cent of the patients achieved complete continence. However, when the number who underwent test stimulation is taken into account, on an intention-to-treat basis, then full continence was achieved in just over 33% of patients.[47] Another study looked at the outcome of 101 patients at 5 years. Sixty of these patients reported a favourable outcome, and 41 reported an unfavourable outcome. Of these, 24 had their implant deactivated or removed. The authors found that age was a negative predictive factor for success. They found that both an improvement in urgency during the test stage and a good outcome at 6 months were predictive of success. This last finding may highlight the problems associated with patient-reported outcome as a way of judging success of test stimulation.[48]

However, this technique is not free of complications, with reported morbidity including implant site pain (28%), paraesthesia (15%), change in sensation of stimulation (12%) and infection (10%), with less than 5% requiring device explantation. A meta-analysis of 34 studies reported an overall complication rate of 15% in permanently implanted patients, with 3% requiring explantation.[49] The latter results were similarly echoed in a separate study, which reported that at a median follow-up of 33 months, 17.6% of patients required explantation of the device or discontinued treatment entirely.[50]

As encouraging as SNS outcomes may be, this modality is expensive and not all patients respond favourably to PNE. A realistic success rate of PNE is thought to be between 65% and 85%. It is unclear what patient factors are likely to preclude a successful outcome. Therefore, patient selection is based on a pragmatic 'trial-and-error' approach, using the PNE test. Test stimulation is indicated not by an underlying physiological condition, but by the existence of an anal sphincter with reduced or absent voluntary squeeze function and intact reflex activity, and nerve–muscle connection.

Contraindications to SNS include pathological conditions of the sacrum preventing adequate electrode placement, skin disease at the area of implantation, severe anal sphincter damage, pregnancy, bleeding risk, psychological instability, low mental capacity and the presence of a cardiac pacemaker or implantable defibrillator.

SNS may be used in those with an anal sphincter defect. A systematic review of the available literature, a total of 119 patients, reported a test stage success rate of 89%. The average number of incontinent episodes per week improved from 12.1 to 2.3 and the Cleveland Clinic incontinent score (CCIS) improved from 16.5 to 3.8.[51]

> ✅✅ SNS is an expensive therapy that requires a dedicated team for an optimal outcome. It can yield dramatic improvement in some, and yet provide no benefit in others.[48,49]

Percutaneous and transcutaneous tibial nerve stimulation

Another form of neurostimulation, known as tibial nerve stimulation, either percutaneous (PTNS) or transcutaneous (TTNS), has been investigated (**Fig. 14.10**). This allows intermittent electrical stimulation of the tibial nerve at the level of the ankle. This has become a popular option for those who have failed to improve with biofeedback, and for whom a sphincter repair is not indicated. The percutaneous method requires a needle electrode, whilst the transcutaneous technique uses an electrode pad. The former requires delivery from the hospital outpatient clinic and is the most reported. The latter is cheaper and may be self-administered at home. It is believed that both techniques work by remote stimulation of the sacral plexus via the tibial nerve. This is then thought to mimic the action of sacral nerve stimulation.

A large number of single group series have been published. All have reported encouraging results for tibial nerve stimulation in the short term. Hotouras and colleagues[52] reported the outcome of 115 patients who had received 12 sessions of PTNS. At a median follow-up of 26 months the median CCIS had improved from 12 to 9.4 (P <0.0001). 'Top-up' treatments were required to maintain efficacy. These were administered at a median of 12 months. The same group[53] reported the outcome of PTNS in those with urge, passive and mixed faecal incontinence; 25 patients had urge incontinence, the mean CCIS improved significantly from 11 to 8 ($P = 0.019$), those with mixed incontinence ($n = 60$) also had a significant improvement in outcome (12.8 to 9.1, P <0.0001). Those with purely passive incontinence ($n = 15$), failed to show a significant improvement in CCIS (11.5 to 9.4, $P = 0.33$).

The effect of transcutaneous tibial nerve stimulation (TTNS) has also been reported. Significant improvements in small group studies were reported by several authors.[54–56] However, a small randomised controlled study attempted to compare PTNS ($n = 11$) with TTNS ($n = 11$) and a sham TTNS ($n = 8$) device.[57] The number of incontinent episodes and urgency improved

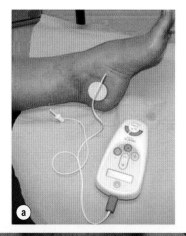

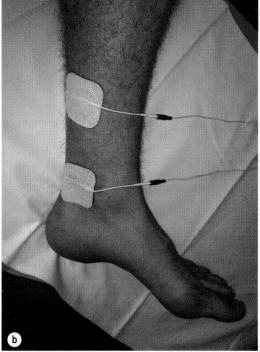

Figure 14.10 • **(a)** Percutaneous tibial nerve stimulation; **(b)** transcutaneous tibial nerve stimulation.

significantly in the PTNS group when compared to the others ($P = 0.035$). The authors suggested that PTNS is likely to be superior to TTNS.

Unfortunately, doubts have been cast on the effectiveness of tibial nerve stimulation by two large randomised controlled trials. Leroi and colleagues[58] compared TTNS with a sham device in a large double-blinded RCT, which investigated 144 patients. No statistically significant difference was seen in the mean number of incontinent episodes. Only 34 (47%) of the active group achieved a reduction of over 30% in a faecal incontinence severity score against 19 (27%) of the sham group (P <0.02). The CONFIDeNT study[59] reported the outcome of a double-blinded RCT to compare PTNS with a sham device. A total of 227 patients were randomised to either group. Only 39 (38%) of the active group achieved a greater than 50% reduction in incontinent episodes compared to 32 (31%) of the sham group (P=0.396). They concluded that PTNS did not confer any benefit over sham treatment.

Despite these findings, a small randomised pilot study compared SNS (n=23) with PTNS (n=17). The authors suggested that both treatment modalities provided some clinical benefit. Eleven out of 18 of those who had received SNS and 7 out of 15 who had received PTNS achieved a greater than 50% improvement in incontinent episodes.[60] More work is needed to establish the place of tibial nerve stimulation in the treatment pathway of faecal incontinence.

Injection therapy

Injectable bulking agents were first described for use in faecal incontinence in 1993. The technique relies on the bulking effect of the injected materials with subsequent fibrosis/collagen deposition helping to enhance continence. These materials are usually injected into either the submucosa or the intersphincteric space. It is not clear if clinical localisation or ultrasound guidance is necessary for optimal placement A variety of materials have been used, including autologous fat, glutaraldehyde cross-linked collagen (Contigen™), pyrolytic carbon beads (Durasphere™) and silicone biomaterial or PTQ™. A recent Cochrane review looked at the published literature to support their use.[61] Five randomised trials were assessed with the outcome in 382 patients reported; no long-term data were available. Four of the five studies were at an uncertain or high risk of bias. The authors reported some benefit from the use of dextranomer in stabilised hyaluronic acid compared to placebo, but this was offset by a greater number of adverse events. Despite the relative simplicity of the procedure, the available data suggest that the effects of bulking agents appear to be short-lived and of limited efficacy.

The most recent addition to this group has been the use of polyacrylonitrile (Gatekeeper™), a shape-memory hydrophilic material that enlarges to seven times its initial diameter of 1.2 mm once in contact with human tissue. An initial single-centre report showed a sustained improvement in incontinence and quality of life scores over a mean follow-up of 33 months.[62] A larger multicentre observational study reported the outcome of this device. At 12 month' follow-up, 30/54(56%) patients achieved a greater than 75% improvement in incontinent symptoms, and 7 (13%) achieved continence. The implant extruded in three patients.[63] Further work is needed to determine the effectiveness of this device in the longer term.

Stoma formation

Antegrade continence enema

This procedure was first described in 1990 for children.[64] The concept of irrigation is to ensure emptying of the colon and/or rectum to prevent seepage of stool. Various procedures have been described to provide an access to the right colon. Initially, the appendix was used to create a continent stoma, an 'appendicostomy', by invaginating the tip of the appendix into the caecum to create a one-way valve. The base of the appendix is then brought out to the abdominal wall and the patient can then introduce antegrade enemas.[64] Other options now include a caecal or ileal tube.[65] This procedure can also be performed percutaneously guided by a colonoscope during which a specially designed catheter (CHAIT Trapdoor™) is introduced into the caecum using the following method: (1) fixation of the caecum to the abdominal wall using anchors, (2) dilatation of the caecostomy site and (3) placement of a CHAIT trapdoor catheter.[66] This minimally invasive approach has been shown to be safe and useful for both paediatric patients and adults.

In a recent long-term review of 75 adult patients, with a median follow-up of 4 years, up to 91% of patients were still performing antegrade enemas, while maintaining a significant reduction in incontinence scores compared to preoperative values.[67] However, some morbidity has been reported with this procedure, the most common being wound infection and leakage from the ministoma.

End stoma

A stoma is appropriate for patients with severe end-stage faecal incontinence in which all other available treatments have failed, are inappropriate because of comorbidities, or when preferred by the patient. While a stoma may be associated with significant psychosocial issues and stoma-related complications, it can allow the patient to resume normal activities and improves quality of life. In a survey of patients who had a colostomy created to manage their faecal incontinence, 83% reported a significant improvement in lifestyle and 84% would choose to have the stoma again.[68] An end sigmoid colostomy without proctectomy is usually recommended as a procedure of choice for patients who elect to have a colostomy. A colostomy, however, can result in its own problems in some patients, such as diversion proctitis and mucus leakage, which may necessitate a secondary proctectomy. The use of laparoscopic surgery has reduced the morbidity associated with this procedure. Recent work suggests that the use of a prophylactic mesh may reduce the, once near certain, chance of a parastomal hernia developing.[69]

> ☑ A colostomy can be a good option for patients who suffer from severe faecal incontinence, offering symptom relief with improved quality of life.

Conclusion

Despite all the currently available treatment procedures presented and discussed above, each patient requires an individualised management approach, taking into account their own needs and preferences. Evidence is unfortunately not robust for most assessment and treatment methods described. Thus, decision-making often relies on expert opinion and personal experience, which should in turn be in the context of a multidisciplinary team of specialists. This is essential for optimising patient outcomes, with the colorectal surgeon being only a part of the support process.

There is active research in this field and new treatments will soon be available. In the future these may involve the use of stem cell therapy and newer sphincter augmentation technologies. Improvement in our understanding of how neuromodulation works will allow more refined electrical stimulation treatments to be developed. A better evidence base is also needed. Large randomised comparative studies are needed to evaluate the new treatments when they emerge.

Key points

- Faecal incontinence (FI) is defined as the involuntary loss of solid or liquid stool.
- The frequency and severity of incontinence episodes and urgency, best assessed with stool diaries, guide the treatment choice.
- FI is multifactorial: the identification of mechanism and cause of FI is key for subsequent management.
- Conservative management including dietary counselling, medication and pelvic floor retraining is first-line. Psychosocial support plays an important role in management of FI.
- Overlapping sphincteroplasty can be offered to patients with significant FI and a documented sphincter injury, frequently due to obstetric trauma. Most patients improve after sphincteroplasty, but outcomes deteriorate over time.
- Sacral nerve stimulation is an effective therapy for patients with significant FI in whom conservative management fails. The technique has the advantage of allowing a therapeutic trial prior to permanent stimulator implantation.
- Colostomy provides restoration of a more normal lifestyle and improves quality of life. An end sigmoidostomy alone is recommended. Antegrade colonic enemas can also be an option in refractory FI.
- New technologies such as the magnetic anal sphincter and the Gatekeeper™ bulking agent may offer an effective treatment option.

▶ Recommended videos:
SNS placement – https://www.youtube.com/watch?v=EnF5NJaQ-3k
    Anal sphincteroplasty – https://www.youtube.com/watch?v=oiiZ0HoeVPc

🌐 Full references available at **http://expertconsult.inkling.com**

Key references

48. Maeda Y, Lundby L, Buntzen S, et al. Outcome of sacral nerve stimulation for fecal incontinence at 5 years. Ann Surg 2014;259(6):1126–31. PMID: 23817505.

    This is one of several studies to demonstrate the efficacy of SNS in the longer term. It also highlights the importance of a positive response to treatment by 6 months to predict a good outcome in the long term. This suggests that good patient selection for SNS is vital.

49. Tan E, Ngo NT, Darzi A, et al. Meta-analysis: sacral nerve stimulation versus conservative therapy in the treatment of faecal incontinence. Int J Colorectal Dis 2011;26(3):275–94. PMID: 21279370.

Functional problems and their surgical management

Nicola S. Fearnhead

Introduction

Pelvic floor pathology tends to be complex and crosses several disciplines. Treatment of urogynaecological pathology in isolation is likely to have an adverse impact on defaecatory function, and vice versa.[1] Ideal care of women with pelvic floor disorders involves input from specialist urologists, gynaecologists and colorectal surgeons, together with allied specialities including radiology, physiotherapy, specialist nursing expertise, physiology, gastroenterology, psychiatry and chronic pain clinics. Preoperative assessment may include questionnaires on obstetric and urogynaecological history, constipation and incontinence scoring, visual analogue scales for pain, quality of life questionnaires, careful clinical examination, proctoscopy with or without colonoscopy, defaecography, transit studies, anorectal physiology and endoanal ultrasound. Increased understanding of the anatomical and functional aspects of pelvic floor problems has led to the establishment of multidisciplinary pelvic floor clinics and teams.[2]

Rectal prolapse

Rectal prolapse or procidentia refers to external protrusion of the rectum through the anus. Prolapse is either mucosal, where only the mucosal layer prolapses, or full-thickness, with circumferential protrusion through the anus of all linings of the rectal wall. Rectal prolapse occurs occasionally in young children but is most common in elderly women.

Risk factors for developing rectal prolapse include connective tissue disorders, for example Marfan's and Ehler's–Danlos syndromes[3] and a history of anorexia nervosa.[4] The latter patients may present some years after resolution of the psychiatric disorder, the prolapse resulting from poor cross-linking of collagen fibres in the pelvic floor musculature during adolescent years. Other risk factors for developing pelvic organ prolapse include high body mass index and high birth-weight during vaginal deliveries.[5,6]

Mucosal prolapse

Mucosal prolapse may occur in isolation but is commonly seen in association with obstructive defaecation syndrome (ODS) and solitary rectal ulcer syndrome (SRUS). It may cause symptoms of perianal discomfort, passage of mucus or blood, constipation and straining at stool. The treatment of mucosal prolapse initially involves bulking agents, increased fibre intake and improving toileting techniques. If surgical intervention is required, outpatient procedures such as suction banding or sclerotherapy or day case procedures such as surgical excision or plication of the prolapse and radiofrequency ablation[7–9] are commonly used. More recently some patients with mucosal prolapse and obstructive defaecation have been treated with the procedure for prolapse and haemorrhoids (PPH) or stapled transanal rectal resection (STARR).[10,11]

Full-thickness rectal prolapse (see Table 15.1)

Although conservative treatment with increased fibre intake and the use of bulking laxatives may improve symptoms to some extent, the definitive

Table 15.1 • Randomised controlled trials in rectal prolapse surgery

Authors	Year	n	Length of follow-up	Trial procedures	Outcomes
Speakman et al.[34]	1991	26	Median 12 months	Open polypropylene mesh rectopexy with division vs preservation of lateral ligaments	Lateral ligament preservation was associated with less postoperative constipation but an increased rate of recurrent prolapse
Luukkonen et al.[43]	1992	30	6 months	Open resection suture rectopexy vs open polyglycolic acid mesh rectopexy	Resection rectopexy resulted in less postoperative constipation
McKee et al.[44]	1992	18	Mean 20 months	Open resection rectopexy vs open suture rectopexy (with division of the lateral ligaments)	Resection rectopexy resulted in less postoperative constipation but less improvement in faecal incontinence
Selvaggi et al.[35]	1993	20	Mean 14 (range 6–24) months	Open Marlex®/Mersilene® rectopexy with division vs preservation of lateral ligaments	Lateral ligament preservation was associated with less postoperative constipation
Winde et al.[40]	1993	49	Mean 50.5 months	Open abdominal rectopexy (with anterior mesh sling) comparing polyglycolic acid vs polyglactin mesh	No significant differences in postoperative complications or recurrence rates
Novell et al.[39]	1994	63	Median 47 (range 44–50) months	Open abdominal Ivalon® sponge rectopexy vs suture rectopexy	No significant difference in recurrence rates Significantly higher incidence of postoperative constipation in Ivalon® sponge group
Deen et al.[28]	1994	20	Median 17 (8–22) months	Altemeier's procedure with pelvic floor repair vs abdominal resection rectopexy with pelvic floor repair	Similar recurrent full-thickness and mucosal prolapse rates Significant postoperative morbidity in both groups Incontinence significantly improved in resection rectopexy group only
Galili et al.[41]	1997	37	Mean 3.7 years	Open abdominal mesh rectopexy (with anterolateral rectal mesh fixation) comparing polyglycolic acid vs polypropylene mesh	No significant differences in postoperative complications or recurrence rates
Boccasanta et al.[48]	1998	21	Mean 29.5 (range 8–45) months	Laparoscopic vs open Marlex®/Mersilene® mesh rectopexy versus open suture mesh (with anterolateral rectal mesh fixation)	No significant difference in recurrence rates
Mollen et al.[36]	2000	18	Mean 3.5 years	Posterior mesh rectopexy with division vs preservation of lateral ligaments	No statistical difference in functional outcome
Solomon et al.[46]	2002	40	Mean 24.2 (range 2–52) months	Laparoscopic vs open abdominal mesh rectopexy	No significant difference in recurrence rate Laparoscopic approach was associated with significantly less morbidity, shorter hospital stays and longer operating times

Table 15.1 • Randomised controlled trials in rectal prolapse surgery—cont'd

Authors	Year	n	Length of follow-up	Trial procedures	Outcomes
Boccasanta et al.[21]	2006	40	Mean 28 months	Altemeier's procedure with levatorplasty comparing monopolar electrocautery dissection and handsewn anastomosis vs harmonic scalpel dissection and circular stapled anastomosis	No significant difference in functional outcomes or recurrence rates Operating time, blood loss and hospital stay were significantly reduced in the stapled group
Karas et al.[29]	2011	252	5 years (10.6% patients lost to follow-up)	Transabdominal rectal mobilisation without rectopexy vs with rectopexy (mesh or sutures)	Significantly higher 5-year recurrence rate in no rectopexy (8.6%) vs rectopexy group (1.5%) ($P=0.003$)
Senapati et al.[17] www.prosper.bham.ac.uk	2013	293	3 years	PROSPER (Prolapse Surgery: Perineal or Rectopexy) trial: First randomisation or surgeon preference to select abdominal vs perineal approach. Second randomisation in abdominal approach of suture vs resection rectopexy and in perineal approach of Delorme's vs Altemeier's operations	49 patients randomised to approach, 78 to abdominal procedures and 213 to perineal procedures Primary endpoint of recurrent prolapse abandoned in favour of secondary endpoints of bowel function and quality of life when recruitment one-third of anticipated No difference in recurrence rates between surgical methods (19% abdominal vs 28% perineal) but overall recurrence rate high
Youssef et al.[27]	2013	82	1 year	Delorme's vs Delorme's with levatorplasty	Significantly higher recurrence rate in Delorme's group (14.3%) vs Delorme's with levatorplasty (2.4%) ($P=0.043$) Greater improvement in faecal incontinence symptoms in Delorme's with levatorplasty arm
Lundby et al.[50]	2016	75	1 year (8 patients withdrew consent for follow-up)	Laparoscopic ventral mesh rectopexy vs posterior rectopexy	Primary outcome of reduction in ODS score at 12 months No significant difference between groups in primary outcome, complication rates or recurrence
Emile et al.[18]	2017	50	18 months	Laparoscopic ventral mesh rectopexy vs Delorme's procedure	No difference in incontinence scores or recurrence rates

ODS, obstructive defaecation syndrome.

treatment for full-thickness rectal prolapse is almost exclusively surgical. The Cochrane Library's review on prolapse surgery failed to identify any trials comparing surgery to non-operative management.[12] Surgical repair may be undertaken either from an abdominal or perineal approach. The systematic reviews of Work Programme 4 of the NIHR-funded CapaCiTY study usefully classify procedures into those involving rectal suspension, rectal excision or reinforcement of the rectovaginal septum.[13]

Choice of abdominal or perineal surgical approaches

The choice of approach has largely been influenced by the preference of the surgeon as well as patient factors including comorbidity, age, gender and sexual activity. Most surgeons used to prefer perineal procedures in elderly or frail patients and abdominal approaches in fit patients irrespective of age,[14] although there has been a shift with increasing evidence that laparoscopic procedures are safe even in the very elderly.[15] The choice of procedure should also take into account the presence of concurrent genital prolapse, constipation, evacuatory difficulties, faecal incontinence and any history of pelvic floor injury.[16] Resection rectopexy has traditionally been recommended for patients who have both constipation and rectal prolapse, although there is little objective evidence to support this practice. Men may prefer perineal procedures in view of the potential for erectile dysfunction resulting from rectal mobilisation during abdominal approaches.

A revised meta-analysis of randomised controlled trials in prolapse surgery was published by the Cochrane Library in 2015 but identified only 15 trials with 1007 patients.[12] The reviewers had set out to address the issues of abdominal versus perineal approaches, rectopexy methods, open versus laparoscopic approaches, and no resection versus resection. The paucity of data, small sample sizes and methodological problems resulted in few useful conclusions being drawn from the analysis. In particular, there was no difference in recurrence rates between abdominal and perineal approaches.[12] Quality of life was poorly reported in all the trials analysed.

The UK's PROSPER trial recruited 293 patients in a pragmatic trial design where randomisation occurred at either one or two steps within the treatment pathway: 48 patients were randomised to abdominal versus perineal approach, 78 to abdominal resection versus suture rectopexy, and 212 to perineal procedure: Delorme's versus Altemeier's.[17] Recurrence rates overall were high, but importantly all procedures were associated with an improvement in quality of life scores. No approach or individual surgical procedure was found to be superior with respect to recurrence of prolapse, quality of life or impact on symptoms of faecal incontinence.[17]

A small trial randomising between laparoscopic ventral mesh rectopexy and Delorme's procedure found no difference in complication rates, incontinence scores or recurrence rates at 18 months but was likely to be under-powered to detect any true difference on its own.[18]

Perineal approaches

The principal perineal approaches are the Delorme's and Altemeier's procedures. Delorme's procedure involves resection of the sleeve of redundant rectal mucosa and plication of the prolapsed muscle wall

without resection.[19] The Altemeier's procedure (perineal rectosigmoidectomy) involves dissection into the peritoneal cavity via the prolapsed peritoneal lining of the pouch of Douglas, followed by excision of the rectum and sigmoid colon and a coloanal anastomosis[20] (Figs 15.1 and 15.2). The latter is usually done by hand but is occasionally described with a circular stapler.[21–23] Pelvic floor repair or levatorplasty may be used in conjunction with perineal procedures to treat symptoms of incontinence.[24]

Delorme's procedure for full-thickness rectal prolapse has remained in favour as it is well tolerated in the elderly, has low morbidity and mortality, and minimal impact on continence and bowel function. Recurrence rates after Delorme's procedure are, however, high, varying between 5% and 26.5%, although the procedure may be repeated.[25–26]

A randomised trial of Delorme's procedure versus Delorme's procedure with levatorplasty in 82 patients found a significant improvement in postoperative symptoms of faecal incontinence, and a non-significant trend to lower recurrence rates at 12 months, in the second group.[27]

Altemeier's procedure carries the potential complication of pelvic sepsis from anastomotic dehiscence, but nevertheless appears well tolerated, even in the elderly. The largest published series report complication rates of 12–14% with very low

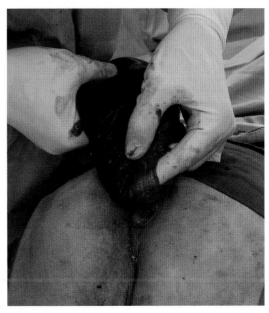

Figure 15.1 • Division of peritoneal reflection during Altemeier's procedure.
Reproduced by permission of Dr Tracy Hull, Cleveland Clinic, Cleveland, Ohio.

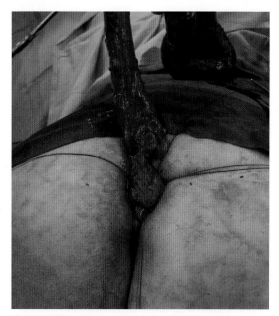

Figure 15.2 • Resection of rectosigmoid prior to coloanal anastomosis during Altemeier's procedure. Reproduced by permission of Dr Tracy Hull, Cleveland Clinic, Cleveland, Ohio.

mortality rates and improved continence in around half of patients, but rates of recurrent prolapse are still high at 10–16%.[25,26]

☑☑ A small randomised trial with a total of 20 participants compared Altemeier's procedure with abdominal resection rectopexy, both procedures being combined with pelvic floor repair.[28] One patient in the Altemeier's arm had recurrent full-thickness prolapse although two patients in each arm also developed mucosal prolapse. Both groups experienced significant postoperative morbidity, but symptoms of incontinence were significantly improved only in the abdominal resection rectopexy group.[28]

Abdominal approaches

Abdominal surgery may be performed either open or laparoscopically. Abdominal rectopexy entails rectal mobilisation and fixation to the sacrum with either sutures or mesh.

☑☑ A randomised trial of 252 patients confirmed the traditional view that fixation of the rectum to the sacrum (rectopexy) is an integral part of the success of prolapse repair by the transabdominal route.[29]

Rectopexy may be performed either posteriorly with Ivalon sponge (Wells' procedure), fascia lata (Orr Loygue operation) or non-absorbable mesh,

or anteriorly with an anterior mesh sling around the rectum to the sacrum (Ripstein's procedure) or ventral mesh rectopexy. Resection during an abdominal rectopexy (Frykman Goldberg procedure) usually involves resection of the sigmoid colon with a handsewn or stapled anastomosis at the sacral promontory.[30]

☑ A multicentre pooled analysis of 643 patients who underwent abdominal procedures for rectal prolapse over a 22-year period found age, gender, surgical technique, means of approach (open or laparoscopic) and method of rectopexy had no impact on recurrence rates.[31] Nevertheless, this study was retrospective and probably not powered to show significant differences between the different surgical techniques of rectal mobilisation only, mobilisation with resection and rectopexy, or mobilisation and rectopexy.[31] Another retrospective meta-analysis using data from six studies on abdominal approaches to rectal prolapse repair again found no difference in recurrence rates with age, sex or surgical technique.[32]

Defaecatory disorders are common after abdominal rectopexy and may present either as novel or worsening constipation, evacuatory difficulties or faecal incontinence. Although many studies include analysis of these problems, the actual extent of the problem is difficult to quantify. A small series of 23 patients undergoing abdominal rectopexy were evaluated prospectively for bowel function: symptoms of incontinence improved in 82%, 36% of patients with preoperative constipation improved with surgery, and 42% developed new onset constipation.[33] Faecal incontinence is reportedly improved in most series of abdominal rectopexy.[26]

Three trials have compared the effects of conservation versus division (with potential rectal denervation) of the lateral ligaments during posterior mesh rectopexy,[34–36] although all studies involved only small numbers of participants. Two of these trials found that preservation of the lateral ligaments was associated with less postoperative constipation,[34,35] although one also found an increased rate of recurrent prolapse with this technique.[34] One small prospective randomised study found that division of the lateral ligaments during posterior Teflon® mesh rectopexy had no impact on postoperative constipation.[36] The latest Cochrane review suggests that lateral ligament division is associated with lower recurrence rates but was inconclusive on the outcome of postoperative constipation.[12]

A number of studies have looked at different methods of rectal fixation during rectopexy. The principal concern with mesh is infection and extrusion. Although the incidence of infection is low,[37,38] the consequences are serious when it occurs. Complete peritoneal closure over non-absorbable meshes may also reduce the incidence of postoperative small-bowel obstruction.

✓✓ A randomised trial in 63 patients comparing Ivalon® sponge to suture rectopexy found no difference in recurrence rates although there was a significantly higher incidence of postoperative constipation in the Ivalon® sponge arm.[39] The authors concluded that there was no need to use prosthetic materials to perform successful rectopexy.

Two trials looking at the relative benefits of different types of mesh in rectopexy surgery found no significant differences in either postoperative complications or recurrence rates with either absorbable or non-absorbable meshes.[40,41]

Resection is usually performed in combination with suture rectopexy in view of the theoretical excess risk of infection if non-absorbable mesh is used for the rectopexy.[38] However, a small series of 35 cases of resection rectopexy with non-absorbable mesh in young patients reported good functional outcomes and no instances of mesh infection or anastomotic leakage.[42]

Three trials with a combined total of 115 patients have examined the impact of concomitant sigmoid resection during open abdominal rectopexy.[17,43,44] One trial randomised patients between resection rectopexy and polyglycolic acid mesh rectopexy[43] and the other two compared resection rectopexy with suture rectopexy.[17,44] If the results of these studies are combined, there is a statistically significant difference in rates of surgically induced constipation, with a lower incidence in the resection arms of each trial.[12] However, one of the trials involved division of the lateral ligaments,[44] which may in itself have contributed to the high incidence of postoperative constipation. When measured, there was no difference in quality of life between the two procedures.[17]

Laparoscopic approaches

Laparoscopic procedures tended to be associated with fewer complications and shorter length of stay in the latest Cochrane review.[12] A meta-analysis conducted to compare open and laparoscopic rectopexy in 688 patients[45] included 12 studies, only one of which was prospective and randomised.[46] The rectopexy techniques included resection, suture and mesh. The meta-analysis concluded that laparoscopic rectopexy was safe, took longer and had comparable recurrent prolapse rates compared to open surgery.[45] Surgeon preference for the laparoscopic abdominal approach has become well-established in the UK.[47]

✓✓ Two small randomised trials have compared open and laparoscopic approaches to mesh rectopexy.[46,48] The first small trial (21 patients) involved anterolateral rectal fixation of non-absorbable mesh to the sacral promontory and found no difference in recurrence rates between the different approaches at just over 2 years.[48] The second trial (40 patients) described full rectal mobilisation with posterior mesh rectopexy to the sacral promontory with a single spiked chromium staple and lateral fixation with hernia staples.[46] It too confirmed no difference in recurrence rates at 2 years (with one recurrence in the open group) but did show that the laparoscopic approach was associated with significantly less morbidity, a shorter hospital stay but a longer operating time.[46]

Improved quality of life is an essential outcome after prolapse surgery but, to date, has only been reported in one trial.[17] Case series suggest that use of the laparoscopic approach may have a significant impact in terms of improving quality of life.[49]

✓✓ Only one Danish trial has compared the laparoscopic procedures of posterior sutured rectopexy and ventral mesh rectopexy: 75 patients with full-thickness prolapse were randomised.[50] The primary outcome selected was change between pre- and postoperative obstructive defaecation syndrome scores. There was no difference in functional outcomes, complication rates or recurrence rates at 12 months.[50] Colonic transit time increased in both groups, but to a significantly lesser extent in the ventral rectopexy arm.[50] Some concern has been raised about the quality of surgery in the ventral mesh rectopexy arm as participating surgeons had performed only ten of these procedures prior to the trial.

A feasibility study has examined the technique of robot-assisted laparoscopic rectopexy and concluded that robotic rectopexy can be safely undertaken with similar functional outcomes but higher recurrence rates than open rectopexy.[51] A small trial of laparoscopic versus robotic ventral mesh rectopexy in 30 patients, of whom only six had full-thickness prolapse, found that the robotic approach was safe and produced good anatomical correction, but without assessing functional outcomes.[52] The additional cost of robotic surgery still needs justification with health economic modelling.[53]

The surgical management of combined rectal and urogenital prolapse is probably best carried out from an abdominal approach and laparoscopic repairs are particularly suitable for repairing abnormalities of the rectum, vagina, bladder and pelvic floor.[54,55]

The advantages of laparoscopic approaches in these patients include nerve-sparing surgery and minimally invasive surgery. A combined approach may also serve to lessen the impact of prolapse repair in one compartment on symptoms in another. If mesh is used, ideally procedures that open the vagina should be avoided to reduce the chances of mesh erosion. Vaginal hysterectomy in the setting of combined rectal and urogynaecological prolapse surgery may be associated with higher morbidity.[56]

Recurrent rectal prolapse

Recurrence rates following rectal prolapse surgery vary widely. As all of the approaches carry a risk of recurrent rectal prolapse, a number of patients will come to a second procedure. There is, however, little in the reported literature on management of recurrent rectal prolapse. Abdominal approaches are used more commonly than perineal approaches for recurrent full-thickness prolapse by some groups,[57] while others point out that perineal procedures can be safely repeated.[58] Recurrent prolapse in more than one compartment may be best treated by an abdominal approach.[59] Irrespective of approach, surgery for recurrent prolapse carries a significant risk of postoperative bowel dysfunction, either with obstructive or incontinent symptoms.[57,58]

Obstructive defaecation, rectocele and rectal intussusception

The cardinal symptoms of obstructive defaecation are straining at stool, a sense of incomplete evacuation and the need for rectal, vaginal or perineal digitation in order to achieve evacuation. Paradoxical contraction of the puborectalis muscle during straining at stool is better termed pelvic floor dyssynergia. The latter is more commonly associated with urogynaecological, gastrointestinal and psychological problems than with slow-transit constipation. Many 'constipated' patients will have improvement in their symptoms with treatment of obstructive defaecation. The treatment is predominantly medical with dietary manipulation, use of laxatives and biofeedback training.[60]

An anterior rectocele and/or rectal intussusception (internal rectal prolapse) are often found in association with obstructive defaecation symptoms. Nevertheless, the syndrome is very complex and symptomatology variable. Symptoms of obstructive defaecation may mask a number of occult disorders including anxiety and depression, gynaecological prolapse, anismus, rectal hyposensitivity and slow-transit constipation. Many problems associated with obstructive defaecation may not be immediately apparent.[61] Recognition and anticipation of occult pathology allows treatment to be tailored to the individual patient.

Objective assessment of the symptoms of obstructive defaecation is particularly important when trying to assess the impact of new surgical interventions for the condition. The Cleveland Clinic Constipation Scoring System is already widely used but is not specific for obstructive defaecation.[62] One, as yet unvalidated, scoring system using a structured questionnaire gives weight to time spent at defaecation, the number of attempts at defaecation each day, use of digitation, use of laxatives and enemas, the presence of incomplete evacuation, straining at stool and stool consistency.[63] The Patient Assessment of Constipation Quality of Life (PAC-QoL) consists of 28 items covering four principal domains: worries and concerns, physical discomfort, psychosocial discomfort and satisfaction.[64] PAC-QoL is currently the validated outcome measure of choice when assessing obstructive defaecation.

Rectocele

A rectocele is a hernia of the anterior rectal wall bulging into the rectovaginal septum. It arises from muscular and nerve damage sustained during vaginal delivery, as a result of hormonal changes following the menopause, or due to paradoxical contraction of puborectalis. Rectoceles occur due to a pressure gradient between the rectum and vagina during coughing and straining and weakness in the puborectalis and bulbocavernosus muscles.[65] Suspensory surgery on the anterior vaginal wall (e.g. anterior colporrhaphy or Burch colposuspension) may predispose to the development of a rectocele.[66] Posterior rectoceles are rarely found, and usually result from traumatic injury or surgical interventions breaching the anococcygeal ligament.

An anterior rectocele is a common finding in patients with obstructive defaecation syndrome, but may also occur in asymptomatic patients. It is often seen on defaecography[67] and magnetic resonance proctography.[68] Symptoms associated with rectocele include difficulty in evacuation, constipation, the need for perineal or vaginal digitation during defaecation and rectal discomfort. Rectoceles vary in size, both in the extent of protrusion into the vagina and in the length of involvement of the rectovaginal septum, but size does not correlate with symptom severity.

The majority of patients with symptoms of obstructive defaecation and an associated rectocele will respond to dietary manipulation and biofeedback.[69-71] Rectocele repair may lead to improved defaecatory symptoms in selected patients who have failed to respond to conservative treatment.[72] Surgical repair by either gynaecologists or colorectal surgeons gives highly variable results and may be performed via transvaginal, perineal, transanal or transabdominal routes. A variety of techniques employ suture plication, mesh reinforcement of the rectovaginal septum, resection of redundant tissue, fixation of the rectum, vagina or perineal body, or reinforcement of the pelvic floor musculature. There has been a recent vogue for repair of rectoceles with laparoscopic ventral rectopexy,[73] or transanal excision using linear[74,75] and circular staplers.

The Block procedure involves full-thickness suture plication of the rectocele with absorbable sutures via a transanal approach.[76] The Sarles procedure consists of an elliptical transanal mucocutaneous flap, plication of the anterior rectal muscle with non-absorbable sutures, resection of redundant mucosa and reapplication of the flap to the anal verge with absorbable sutures[77] (much like an anterior Delorme's operation). Transanal approaches may compromise the integrity of the sphincter complex with consequent faecal incontinence,[78,79] although other studies have shown no effect on continence or sexual function.[80]

Abdominal repair may be performed by open or laparoscopic approaches and involve dissection of the rectovaginal septum via the pouch of Douglas; repair of the rectocele can then be carried out with or without concomitant rectopexy or sacrocolpopexy.

Although a number of authors report series of varying numbers, there have been very few prospective randomised controlled trials (Table 15.2).

✅ A retrospective multicentre study examined the results of rectocele repair in 317 patients by transanal approaches (n = 141), perineal levatorplasty (n = 126) or combined transanal repair and perineal levatorplasty (n = 50).[81] None of the procedures was functionally superior, but bleeding complications were more common in transanal procedures, and dyspareunia and delayed perineal wound healing were more frequent after perineal levatorplasty. About half of the patients studied who had preoperative faecal incontinence and who underwent perineal levatorplasty had improved continence scores postoperatively.[81]

✅✅ Two small randomised trials (see Table 15.2) have compared transanal rectocele repair with posterior colporrhaphy in 57 and 30 patients, respectively,[82,83] with both trials favouring the vaginal approach. Limited evidence reported in a recently updated Cochrane review suggested that vaginal approaches to rectocele repair may offer better

anatomical restoration than transanal repair but the functional outcomes remain uncertain.[84] Use of mesh is associated with less awareness of prolapse but there is a significant mesh erosion rate.[84]

A recent trial did not find in favour of using biological mesh to augment rectocele repair.[85] A randomised trial in multiparous women with obstructed defaecation randomised patients to three different types of rectocele repair: transperineal repair with or without levatorplasty and transanal repair. All three methods improved the anatomical appearances of rectocele on defaecography but transperineal repair with levatorplasty was associated with the best functional outcome.[86]

Rectal intussusception

Rectal intussusception refers to the invagination of the rectal wall during the act of defaecation. The bowel wall will descend to a varying degree which is classified according to the leading edge of the intussusception. The intussusception may remain entirely within the rectum, reach the dentate line, protrude into the anal canal or (in the case of full-thickness prolapse) protrude through the anus. There is, however, little correlation between the degree of intussusception seen on evacuation defaecography and the symptoms experienced by the patient. Rectal intussusception is also seen in asymptomatic individuals.

Rectal intussusception may be associated with symptoms of obstructive defaecation. It may be diagnosed at rigid sigmoidoscopy by an experienced practitioner on asking the patient to strain during withdrawal of the sigmoidoscope. It is more commonly seen during contrast or MR defaecography. Internal rectal intussusception is initially treated with conservative measures. Surgical procedures in the event of failure of conservative management have included abdominal rectopexy,[90,91] an internal Delorme's procedure,[92] laparoscopic ventral rectopexy[93,94] and the STARR procedure.[95,96]

✅✅ Although there was initial interest in sacral nerve stimulation as a treatment for constipation, the evidence suggests that there is no benefit from using neuromodulation in this context.[97,98]

The external pelvic rectal suspension (EXPRESS) procedure was developed as an alternative surgical repair for patients with symptoms of obstructive defaecation in conjunction with rectal intussusception with or without a rectocele. The procedure was first described using Gore-Tex® mesh[99] and then Permacol[100] but has never been adopted in widespread practice.

Table 15.2 • Randomised controlled trials in rectocele surgery

Authors	Year	n	Length of follow-up	Procedures	Outcomes
Kahn et al.[82]	1999	63	25 months	Posterior colporrhaphy (n=24) vs transanal repair (n=33)	Longer length of stay and higher narcotic usage in vaginal approach group Successful repair higher in vaginal group (87.5%) vs transanal group (69.7%)
Sand et al.[87]	2001	160	12 months	Anterior and posterior colporrhaphy without vs with Vicryl™ mesh (Ethicon)	No difference in rates of recurrent rectocele at 1 year 10% vs 8.2% (P=0.71) Cystocele recurrence greater in group without mesh (43%) than with mesh (25%) (P=0.02)
Boccasanta et al.[88]	2004	50	23.4±5.1 months vs 22.3±4.8 months	Stapled transanal prolapsectomy with perineal levatorplasty vs STARR procedure	STARR group had less postoperative pain (P<0.0001) and greater decrease in rectal sensitivity threshold volume (P=0.012) No differences in functional outcomes or early and late complication rates Significantly higher incidence of dyspareunia in prolapsectomy with levatorplasty group (20%) over STARR group (none) (P=0.018)
Nieminen et al.[83]	2004	30	12 months	Posterior colporrhaphy (n=15) vs transanal repair (n=15)	Improved defaecatory function 93% vs 73% (P=0.08) Recurrent symptomatic rectocele/enterocele 7% vs 40% (P=0.04)
Paraiso et al.[89]	2006	106	17.5±7 months	Posterior colporrhaphy (n=37) vs site-specific rectocele repair (n=37) vs site-specific rectocele repair with graft augmentation (n=32)	No difference in symptom improvement among groups (15% functional failure rate overall) Anatomical failure rate 46% in graft augmentation group compared to 14% and 22% in other groups (P=0.02) No differences in improvement in sexual function or dyspareunia rates Bowel symptoms at 12 months were improved significantly in all groups[62]
Farid et al.[86]	2010	48	6 months	Transperineal repair with levatorplasty (n=16) vs transperineal repair without levatorplasty (n=16) vs transanal repair (n=16)	Significant reduction in rectocele size on defaecography in all groups Best functional outcome in transperineal groups with levatorplasty giving best outcomes
Sung et al.[85]	2012	160	12 months	Transvaginal rectocele repair with vs without augmentation of biological mesh SurgiSIS™ (Cook, Biotech)	No impact of use of mesh on anatomical or functional outcomes

ODS, obstructive defaecation syndrome; QoL, quality of life; SAE serious adverse event; STARR, stapled transanal resection rectopexy.

✅ A recent survey of European pelvic floor surgeons confirmed that the majority would offer surgery for symptoms of obstructed defaecation in selected patients and that there was a trend over time moving away from offering stapled transanal resection rectopexy (STARR) towards abdominal rectopexy with just half of experts still offering transanal procedures in 2016.[101]

Laparoscopic ventral rectopexy

Working on the premise that rectal prolapse is always initiated by anterior rectal wall intussusception, ventral rectosacropexy with no other rectal mobilisation was introduced. The operation can be performed open or laparoscopically. Laparoscopic ventral rectopexy involves peritoneal mobilisation over the pouch of Douglas to gain access via the rectovaginal septum to the pelvic floor, mesh fixation to the septum distally and with either sutures or a ProTack™ stapling device proximally to the sacrum, and extraperitonealisation of the mesh by full peritoneal closure.[55] A simultaneous colporrhaphy to treat an enterocele or vaginal prolapse may be performed by anchoring the posterior vagina to the mesh with sutures.

Proponents of ventral rectopexy for full-thickness rectal prolapse propose that avoidance of posterior mobilisation reduces rectal denervation and may lessen postoperative symptoms of constipation.[102,103] Improvement of constipation symptoms after rectopexy in patients with external prolapse has led to the introduction of ventral rectopexy as a treatment for other disorders associated with obstructed defaecation, including internal rectal intussusception and rectocele.[73,92,93,102,104]

✅ A systematic review on ventral rectopexy for rectal prolapse and intussusception examined the outcomes of 728 patients in 12 case series. Recurrence rates appeared reasonable at 0–15.6%. Avoidance of posterior mobilisation appeared to reduce the postoperative incidence of new onset constipation or faecal incontinence, but the review emphasised the heterogeneity of the studies included and the relatively short follow-up.[105]

While laparoscopic mesh ventral rectopexy may benefit patients with obstructive defaecation, it is also associated with a significant learning curve effect in terms of optimising outcomes.[106] Robotic ventral mesh rectopexy has been carried out with equivalent functional outcomes[107] but has yet to be evaluated within a health economic setting.

Stapled transanal rectal resection (STARR)

Stapled transanal rectal resection (STARR) was first used in obstructive defaecation following the introduction of the procedure for prolapse and haemorrhoids (PPH) technique. The latter uses a circular stapling device called Proximate PPH-01™ made by Ethicon Endo-Surgery®. The STARR technique was described by Altomare et al. in 2002,[108] who combined dissection of the rectovaginal septum through a perineal incision with a single transanal firing of the PPH-01™ stapling gun. The PPH technique was modified for STARR by using a purse-string suture which was full-thickness anteriorly and only mucosal posteriorly. The initial study described the results in eight female patients, all of whom had symptoms of obstructive defaecation in association with an anterior rectocele.[108] The PPH-03™ (Ethicon Endo-Surgery®) stapling device has been modified to reduce the risk of haemorrhagic complication during STARR.[109]

STARR is normally carried out in the Lloyd–Davies position, although some surgeons prefer the prone jack-knife or Kraske position. STARR consists of a full-thickness circumferential resection of the lower rectum using stapling devices, either with a PPH technique with protection of the rectovaginal septum, or a circumferential technique involving four or five firings of a curved linear stapler (Contour Transtar™, Ethicon Endo-Surgery®).[110] With either method the end result should be a circumferential row of staples. Any bleeding points are oversewn manually with an absorbable suture.

✅✅ Two randomised trials have compared use of the double firing PPH stapling technique to Transtar.[111,112] Both studies showed an improvement in functional outcome at 12 months but there was a higher rate of recurrent symptoms of obstructed defaecation in the PPH groups in both studies. One of the studies reported a significantly higher incidence of postoperative faecal urgency in the PPH group[111] (see Table 15.3). Another trial assessing the technical difficulty of using Transtar or a combination of linear and circular staplers to perform Transtar had comparable outcomes while favouring the combination technique.[113]

One of the major concerns about the STARR technique is that it is performed blind and so poses a potential threat to structures lying anterior to the rectal wall in the pouch of Douglas. As an enterocele is a fairly common finding in patients with pelvic floor disorders, it is important to establish the presence of an enterocele with

Table 15.3 • Randomised controlled trials of stapled transanal rectal resection (STARR)

Authors	Year	n	Length of follow-up	Procedures	Outcomes
Boccasanta et al.[88]	2004	50	23.4±5.1 months vs 22.3±4.8 months	Stapled transanal prolapsectomy with perineal levatorplasty vs STARR procedure	STARR group had less postoperative pain (P <0.0001) and greater decrease in rectal sensitivity threshold volume (P=0.012) No differences in functional outcomes or early and late complication rates Significantly higher incidence of dyspareunia in prolapsectomy with levatorplasty group (20%) over STARR group (none) (P=0.018)
Lehur et al.[114]	2008	119	12 months	STARR (n=59) vs biofeedback therapy (n=60) for women with ODS, rectocele and rectal intussusception	Only 54 STARR patients and 39 biofeedback patients completed the follow-up period ODS and QoL scores improved significantly in both groups (P=0.0001) Successful functional outcomes were observed in 44 (81.5%) STARR vs 13 (33.3%) biofeedback patients (P <0.0001) Complications occurred in 8 (15%) STARR patients (including 1 SAE – bleeding) and in 1 (2%) biofeedback patient who experienced anal pain
Boccasanta et al.[111]	2011	100	3 years	STARR with double firing PPH-01™ vs CCS-30 Contour Transtar™	Functional outcomes improved significantly in both groups (P <0.001) Operating time was significantly shorter in STARR group (P=0.008) Faecal urgency incidence was 34.0% in STARR group and 14.0% in TRANSTAR group (P=0.035) Recurrence rates at 3 years were 12.0% in STARR group and none in TRANSTAR group (P=0.035)
Renzi et al.[112]	2011	63	2 years	STARR with double firing PPH-01™ vs CCS-30 Contour Transtar™	Functional outcomes improved significantly in both groups at 12 months (P <0.0001) Improvement in functional outcome was only maintained in Transtar group at 24 months No significant differences in length of stay or complication rates
Gentile et al.[115]	2014	66	12 months	Internal Delorme's procedure with levatorplasty vs STARR	Similar rates of improvement in function Low complication rates for both Delorme's procedure was cheaper
Renzi et al.[113]	2016	270	12 months	STARR performed with CCS-30 Contour Transtar™ vs combined use of curved and linear staplers	Primary outcome was technical difficulty in performing surgery; the trial favoured the combined use of linear and curved staplers Complications and efficacy were similar between groups

ODS, obstructive defaecation syndrome; QoL, quality of life; SAE, serious adverse event STARR, stapled transanal resection rectopexy.

defaecography or MRI prior to performing a STARR procedure. A German group has advocated the use of laparoscopic surveillance during the STARR procedure in patients known to have an enterocele preoperatively.[116] Early concern about the STARR procedure arose from a report of 29 patients of whom half had severe postoperative complications or recurrent symptoms.[117] The authors discussed potential errors in technique, including the possibility of stapling too close to the dentate line, undetected co-pathology including pelvic floor dyssynergia, or poor patient selection, and suggested that parity, pelvic floor dyssynergia and anxiety states were risk factors predisposing to failure of STARR.[117] Small rectal diameter, marked pelvic floor descent and low sphincter pressures are also poor prognostic indicators for STARR, whereas rectocele, enterocele and intussusception are positive predictors for a favourable outcome.[118]

The Milan group reported a randomised controlled trial between single stapled transanal prolapsectomy with perineal levatorplasty and the STARR procedure.[119] The STARR group had consistently lower postoperative pain scores but there were otherwise no differences in operative time, hospital stay or return to work. The stapled prolapsectomy group had improvement in constipation symptoms in 76% as compared to 88% in the STARR group. Both groups experienced similar complication rates, with a significant incidence of delayed perineal wound healing in the prolapsectomy group. Late complications were again similar, with urgency of defaecation, incontinence to flatus and anal stenosis occurring in both groups. Dyspareunia affected 20% of the prolapsectomy group but did not occur within the STARR group.[119]

STARR became widely used without good published evidence for its efficacy and safety, raising concerns in the surgical press about the need for evidence-based practice.[120] International registries were established to address these concerns. In 2009, the European STARR registry reported the combined UK, Italian and German 1-year follow-up results of 2224 patients who had undergone a STARR procedure.[121] The mean age for undergoing a STARR procedure was 54.7 years and 83.3% of patients were female. While significant improvements were seen in obstructive defaecation and symptom severity scores, and in quality of life assessment, the complication rate was high at 36%. Reported complications included urgency (20%), persistent pain (7.1%), urinary retention (6.9%), postoperative bleeding (5%), sepsis (4.4%), staple line complications (3.5%) and incontinence (1.8%). Single cases each of rectal necrosis and rectovaginal fistula were reported although there was no perioperative mortality. The conclusions

urged better methods of patient selection and optimisation of technique to reduce postoperative defaecatory urgency and pain.[121] A more recent report of the outcomes after Transtar suggests a lower complication rate of 11%.[122]

Reports of significant complication rates persist, a particular concern in surgery for benign disease. While initial reports may have overestimated risks, the value of the procedure is also difficult to quantify, as a variety of mostly unvalidated scoring systems makes analysis difficult,[123] and concern persists that the STARR procedure may be associated with a marked tendency to cause faecal urgency.[13]

> ✅✅ A meta-analysis of outcomes after the STARR procedure included 26 papers and 1298 patients with a median follow-up of 12 (range 3–42) months. The analysis was confounded by a variety of scoring systems but overall there was a significant improvement in symptoms of obstructive defaecation yielding a combined standardised effect size of 3.8. However, marked heterogeneity, shortcomings in methodology and the variety of scoring systems used across the studies all suggest that the effect size may well be an overestimate.[123]

Solitary rectal ulcer syndrome (SRUS)

Solitary rectal ulcer syndrome (SRUS) may be caused by paradoxical contraction of the anal sphincter muscle during defaecation, is frequently associated with anal digitation and results in anterior mucosal trauma and ulceration. It is characterised by classical symptoms, endoscopic findings and histopathological changes.[124] Treatment involves dietary changes, bulking agents and biofeedback to reverse the underlying defaecatory disorder.[125] Surgical intervention is only rarely indicated and should only be used for patients with concomitant demonstrable prolapse or intractable symptoms refractory to conservative management. A number of surgical options have been described in SRUS management, including transanal excision of the ulcer, stapled mucosal resection, modified anterior Delorme's procedure, abdominal rectopexy and colostomy formation.[126] Simple resection of the ulcer without biofeedback does not resolve the symptoms.[127] Laparoscopic mesh rectopexy may offer some hope for these patients with improvement in symptoms in around three-quarters of patients.[128,129]

Key points

- Patients being considered for surgical management of functional disorders of defaecation are best managed within the setting of a multidisciplinary clinic or team.
- The management of full-thickness prolapse is almost exclusively surgical.
- Correcting full-thickness rectal prolapse results in improved quality of life.
- There is no current evidence to support the superiority of abdominal or perineal approaches to rectal prolapse repair.
- Laparoscopic approaches to abdominal rectopexy are as effective as open approaches, and may have benefits in terms of recovery times and lower morbidity.
- Further evidence is needed to determine whether laparoscopic ventral rectopexy is superior to posterior rectopexy in terms of functional outcomes, as only a single trial has been carried out comparing the two procedures.
- Laparoscopic surgery may have particular benefits for management of combined genital and rectal prolapse.
- Rectocele repairs should only be offered to patients who remain symptomatic after conservative management of obstructed defaecation with dietary manipulation, bulking agents and biofeedback, and who digitate vaginally or perineally (i.e. not anal digitators).
- Surgery may offer symptomatic relief in carefully selected patients with obstructive defaecation syndrome.
- The Transtar technique of STARR may be associated with less postoperative faecal urgency and more sustained long-term results.

▶ Recommended video:

- Ventral mesh rectopexy – https://tinyurl.com/y96yjasm

🌐 Full references available at **http://expertconsult.inkling.com**

Key references

12. Tou S, Brown SR, Nelson RL. Surgery for complete (full thickness) rectal prolapse in adults (Review). Cochrane Database Syst Rev 2015;(4): CD001758. PMID: 26599079.
    Cochrane meta-analysis of randomised controlled trials in prolapse surgery identified 15 trials with 1007 patients. There was no difference in recurrence rates between abdominal and perineal approaches.

17. Senapati A, Gray RG, Middleton LJ, et al. PROSPER: a randomised comparison of surgical treatments for rectal prolapse. Colorectal Dis 2013;15(7):858–68. PMID: 23461778.
    The largest reported randomised study in rectal prolapse surgery did not favour any specific procedure or approach, but did demonstrate an improvement in quality of life after prolapse repair. Recurrence rates overall were higher than anticipated.

27. Youssef M, Thabet W, El Nakeeb A, et al. Comparative study between Delorme operation with or without postanal repair and levatorplasty in treatment of complete rectal prolapse. Int J Surg 2013;11(1):52–8. PMID: 23187047.
    Showed significant improvement in faecal incontinence with levatorplasty

28. Deen KI, Grant E, Billingham C, et al. Abdominal resection rectopexy with pelvic floor repair versus perineal rectosigmoidectomy and pelvic floor repair for full-thickness rectal prolapse. Br J Surg 1994;81(2):302–4. PMID: 8156369.
    A randomised controlled trial of Altemeier's procedure with pelvic floor repair compared to abdominal resection rectopexy with pelvic floor repair. Similar recurrent prolapse rates and significant postoperative morbidity were observed in both groups. Incontinence significantly improved in the resection rectopexy group only.

29. Karas JR, Uranues S, Altomare DF, et al. No rectopexy versus rectopexy following rectal mobilization for full-thickness rectal prolapse: a randomized controlled trial. Dis Colon Rectum 2011;54(1):29–34. PMID: 21160310.
    A randomised trial of 252 patients confirmed that fixation of the rectum to the sacrum (rectopexy) is an integral part of the success of prolapse repair.

39. Novell JR, Osborne MJ, Winslet MC, et al. Prospective randomized trial of Ivalon sponge versus sutured rectopexy for full-thickness rectal prolapse. Br J Surg 1994;81(6):904–6. PMID: 8044618.

A prospective randomised trial comparing Ivalon® sponge to suture rectopexy found no difference in recurrence rates, although there was a significantly higher incidence of postoperative constipation in the Ivalon® sponge arm.

46. Solomon MJ, Young CJ, Eyers AA, et al. Randomized clinical trial of laparoscopic versus open abdominal rectopexy for rectal prolapse. Br J Surg 2002;89(1):35–9. PMID: 11851660.
No significant difference was found in recurrence rates but the laparoscopic approach was associated with significantly less morbidity, shorter hospital stays and longer operating times.

50. Lundby L, Iversen L, Buntzen S, et al. Bowel function after laparoscopic posterior sutured rectopexy versus ventral mesh rectopexy for rectal prolapse: a double-blind, randomised single-centre study. Lancet Gastroenterol Hepatol 2016;1(4):291–7. PMID: 28404199.
Randomised trial that showed equivalent functional outcomes for laparoscopic mesh rectopexy and posterior rectopexy.

84. Maher C, Feiner B, Baessler K, et al. Surgical management of pelvic organ prolapse in women. Cochrane Database Syst Rev 2013;(4):CD004014. Review. Update in: Cochrane Database Syst Rev 2016 Nov 30;11:CD004014. PMID: 23633316.
Cochrane review that analyses trials comparing transanal rectocele repair with posterior colporrhaphy. Outcomes favour the transvaginal approach. Mesh erosion rates are high.

97. Thaha MA, Abukar AA, Thin NN, et al. Sacral nerve stimulation for faecal incontinence and constipation in adults. Cochrane Database Syst Rev 2015;(8): CD004464. PMID: 26299888.
Two trials of SNS for constipation failed to show improvement in symptoms of constipation and high rate of adverse events.

113. Renzi A, Brillantino A, Di Sarno G, et al. Evaluating the surgeons' perception of difficulties of two techniques to perform STARR for obstructed defecation syndrome: a multicenter randomized trial. Surg Innov 2016;23(6):563–71. PMID: 27370308.

123. Van Geluwe B, Stuto A, DaPozzo F, et al. Relief of obstructed defecation syndrome after stapled transanal rectal resection (STARR): a meta-analysis. Acta Chir Belg 2014;114(3):189–97. PMID: 25102709.

16

Functional problems and their medical management

Anton V. Emmanuel

Introduction

Symptoms related to functional gastrointestinal disorders (FGIDs) are highly prevalent. In community-based studies, up to 22% of 'normal' UK subjects can be diagnosed as having irritable bowel syndrome (IBS) and up to 28% have functional constipation.[1] These disorders are constellations of symptoms – they are not diseases. As such, the emphasis of management of these patients is based on simple principles: the exclusion of organic disease, making a confident diagnosis, explaining why symptoms occur, alteration of lifestyle where appropriate and avoidance of surgery. Education about healthy lifestyle behaviours, reassurance that the symptoms are not due to a life-threatening disease such as cancer and establishment of a therapeutic relationship are essential, and patients have a greater expectation of benefit from lifestyle modification than drugs. This chapter will deal primarily with IBS and functional constipation, leaving the treatment of faecal incontinence to Chapter 14. Similarly, rectal prolapse, which is a frequent comorbidity of chronic constipation, is dealt with in Chapter 15.

The prevalence of functional disorders depends on the exact diagnostic criteria used; the current standards are the Rome IV criteria.[2] These have updated the previous core diagnostic criteria for IBS: namely the presence of abdominal pain, altered bowel function (in terms of altered stool form or frequency) and a temporal relationship between pain and function. The new criteria require 'pain' rather than just 'discomfort' and that the pain is present at least once a week. The definition of functional constipation requires the presence of at least two of the following: less than three bowel actions a week, need to strain or manually assist evacuation on over 25% of occasions, passage of hard stools on over 25% of occasions or a sensation of abnormal evacuation on over 25% of occasions. These symptoms need to be chronic, and organic disease needs to have been excluded. Although these criteria can be criticised for being over-inclusive, what is clear is that FGIDs represent a major burden on secondary and tertiary outpatient clinics and IBS is the commonest diagnosis in gastrointestinal clinics.[3] An important confounding factor to be borne in mind when reviewing the literature on FGIDs is that the overwhelming majority of studies originate from tertiary centres. Patients attending such institutions are known to have disproportionately high scores on scales of depression, health-related anxiety and somatisation,[4] representing a potentially biased, self-selected group. One further compounding variable in assessing studies of FGIDs is that there is a notoriously high placebo response, ranging from 30% to 80%.[5]

Irritable bowel syndrome

The key to successful management of IBS is empathic reassurance. This will need to be individually directed according to the patient's symptoms, beliefs and anxieties.[6] Early and positive diagnosis is essential. Helpful factors in establishing a diagnosis are: (i) presence of symptoms for more than 6 months; (ii) frequent consultations for non-gastrointestinal symptoms; (iii) self-reporting that stress aggravates symptoms.

A key component of the reassurance is provision of a simple explanation of the benign nature and prognosis of the condition. Patients should be advised that no more than 2% of patients need their diagnosis of IBS to be revised at 30 years of follow-up.[1] Equally, it is important to remember that 88% of patients have recurring episodes of gastrointestinal symptoms, and so reassurance should be allied to advice about the need for long-term symptom control.[1]

Investigation

The presence of alarm features such as symptom onset after age 50, rectal bleeding, significant weight loss or abdominal mass mandates serological and luminal investigation to exclude organic disease. Investigations in these frequently young patients (the majority of patients at presentation are aged less than 35 years[1]) should otherwise be avoided since they may both exacerbate patients' anxieties and undermine their confidence in the clinician. The search for a simple diagnostic test of IBS remains, and faecal calprotectin has emerged as a possible candidate to differentiate IBS from an organic cause of diarrhoea.[7]

☑☑ An important diagnosis to consider, especially in the presence of low-grade anaemia, is coeliac disease.[8]

☑ Microscopic colitis should be a differential diagnosis in an older patient with diarrhoea (especially if nocturnal), weight loss and a history of autoimmune disease and recent commencement of a non-steroidal or proton pump inhibitor.[9]

Approximately 5% of patients fulfilling IBS diagnostic criteria will have histological evidence of coeliac disease compared to 0.5% of controls without IBS symptoms.[8]

Treatment

Lifestyle modification

The low FODMAPs diet has emerged in a series of randomised clinical trials as an effective treatment for patients with IBS, especially for the symptoms of bloating, flatulence and abdominal discomfort.[10] Careful dietary adherence supported by specialised dietitians appears to be vital for the success of the diet. Long-term data with the low FODMAPs diet are not available and strict FODMAP restriction is associated with inadequate nutrient intake (e.g. calcium) and

potential alteration of gut microbiota.[10] Another helpful dietary intervention worth considering in diarrhoea-predominant IBS patients (d-IBS) is reduction of excess caffeine and sorbitol (found in chewing gum and sweeteners).[11]

Studies have been carried out on the effect of dietary fibre augmentation in some constipation-predominant IBS (c-IBS) patients.[12,13] Early placebo-controlled crossover studies showed some acceleration of transit but no significant effect on symptoms.[12] Later studies have corroborated the absence of beneficial effect on symptoms and suggested that there is an increase in abdominal bloating, discomfort and flatulence during dietary fibre supplementation.[13] In summary, the effect of dietary fibre in IBS is not significantly beneficial, and the diet is frequently difficult to adhere to in the long term.[14] Current UK national guidelines generally recommend avoiding fibre supplementation in IBS patients.[15]

Pharmacological treatments

Most patients with FGIDs do not need regular drug therapy. The strongest evidence for a single agent in IBS patients is in d-IBS, where loperamide is a well-tolerated and effective treatment of diarrhoea and urgency.[16]

The popular aetiological theory that IBS symptoms relate to gut spasm has led to a huge number of uniformly low-quality studies of antispasmodics in IBS patients. These have been subject to meta-analysis.[17] In essence, what can be concluded is that, even allowing for publication bias in favour of positive studies, the evidence is of only modest benefit for anticholinergic (such as dicycloverine, hyoscine) or antispasmodic drugs (mebeverine, peppermint) over placebo in treating the symptoms of IBS.

☑☑ In contrast, the data for the efficacy of tricyclic antidepressants show unequivocal benefit in favour of low-dose usage of these agents.[18] Doses of amitriptyline or nortriptyline of 10–50 mg act at both the central (anxiety and depression) and peripheral (neuromodulatory) mechanisms of IBS.

The putative mechanism of action of tricyclic agents is through an effect on gut serotonin receptors and visceral sensitivity.

☑☑ Many drugs that agonise or antagonise serotonin receptors have been developed, and the effect of all these drugs amounts to about 20% advantage over placebo.[19]

Whilst none of these agents is licensed for use in the UK at the time of writing, with some having been withdrawn due to safety concerns, there is good evidence supporting the use of ondansetron for diarrhoea-predominant IBS.[20] Serotonin agents are amongst a number of emerging agents targeting enteric neurotransmitter receptors, some of which may have a role in relieving the sensory symptoms of IBS.[19] In contrast to studies of low-dose tricyclics, standard doses of newer antidepressants (selective serotonin reuptake inhibitors) lead to a less impressive improvement in IBS, and at greater cost.[18,21] Finally, early evidence suggests the possibility that some probiotic strains of bacteria may have a beneficial influence in patients with IBS, though this is very much emerging information.[22]

Psychological treatments

✓✓ Cognitive behavioural therapy directed towards bowel symptoms, and gut-focused hypnotherapy are effective in treating women with IBS, with a 'number needed to treat' of 3.[18,23]

The essence of such treatment is that it is gut-focused, since general cognitive behavioural and relaxation therapies are no more effective than standard care. A study by Creed also showed that such treatment is cost-effective and beneficial in the long term.[23]

✓✓ A number of studies in the literature show the value of hypnotherapy in IBS with benefit in the long-term setting, at up to 6 years following the cessation of therapy.[18]

In brief, three-quarters of patients report symptom alleviation after hypnotherapy, and over 80% of these responders remain well at a median follow-up of 5 years.[18,24]

Surgery

Patients with IBS are disproportionately more likely to undergo abdominal and pelvic surgery than age- and sex-matched controls.[25,26] IBS patients have a prevalence of cholecystectomy of 4.6% compared with 2.4% in controls, and a prevalence of hysterectomy of 18% versus 12% in controls. There is also evidence that IBS patients are more likely to undergo appendicectomy (35% prevalence compared to 8% in control patients with ulcerative colitis [which is lower than the normal prevalence of appendicectomy]).[26] Furthermore, these are more likely to yield normal findings macroscopically and histologically in IBS patients.[6]

✓✓ Recent years have seen the re-emergence of the SeHCAT test to assess for bile acid malabsorption as a cause of symptoms in some patients with IBS, especially when there are symptoms of nocturnal diarrhoea and faecal incontinence in a patient with previous biliary disease.[27]

Abdominal or pelvic surgery may predispose to the development of functional symptoms through mechanical, neural or hormonal impairments. Heaton et al. reported that 44% of subjects develop new symptoms of urgency after cholecystectomy and 27% report constipation symptoms beginning after hysterectomy.[28] In contrast, women undergoing gynaecological surgery for non-pain indications did not develop IBS more often than non-operated controls.[29] What these studies do highlight is the key importance of trying to minimise surgery in patients with FGIDs. In those patients who do undergo an operation it is implicit that there is complete explanation of the possibility of developing new symptoms postoperatively. The corollary of this is that patients in whom there is a high suspicion of FGID (based on symptoms and normal investigations) should be dissuaded from undergoing diagnostic laparoscopy, which is not usually revealing and which may result in new complaints.

Functional constipation

Estimates from the USA suggest that 1.2% of the population consult a physician every year with the complaint of constipation.[30] Healthcare costs are high (over $7500 per year at 2007 levels) since 85% of these consultations result in the prescription of a laxative.[31] This figure does not include the cost of over-the-counter laxatives nor the costs of specialist investigation and work absenteeism. What these figures reflect is the importance of the role of the hospital specialist in identifying appropriate patients to put through further investigation and specific treatments.

In terms of pathophysiology, functional constipation is considered to be due to either slow whole-gut transit ('colonic inertia'), rectal evacuatory dysfunction or a combination of both of these abnormalities. The commonest cause of slow transit in general practice is as a side-effect of drug therapy for other reasons. The commonest culprit drugs are opiates, anticholinergics, antihypertensives, iron supplements, antacids and non-steroidal anti-inflammatory drugs.[32]

Investigation

As in the case of patients with IBS, luminal investigation is reserved for patients with a short history or alarm symptoms, in whom there is the need to exclude colorectal cancer. In addition to the drug causes listed above, which can be identified from careful history-taking, the other common associations are with neurological disease (multiple sclerosis, Parkinson's disease and diabetic autonomic neuropathy). Causes of constipation that can be identified from simple serological testing include hypothyroidism, hypercalcaemia and hypokalaemia.

Whereas the diagnosis of IBS is one of exclusion, there are investigations available both to define the pathophysiological abnormality and confirm the presence of constipation. Colonic transit can be simply measured by use of radio-opaque markers followed by a plain abdominal X-ray. One well-described assessment comprises ingestion of three sets of radiologically distinct markers that are ingested at 24-hour intervals and an abdominal X-ray taken 120 hours after the first ingestion; retention of more than the normal range for any one of the three sets of markers reflects slow transit. The test is cheap, sensitive and reproducible, and provides clinically helpful information in the management of patients with constipation.[33]

Defecating proctography (using barium or magnetic resonance contrast gel) and the balloon expulsion test are means of quantifying the anatomical and physiological disturbances of rectal evacuation in patients with functional constipation. Abnormalities such as paradoxical anal sphincter contraction, impaired pelvic floor relaxation, anal intussusception and rectal prolapse can be demonstrated by these techniques.[33] No firm evidence exists as to the value of identifying these abnormalities in the management of patients with constipation.[33] The place of anorectal manometry in patients with chronic constipation is primarily in the exclusion of Hirschsprung's disease.[33]

Treatment

Dietary fibre supplementation

This is the traditional first line of therapy for chronic constipation, and by the time of specialist referral most patients would have already undertaken trials of such therapy. Fibre supplementation increases gut transit and stool bulk by a fraction of the starting value, and as such is only effective in patients with mild constipation.[34] In those small numbers of patients seen in hospital who have not tried fibre supplementation, advice needs to be offered about a gradual stepwise increase in fibre intake. Patients need to be counselled that the effect is not apparent until therapy has been established for several weeks.

> ✔ Patients need to continue with the diet in the long term,[35] and there is evidence that this can be difficult for a significant proportion. Increasing liquid intake and attempting to maintain regular meal-time patterns seem also to have a place in improving symptoms, although the evidence is strongest in the elderly.[34]

Laxatives, suppositories, enemas and novel prokinetics

There are widely held misconceptions of the danger of 'self-poisoning' without a daily bowel action. Given the limited evidence base for the use of laxatives, the first step in the management of constipation is to discourage laxative overuse.[32] The effect of laxatives in chronic constipation is modest at best. Only a very small number of trials have compared a laxative regimen with placebo, and meta-analysis would not be statistically or clinically meaningful.[32] Compared to the dearth of placebo-controlled studies, there are a number of open and blinded comparisons between different laxatives. These have been reviewed,[32] and as might be predicted the opinion of the reviewers is that methodological flaws and inconsistencies prevent meaningful conclusions being drawn. The conclusions that can be drawn are listed below. Overall there is an increase in stool frequency with bulking agents of 1.4 bowel movements per week, and with other laxative classes of 1.5 bowel movements per week.

Bulk laxatives have a limited role in chronic constipation. They should be reserved for patients who are unable to consume adequate dietary fibre. They have no role in either patients with severe constipation or those who need rapid relief of symptoms.

> ✔ **Osmotic agents** comprise either poorly absorbed ionic salts or non-absorbed sugars and alcohols. Dose titration is possible with osmotic laxatives, which have a particular place in the management of megacolon and megarectum once the patient has been disimpacted.

> ✔ **Stimulant laxatives** (anthranoid compounds such as senna, or polyphenolic compounds such as bisacodyl) usually have an effect on stool output within 24 hours of ingestion, and are most suitable for occasional, rather than regular, use.

The effect of these drugs is unpredictable and dose escalation is often required. Nevertheless, they appear to be harmless and are frequently used in chronic severe constipation. What is clear is that the previous fears that chronic use of anthranoid laxatives may result in enteric nerve damage is highly unlikely.[36] **Stool softeners** and **compound mixtures** of the above classes of laxative are also commonly used, although their efficacy has not been rigorously demonstrated.

Some **suppositories** induce a chemically induced reflex rectal contraction. **Enemas** act either by stimulating rectal contraction or by softening hard stool.[37]

> ✔ Suppositories and enemas can be effective in alleviating the symptoms of evacuation difficulty if dietary modification and behavioural therapy have been unsuccessful. Used on an as-required basis, enemas have a particular place in managing rectal impaction.

Prucalopride is an effective **prokinetic** for patients with chronic constipation refractory to laxative therapy.[38] Chloride channel agents such as linaclotide and lubiprostone have also been shown in large-scale randomised trials to have efficacy in similar populations.[39] All these drugs improve transit and pain/bloating symptoms, although the optimal duration of treatment remains uncertain. There seems to be efficacy in patients with transit delay as well as those with pelvic floor dyssynergia.[39] Peripherally acting mu-opioid receptor antagonists have also been developed with a beneficial effect on patients with opioid induced constipation.[39]

> ✔✔ In laxative-refractory patients, novel prokinetic and secretagogue drugs offer a therapeutic alternative to behavioural therapy or surgery.[38,39]

Behavioural therapy (biofeedback)

Gut-directed behavioural therapy, biofeedback, is now an established therapy for functional constipation, and in a number of specialist centres is first-line therapy for new referrals.[40,41] Biofeedback is a learning strategy based on operant conditioning. The main focus is on abdominal and pelvic coordination and it is undoubtedly beneficial in patients with dyssynergic evacuation,[40] but it also seems beneficial in patients with slow transit.[41]

> ✔✔ Short- and long-term benefit is evident in over 60% of unselected patients in specialist centres.[9,41,42]

The effect of treatment is seen not only in symptoms (improved bowel frequency, reduced need to strain), but also in terms of reduced laxative use and improved quality of life scores.[9]

Biofeedback seems to have its effect through alteration of a variety of pathophysiological disturbances. There is evidence that successful outcome with biofeedback is associated with specifically improved autonomic innervation to the colon, and improved transit time for patients with slow and normal transit.[9]

> ✔ Additionally, treatment may improve pelvic floor coordination,[41] thereby allowing antegrade peristalsis and preventing retrograde movement of colonic content. What is important is that biofeedback is successful not just in patients with mild symptoms, but also in those with intractable symptoms who are being considered for surgery.[42]

Surgical treatment for constipation

Surgery for rectal evacuation symptoms in the context of structural anorectal disturbance is described elsewhere in this book. In those patients with proven slow transit who have failed to respond to dietary modification, biofeedback, long-term trials of laxatives and prokinetics, the traditional algorithm dictates consideration of a surgical approach. The standard surgical procedure has been total colectomy (performed to the level of the sacral promontory) and ileorectal anastomosis.[43] Ileorectostomy is reported as being more successful than ileosigmoidostomy in terms of successful relief of constipation and, providing greater than 7–10 cm of rectum is left intact, then bowel frequency and urgency are not unacceptably frequent.[43]

Almost every major colorectal institution and a huge number of other centres have published on their experience of subtotal colectomy for slow transit constipation. Results vary widely, with satisfaction rates varying from 39% to 100%.[41] Whilst median scores of bowel frequency tend to show statistically significant improvements, what these composite figures mask are the facts that, firstly, approximately one in three patients do not improve at all and, secondly, that some patients develop diarrhoea.

> ✔✔ The strongest argument against colectomy for slow transit constipation is that the disorder is a pan-enteric one, and so mere removal of the colon is unlikely to yield sustained benefit.[44,45]

There are two unequivocal conclusions that come out of the welter of small studies in the literature. Firstly, adverse effects occur in over half of all patients. Most common is episodic subacute small bowel obstruction (occurring in up to two-thirds in some series), need for further abdominal surgery (in up to one-third of patients), persisting constipation (in up to one-quarter), diarrhoea (in up to one-quarter) and faecal incontinence (in up to 10%).

> ✔ The second conclusion, related to the incidence of adverse events, is the importance of careful patient selection.

Thus, of the many patients complaining of constipation in the community, only a tiny proportion (approximately 1%) are referred to tertiary care, of whom only a small fraction (less than 5%) might benefit from surgical treatment.[46] Patient selection must initially be on clinical grounds (including careful consideration of potential psychiatric disorders) and the physiological demonstration of slow transit. Some authors have recommended extensive anorectal sensory and motor physiological testing, defecating proctography and upper gut motility studies to aid identification of subgroups in whom surgery may be more successful.[47] In contrast, Rantis et al.[48] identified only 23% of patients in whom such extensive testing altered clinical management; additionally, the cost of this testing was great (US $140 000 in 1997).

In view of the controversy about subtotal colectomy, a vogue for alternative surgical therapies arose. Two particular surgical approaches have received sustained study: stoma formation and segmental colonic resection. However, the data on efficacy and morbidity of these techniques are little different and no less controversial than those for subtotal colectomy.[49] There is unequivocally no place for division of the puborectalis in an attempt to treat rectal evacuatory dysfunction.[50]

A less invasive surgical approach to functional constipation has been the antegrade continence enema (the Malone procedure). Initially used in patients with constipation secondary to neurological disease, the technique has been widely reported in functional constipation.[51] Patients intubate their stoma (appendix or plastic conduit) and irrigate with either water, a stimulant or osmotic laxative. Although there are stomal complications in over 50% of patients (stenosis, mucus leak, pain), three-quarters of patients report 'high' or 'very high' satisfaction with the procedure.[51]

Current trials of medical therapy for FGIDs require quality-of-life data to complement conventional efficacy data. The surgical literature to date shows that although stool frequency may improve, gut-specific quality of life does not.[52]

Putative treatments for constipation

> ✔ Recent surgical developments have looked at modifications of subtotal colectomy. Small, short-term studies have shown that ileosigmoid or antiperistaltic caecorectal anastomoses may improve bowel frequency and quality of life.[53]

In some patients with constipation, the presence of intussusception on proctography may provoke the decision to undertake laparoscopic ventral mesh rectopexy. Long-term data are not available, and it is evident that there are mesh-related complications,[54] so at this time, caution is advocated.

Sacral nerve stimulation for constipation has been studied, but disappointing long-term data have meant that the treatment is no longer supported for this indication.[55]

Idiopathic megarectum and megacolon

Megarectum and megacolon are uncommon clinical conditions of unknown aetiology that present typically, but not exclusively, with intractable constipation in the first two decades of life.[56] Other conditions presenting with constipation in the context of gut dilatation (e.g. Hirschsprung's disease, chronic intestinal pseudo-obstruction) are not included since the aetiology of these disorders is known. Patients with idiopathic megarectum tend to present with faecal incontinence in the context of recurrent faecal impaction frequently requiring surgical disimpaction. In contrast, patients with idiopathic megacolon more frequently present with abdominal pain and distension in the context of chronic constipation.[56]

> ✔ The majority of patients with idiopathic megarectum and megacolon can be successfully managed by disimpaction followed by the use of osmotic laxatives. The osmotic agent needs titration in order that the patient obtains a semiformed ('porridgey') stool that is passed three times a day. Occasionally, rectal evacuation techniques (such as suppository use or biofeedback therapy) are required actually to empty the rectum of the semiformed stool.[57]

When medical therapy fails (due to compliance failure or lack of success in avoiding recurrent impaction), surgical therapy is warranted. A number of surgical procedures have been performed, with variable reports of success. As with reports of surgery for idiopathic constipation, the longer the duration of follow-up, the worse the documented outcome. Anorectal physiology, whole-gut transit studies and evacuation proctography do not help identify patients who may benefit or help with choice of surgical procedure.[58] Anorectal physiology testing does have a role in identifying the presence of a rectoanal inhibitory reflex, which excludes the differential diagnosis of Hirschsprung's disease.

✓✓ With regard to resectional surgery, colectomy offers good results in the majority of patients (80%), with ileorectal anastomosis yielding the greatest levels of patient satisfaction.[58]

Outcomes with the Duhamel procedure, anal myomectomy and restorative proctocolectomy are also favourable in the majority of cases, approaching 70% in the majority of series. Restorative proctocolectomy is suitable in patients with dilatation of both the colon and rectum, whilst the recent procedure of vertical reduction rectoplasty has been proposed for those with dilatation confined to the rectum.[58]

✓ In situations where initial surgery has failed, formation of a stoma (colostomy or ileostomy) is associated with excellent results.[59]

Stoma formation as a primary procedure is also successful in the vast majority of cases.[59] The ultimate choice of surgical procedure will depend on available expertise, patient physical and psychological factors, and the patient's choice.

Key points

- Dietary manipulation is rarely helpful in managing symptoms in hospital-referred patients with functional disorders.
- There is an expanding differential before making a diagnosis of IBS – coeliac disease, bile acid malabsorption and microscopic colitis.
- Drug therapy is rarely needed in treating patients with IBS.
- Loperamide is unequivocally beneficial in patients with loose stools and urgency.
- Low-dose tricyclic antidepressants are effective in relieving functional abdominal pain.
- A comprehensive approach to therapy of functional disorders requires close liaison with psychological services.
- Tailored laxatives are preferable to empiric treatment of particular agents.
- Novel prokinetic and secretagogue drugs offer an alternative therapy in laxative refractory cases.
- Biofeedback is effective in almost two-thirds of patients with constipation, whether due to slow transit or evacuatory dysfunction.
- Subtotal colectomy and ileorectal anastomosis is beneficial in a small number of highly selected patients, although surgical morbidity is fairly high.
- The majority of patients with idiopathic megarectum and megacolon can be managed by disimpaction and initiation of osmotic laxatives.

🌐 Full references available at **http://expertconsult. inkling.com**

Key references

8. Sanders DS, Carter MJ, Hurlstone DP, et al. Association of adult coeliac disease with irritable bowel syndrome: a case control study in patients fulfilling the Rome II criteria referred to secondary care. Lancet 2001;358:1504–8. PMID: 11705563.
9. Emmanuel AV, Mason HJ, Kamm MA. Response to a behavioural treatment, biofeedback, in constipated patients is associated with improved gut transit and autonomic innervation. Gut 2001;49:209–13. PMID: 11454796.
18. Ford AC, Quigley EM, Lacy BE, et al. Effect of antidepressants and psychological therapies, including hypnotherapy, in irritable bowel syndrome: systematic review and meta-analysis. Am J Gastroenterol 2014;109:1350–65. PMID: 24935275. Meta-analysis of studies using a variety of tricyclic antidepressants in varying doses in patients with FGIDs showing clear benefit for low-dose tricyclics over placebo.

19. Spiller R, Aziz Q, Creed F, et al. Guidelines on the irritable bowel syndrome: mechanisms and practical management. Gut 2007;56:1770–98. PMID: 17488783. Practical review of management options available for IBS, encompassing minimum investigation, pharmacological, dietary and lifestyle treatment.
23. Creed F, Fernandes L, Guthrie E, et al. The cost-effectiveness of psychotherapy and paroxetine for severe irritable bowel syndrome. Gastroenterology 2003;124:303–17. PMID: 12557136.
27. Slattery SA, Niaz O, Aziz Q, et al. Systematic review with meta-analysis: the prevalence of bile acid malabsorption in the irritable bowel syndrome with diarrhoea. Aliment Pharmacol Ther 2015;42(1):3–11. PMID: 25913530.

38. Emmanuel AV, Cools M, Vandeplassche L, et al. Prucalopride improves bowel function and transit time in patients with chronic constipation: an integrated analysis. Am J Gastroenterol 2014;109(6):887–94. PMID: 24732867.

39. Emmanuel AV, Tack J, Quigley EM, et al. Pharmacological management of constipation. Neurogastroenterol Motil 2009;21(Suppl. 2):41–54. PMID: 19824937.
A pragmatic approach to using laxatives, based on a combination of what is known about mechanism of action and the available literature on evidence.

41. Chiotakakou-Faliakou E, Kamm MA, Roy AJ, et al. Biofeedback provides long term benefit for patients with intractable slow and normal transit constipation. Gut 1998;42:517–21. PMID: 9616314.
Demonstration of long-term efficacy of biofeedback in patients who have an initially good response to treatment.

42. Emmanuel A, Kamm MA. Response to a behavioural treatment, biofeedback, in constipated patients is associated with improved gut transit and autonomic innervation. Gut 2001;49(2):214–9. PMID: 11454797.

44. Knowles CH, Scott M, Lunniss PJ. Outcome of colectomy for slow transit constipation. Ann Surg 1999;230:627–38. PMID: 10561086.
Systematic review of most of the small reports of subtotal colectomy showing that efficacy is inversely related to duration of follow-up. A rationale for patient selection is presented.

58. Gladman MA, Scott SM, Lunniss PJ, et al. Systematic review of surgical options for idiopathic megarectum and megacolon. Ann Surg 2005;241:562–74.
A definitive systematic review of the published data on surgical procedures for idiopathic megacolon and megarectum in adults.

17

Anal fistula: evaluation and management

Phil Tozer
Robin K.S. Phillips

Introduction

Anorectal sepsis is common, presenting as either an acute abscess or a chronic anal fistula. Treatment in most involves only a small risk of minor complications, but a minority can present a major challenge to both sufferer and surgeon.

Although fistula-in-ano may be found in association with a variety of specific conditions, the majority in the UK are idiopathic or crypto-glandular, their exact aetiology having not been fully proven, although the diseased anal gland in the intersphincteric space is considered central. Research interest in factors encouraging fistula formation and persistence is growing. Fistulas may either be seen in association with or confused with Crohn's disease, tuberculosis, pilonidal disease, hidradenitis suppurativa, lymphogranuloma venereum, presacral dermoid/rectal duplication, actinomycosis, trauma and foreign bodies.[1] An important association is malignancy, which may manifest as a discharging opening on the perineum from a pelvic source, but which may (very rarely) also arise in long-standing fistulas, whether cryptoglandular, or associated with Crohn's disease or hidradenitis suppurativa.

The incidence is not known, as most data come from tertiary referral centres. Perhaps the most accurate information comes from Scandinavia, where incidences of between 8.6 and 10 per 10 000 have been reported. There is a male predominance, most series reporting a male to female ratio between 2:1 and 4:1. No sex differences in histology or distribution of anal glands has been found, and there seem to be no differences in circulating sex hormone concentrations between sufferers of either sex and healthy controls. Evidence supporting a hormonal explanation, via various mechanisms, for the observed gender difference has been published.[2] Anal fistulas most commonly afflict people in their third, fourth or fifth decades.[3-5]

The overall morbidity from fistula is difficult to assess in either individual or economic terms. For the majority of patients with simple fistulas, the time spent off work with the initial abscess and subsequent fistula management may be relatively short. However, it is not uncommon for a patient with a complex fistula to have had multiple hospital admissions over several years, loss of bowel control or a permanent stoma, or even be permanently incapacitated. For these patients, tertiary referral centres with the necessary expertise are essential, expertise lying in the hands not only of the surgeons, but also the nurses, radiologists, physiologists and psychologists.

Aetiology

Anal glands and their link with anal fistulas have been recorded since the end of the 19th century; their function is uncertain. They have been shown to secrete mucin, but this has a different composition from that secreted by rectal mucosa. Current thinking blames anal glands situated in the intersphincteric space; these may constitute one-third to two-thirds of the total number of anal glands found in an anal canal.[4]

✅ Eisenhammer[6] considered all non-specific abscesses and fistulas to be the result of extension of sepsis from an intramuscular or intersphincteric anal gland, the sepsis being unable to drain spontaneously into the anal lumen because of infective obstruction of its connecting duct across the internal sphincter.

✅ Parks[7] proposed that, should the initial abscess in relation to the intersphincteric anal gland subside, the diseased gland might become the seat of chronic infection with subsequent fistula formation. The fistula is thus a granulation tissue-lined track kept open by the infective source, which is the abscess around a diseased anal gland in the intersphincteric space. Parks[7] studied 30 consecutive cases of anal fistula and found cystic dilatation of anal glands in eight, which he attributed to acquired duct dilatation or more probably a congenital abnormality, a precursor to infection within a mucin-filled cavity.

Few studies have examined the cryptoglandular hypothesis. Goligher et al.[8] found intersphincteric space sepsis in only 8 of 28 cases of acute anorectal sepsis; of 32 cases of anal fistula, only 14 had evidence of either intersphincteric sepsis or the track travelling within (rather than simply across) the intersphincteric space. However, Goligher et al. failed to acknowledge that a proportion of cases of acute sepsis have nothing to do with fistula and that some common fistulas (e.g. superficial fistulas and those arising from a chronic anal fissure) have an aetiology separate from that postulated by Parks.

The importance of bacterial infection in fistula aetiology or persistence remains unclear. Although infection and its effective drainage are the primary problems in the acute stage, and although failure to treat secondary extensions and abscesses will inevitably lead to recurrence, the possibility that the anal gland becomes the seat of chronic infection in the established fistula has found little support in the only two studies directed at this aspect of the hypothesis.[9,10] Subsequent assessments of the fistula track microbiota using molecular techniques have also failed to demonstrate live bacteria but have found evidence of inflammation derived from the lumen, and of antibodies to and macrophages containing bacterial cell wall products.[11,12] Another aspect explaining why idiopathic fistulas might persist is that they become (at least partly) epithelialised, a factor responsible for failure of healing of fistulas at other sites in the body. A histological study of the intersphincteric component of 18 consecutive idiopathic anal fistulas showed that although an association between anal gland and fistula may be demonstrated in a minority of

cases, epithelialisation from either or both ends of the fistula track is a more common finding.[13]

Spread of sepsis from an acutely infected anal gland may occur in any of the three planes, vertical, horizontal or circumferential. Caudal spread is the simplest and most usual way by which infection is thought to disseminate to present acutely as a perianal abscess (labelled (a) in **Fig. 17.1**). Cephalad extension in the same space will result in a high intermuscular abscess (labelled (b) in **Fig. 17.1**) or a supralevator pararectal (or pelvirectal) abscess (labelled (c) in **Fig. 17.1**), depending on the relation of the sepsis to the longitudinal muscle layer. Lateral spread across the external sphincter will reach the ischioanal fossa (labelled (d) in **Fig. 17.1**), where further caudal spread will result in the abscess pointing at the skin as an ischioanal abscess; upward spread may penetrate the levators to reach the supralevator pararectal space. Circumferential spread (**Fig. 17.2**) may occur in any of the three planes: intermuscular (synonymous with intramuscular and equivalent to intersphincteric but with no restriction to a level beneath the anorectal ring), ischioanal or supralevator. All those conditions that Eisenhammer[14] considered not to be of cryptoglandular origin he placed into

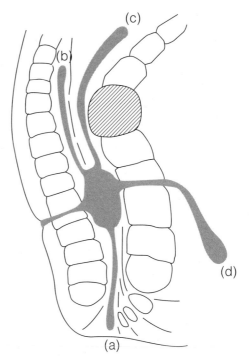

Figure 17.1 • The possible courses of spread of sepsis from the diseased anal gland in the intersphincteric space. See text for explanation.
Reproduced from Parks AG. The pathogenesis and treatment of fistula-in-ano. Br Med J 1961;i:463–9. With permission from BMJ Publishing Group Ltd.

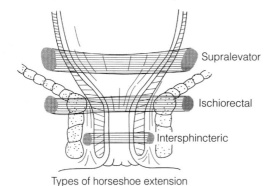

Types of horseshoe extension

Figure 17.2 • The three planes in which sepsis may spread circumferentially.
Reproduced from Parks AG, Gordon PH, Hardcastle JD. A classification of fistula-in-ano. Br J Surg 1976;63:1–12. © British Journal of Surgery Society Ltd. Permission is granted by John Wiley & Sons Ltd on behalf of the BJSS Ltd.

the miscellaneous group of acute anorectal non-cryptoglandular non-fistulous abscesses (**Fig. 17.3**). These included the submucous abscess (arising from an infected haemorrhoid, sclerotherapy or trauma), the mucocutaneous or marginal abscess (infected haematoma), the perianal abscess (follicular skin infection), some ischiorectal abscesses (primary infection or foreign body) and the pelvirectal supralevator abscess originating from pelvic disease.

Management of acute sepsis

The majority of chronic anal fistulas are preceded by an episode of acute anorectal sepsis, although acute sepsis does not inevitably lead to fistula formation.[15] The reported rates of recurrent abscess or fistula development following simple incision and drainage range from 17% to 87%. Hospital Episode Statistics (HES) data suggest that the rate is 17%. The optimal management of acute sepsis should reside in an understanding of aetiology. Pilonidal infection, hidradenitis and perianal Crohn's disease are usually fairly easy to recognise by history and examination, although it is worth noting that 10% of perianal disease in Crohn's presents before luminal symptoms and that a 14-month delay between abscess drainage and Crohn's diagnosis has also been reported based on HES data.[16] Pus in the perianal space may result from caudal spread of intersphincteric (cryptoglandular) infection or from simple skin appendage infection. Similarly, pus in the ischioanal space may or may not be related to anal gland disease.

Patients with acute anorectal sepsis usually present to the accident and emergency department rather than the outpatient clinic. Those with perianal sepsis tend to present early, 2 or 3 days after onset of symptoms, with pain and a tender lump close to

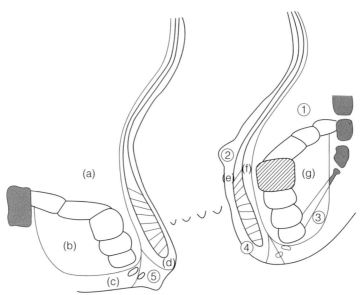

Figure 17.3 • The acute anorectal non-cryptoglandular non-fistulous abscesses of Eisenhammer: (a) pelvirectal supralevator space; (b) ischiorectal space; (c) perianal or superficial ischiorectal space; (d) marginal or mucocutaneous space; (e) submucous space; (f) intermuscular (syn. intersphincteric) space; (g) deep postanal space. 1, Pelvirectal supralevator abscess; 2, submucous abscess; 3, ischiorectal abscess; 4, mucocutaneous or marginal abscess; 5, perianal or subcutaneous abscess.
Reproduced from Eisenhammer S. The final evaluation and classification of the surgical treatment of the primary anorectal cryptoglandular intermuscular (intersphincteric) fistulous abscess and fistula. Dis Colon Rectum 1978;21:237–54. With permission from Lippincott, Williams & Wilkins.

the anal margin, and usually with no constitutional symptoms. Patients with ischioanal abscesses tend to present later with vague discomfort, but because much more pus may accumulate in the large relatively avascular loose areolar tissue of the ischioanal fossa, they often have fever and constitutional upset. Examination may reveal tender induration over the abscess rather than an exquisitely tender, well-defined lump. Sepsis higher up in the sphincter complex may present with rectal pain, and possibly disturbance of micturition, and there may be no external signs of pathology.

It was previously said that clues as to the aetiology of perineal sepsis may be gleaned from microbiology of the drained pus,[17,18] and that if skin organisms alone are cultured and the acute abscess is adequately drained, neither recurrence nor a fistula will result. Conversely it was said that if gut organisms are cultured, it is probable but not inevitable that there is an underlying fistula. In practice, microbiological assessment is rarely undertaken at the time of incision and drainage as the findings of such assessment would not change management and the evidence base underpinning these assertions is limited.

Determination of the presence or absence of sepsis in the intersphincteric space (irrespective of the site of the main abscess or whether an internal opening is demonstrable) has been shown to be the most accurate way of determining the presence of an underlying fistula,[19] although the clinical value of this determination remains disputed.

Those who advocate a more aggressive approach to acute sepsis do so on the basis that incision and drainage can only be effective if the abscess is not cryptoglandular,[14] that definitive treatment in the initial stage obviates further surgery, and that such a policy reduces the incidence of complex fistulas arising due to incompletely drained sepsis. The reported recurrence/fistula rate following primary fistulotomy (0–7%) supports this. There are drawbacks, however: internal openings are evident in only about one-third of cases; the acute situation facilitates creation of false tracks and internal openings; and the unknown proportion of patients with cryptoglandular sepsis who might be cured by incision and drainage alone would not be well served by a procedure associated with a greater risk of flatus incontinence and soiling. The randomised controlled trials of immediate fistula treatment (reviewed in references 20, 21) have a control arm of simple drainage in which 9–29% of patients presented postoperatively with a persistent fistula whereas 83–100% of patients in the fistula treatment arms were found to have a track that was treated at the initial procedure. Iatrogenic injury may account for this difference but, more likely, is an appreciation of the difference between aetiology

and persistence. Unnecessary fistulotomy or seton insertion ensures that patients will be exposed to the risks of fistula surgery without any benefit to them and only a minimal benefit to those who would develop a persistent fistula and could then be treated with the same operation at a later date.

✅✅ Meta-analysis of these trials[20,21] concluded that fistulotomy resulted in reduction in risk of recurrence at final follow-up but was associated, in the analysis by Quah et al., with a tendency to a higher risk of flatus incontinence and soiling (RR 2.46, 95% CI 0.75–8.06, $P = 0.14$). It is our view that these reviews conflate two groups of patients: those who will go on to suffer with a chronic fistula and those that would never suffer again after abscess drainage, and that therefore the latter group is put at an unnecessary risk.

Some advocate a policy (in experienced hands) of simple incision when a fistula is not evident, and primary fistulotomy when a fistula is evident and low (or a draining loose seton placed if there is any doubt about the level, or concern about continence), as long as the patient has been adequately counselled. However, we consider it more sensible to avoid fistula treatment in any form unless a chronic track in the context of recurrent abscess formation is found. In these circumstances, spontaneous regression seems unlikely and fistula treatment (after adequate counselling) will not be disadvantageous.

Classification of anal fistula

Successful surgical management of anal fistula depends upon accurate knowledge of anal sphincter anatomy and the fistula's course through it.

✅ The most comprehensive, practical and widely used classification is that devised by Sir Alan Parks at St Mark's Hospital, based on a study of 400 fistulas treated there.[22]

The cryptoglandular hypothesis and the presence of intersphincteric sepsis is central to this classification. Four main groups exist: intersphincteric, transsphincteric, suprasphincteric and extrasphincteric. These can be further subdivided according to the presence and course of secondary extensions.

Intersphincteric fistulas (**Fig. 17.4**; 45% of the original St Mark's series) are usually simple; however, others have a high blind track, or a high opening into the rectum or no perineal opening, or even have pelvic extension, or arise

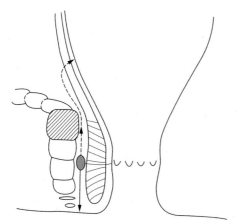

Figure 17.4 • The possible courses of an intersphincteric fistula.
Reproduced from Marks CG, Ritchie JR. Anal fistulas at St Mark's Hospital. Br J Surg 1977; 64:84–91. © British Journal of Surgery Society Ltd. Permission is granted by John Wiley & Sons Ltd on behalf on the BJSS Ltd.

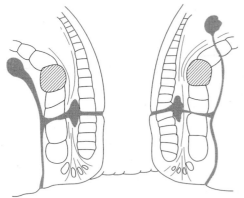

Figure 17.5 • A trans-sphincteric fistula with blind infralevator ischiorectal extension (*left*) and supralevator pararectal extension (*right*).
Reproduced from Parks AG, Gordon PH, Hardcastle JD. A classification of fistula-in-ano. Br J Surg 1976; 63:1–12. © British Journal of Surgery Society Ltd. Permission is granted by John Wiley & Sons Ltd on behalf on the BJSS Ltd.

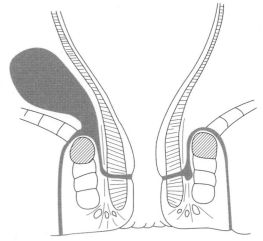

Figure 17.6 • Simple suprasphincteric fistula (*right*) and more complex form with associated secondary pelvic abscess (*left*).
Reproduced from Parks AG, Gordon PH, Hardcastle JD. A classification of fistula-in-ano. Br J Surg 1976;63:1–12. © British Journal of Surgery Society Ltd. Permission is granted by John Wiley & Sons Ltd on behalf on the BJSS Ltd.

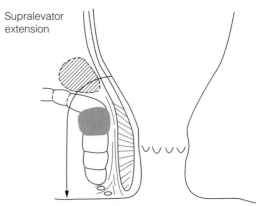

Supralevator extension

Figure 17.7 • Extrasphincteric fistula running without relation to the sphincter complex.
Reproduced from Marks CG, Ritchie JK. Anal fistulas at St Mark's Hospital. Br J Surg 1977;64:84–91. © British Journal of Surgery Society Ltd. Permission is granted by John Wiley & Sons Ltd on behalf on the BJSS Ltd.

from pelvic disease. Trans-sphincteric fistulas (**Fig. 17.5**; 29%) have a primary track that passes through the external sphincter at varying levels into the ischioanal fossa. Such fistulas may be uncomplicated, consisting only of the primary track, or can have a high blind track that may terminate below or above the levator ani muscles. Suprasphincteric fistulas (**Fig. 17.6**; 20%) run up to a level above puborectalis and then curl down through the levators and ischioanal fossa to reach the skin. Extrasphincteric fistulas (**Fig. 17.7**; 5%) run without relation to the sphincters and

are classified according to their pathogenesis. In addition to horizontal and vertical spread, sepsis may spread circumferentially in the intersphincteric, ischioanal or pararectal spaces.

The St Mark's classification does have drawbacks but these are of little clinical significance. Superficial fistulas and those associated with bridged fissures are not acknowledged by a classification whose emphasis is the intersphincteric space. There can be clinical difficulty in differentiating between a simple intersphincteric fistula and a very low trans-sphincteric fistula that crosses the lowermost fibres of the external sphincter. And some argue whether suprasphincteric tracks can be part of a classification based on cryptoglandular pathology (arguing that many are iatrogenic). The extreme rarity of suprasphincteric fistulas and the difficulty of distinguishing them from high trans-sphincteric tracks raise doubts about their very existence. However, clinical differentiation from high trans-sphincteric fistulas is in most cases immaterial since the same methods of treatment are employed.

Assessment

Clinical

A full history and examination, including proctosigmoidoscopy, are essential to exclude any associated conditions. The normal bowel habit and any risk of deterioration in the future (such as the presence of irritable bowel syndrome, inflammatory bowel disease or simply a tendency towards a loose stool) should be identified. A patient who passes a hard stool twice a week will tolerate a greater degree of sphincter disturbance than another who opens their bowel three times a day to a loose stool. Clinical assessment of the fistula involves five essential points, enumerated by Goodsall and Miles:

1. location of the internal opening;
2. location of the external opening;
3. course of the primary track;
4. presence of secondary extensions;
5. presence of other diseases complicating the fistula.

The relative positions of the external and internal openings indicate the likely course of the primary track, and the presence of any palpable induration, especially supralevator, should alert the surgeon to a secondary track. The distance of the external opening from the anal verge may assist in differentiating an intersphincteric from a trans-sphincteric fistula; also, the greater the distance the greater the likelihood of a complex cephalad extension.[4] Goodsall's rule generally applies in that the likely site of the internal opening can be predicted by the position around the anal circumference of the external opening. Exceptions to this rule include anteriorly located openings more than 3 cm from the anal verge (which may be anterior extensions of posterior horseshoe fistulas) and fistulas associated with other diseases, especially Crohn's and malignancy.

The first is to identify the position of the external opening(s). Next, the perianal area should be

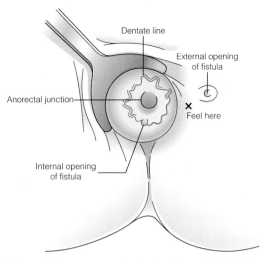

Figure 17.8 • Palpating for the direction and depth of the primary tract.
Reproduced from Phillips RKS. Operative management of low cryptoglandular fistula-in-ano. Operat Tech Gen Surg 2001;3(3):134–41. With permission from Elsevier.

carefully palpated with a well-lubricated finger to feel for the presence and direction of induration, which will indicate the course of the primary track (**Fig. 17.8**). If the track is not palpable, it is likely the fistula is not intersphincteric or low trans-sphincteric. Digital examination within the anorectal lumen is then performed to locate indentation/induration marking the site of the internal opening. Asking the patient to contract the anal sphincters allows assessment of the position of the primary track in relation to the puborectalis sling (posteriorly) or upper border of the external anal sphincter (anteriorly), although it must be remembered that in trans-sphincteric fistulas the level of the internal opening may not be the same as that at which the primary track crosses the external sphincter (which may be higher, especially if the internal opening is above the dentate line). The finger is then advanced into the rectum and supralevator induration sought (it feels like bone and is easier to notice when it is unilateral as there will be asymmetry; **Fig. 17.9**). Digital assessment of the primary track by an experienced coloproctologist has been shown to be 85% accurate.[23]

Examination under anaesthesia complements examination in the awake patient. The internal opening may be easily seen at proctoscopy, aided if necessary by gentle downward retraction of the dentate line, which may expose openings concealed by prominent valves or papillae. Lateral traction of an opened Eisenhammer proctoscope may reveal dimpling at the internal opening due to its underlying fibrous inelasticity. Massage of the track may reveal the site of the internal opening as a bead

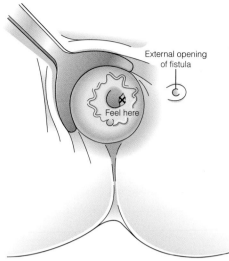

Figure 17.9 • Palpating for the presence of induration, indicating either a high primary tract or secondary extension in the roof of the ischiorectal fossa or supralevator space.
Reproduced from Phillips RKS. Operative management of low cryptoglandular fistula-in-ano. Operat Tech Gen Surg 2001;3(3):134–41. With permission from Elsevier.

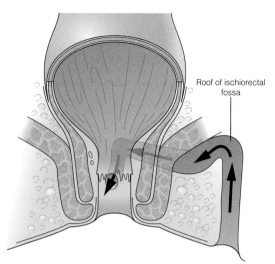

Figure 17.10 • Trans-sphincteric horseshoe fistulas may have several sharp bends along their course, preventing exact delineation unless the ischiorectal fossa is opened widely (to reach the acute bend in the roof of the ischiorectal fossa), and often necessitating dislocation of the posterior sphincter from its ligamentous attachments (to ascertain the site at which the tract crosses the external sphincter).
Reproduced from Phillips RKS. Operative management of low cryptoglandular fistula-in-ano. Operat Tech Gen Surg 2001;3(3):134–41. With permission from Elsevier.

of pus. If the track is simple, a probe may traverse its entire length, but if the probe comes to lie above or remote from the dentate line, a direct association between the track and the adjacent anoderm cannot be assumed.[24] Instillation of dilute hydrogen peroxide is the easiest way of locating the internal opening, as staining (for example with methylene blue) is avoided.[24,25]

Careful probing can delineate primary and secondary tracks. If the internal and external openings are easily detected but the probe cannot traverse the track, it is possible that there is a high extension, and a probe passed from each opening may then delineate the primary track. Failure to negotiate probes around a horseshoe posterior trans-sphincteric fistula suggests at least one acute bend in the track, within the intersphincteric space and crossing the external sphincter, or in the roof of the ischioanal fossa, in which case anatomy will only be defined once surgery is under way (**Fig. 17.10**). Persistence of granulation tissue after curettage during the operation is an indication of a secondary extension.[25]

Imaging

Previous surgery leads to scarring and deformity, as well as the creation of unusual tracks, which can make clinical assessment extremely difficult. Also, some techniques such as 'ligation of the intersphincteric fistula tract' (LIFT) or 'fistula tract laser closure' (FiLaC), rely on a simple, single track and confirmation of the anatomy is sensible to reduce the risk of failure due to occult extensions. The advent of endoanal ultrasound (EAUS) and magnetic resonance imaging (MRI), however, has resulted in a plethora of reports assessing and comparing imaging modalities, which have been comprehensively reviewed.[26]

These modalities have rendered fistulography almost obsolete, but it should be considered if an extrasphincteric track is possible. Computed tomography (CT) is indicated only when the fistula arises from an intra-abdominal or pelvic source.

EAUS is relatively cheap and easy to perform, but operator-dependent with limited focal range, making evaluation of pathology beyond the sphincters (laterally or above) difficult. These are the same areas from which difficulty in clinical assessment often arises. Also, sepsis and scarring from prior surgery can confuse fistula assessment. EAUS is superior to MRI in assessing sphincter integrity. Although the use of endoanal MRI coils has been favoured by some, they are not widely available. 3D EAUS is practised successfully by some surgeons in the clinic and the operating room, however we find the repeatability and accessibility of MRI make it the most useful modality. 3D

MRI, volume and activity assessment are under investigation and may enhance the value of MRI further in education, surgical planning and medical treatment monitoring.

Short tau inversion recovery (STIR) sequencing (a fat-suppression technique) to highlight the presence of pus and granulation tissue without the need for any contrast media[27] was used in a prospective study involving 35 patients at St Mark's Hospital that favourably compared MRI interpretations with the independently documented operative findings.[28] Schwartz et al. compared the accuracy of MRI, EAUS and EUA in a prospective cohort and found that a combination of any two yielded accuracy of 100%.[29]

Further prospective studies have confirmed that the technique certainly challenges operative assessment by an experienced coloproctologist as the gold standard. A prospective study has demonstrated a therapeutic impact of MRI in the management of patients treated for primary anal fistulas,[30] although the therapeutic impact is much greater when used to assess recurrent fistulas.[31]

✔ There is strong evidence that all recurrent fistulas should be examined using MRI preoperatively, and that the surgeon should use the scans to aid surgery. The accuracy of MRI also means that we are now able to refute or confirm the presence of sepsis in those patients with symptoms but in whom clinical examination is unrewarding, and in the prospective assessment of newer methods of attempted fistula eradication.

Physiological

The correlation between subjective assessment of an individual's continence and physiological measurements recorded in a laboratory is debatable. Some argue for physiological assessment (anal canal length, pressures along it, anorectal sensitivity, sphincter integrity and pudendal nerve conduction studies) in the clinical context of a patient with a complex fistula (or at risk of functional compromise); others (including the authors) find little or no value in it.

✔ Milligan and Morgan[32] stressed the importance of the anorectal ring in fistula surgery: 'If this ring be cut, loss of control surely results, yet as long as the narrowest complete ring of muscle remains, control is preserved. All the anal sphincter muscles below this ring may be divided in any manner without harmful loss of control.' This is substantially true.

Complete division of the puborectalis sling in suprasphincteric and extrasphincteric fistulas results in total incontinence. It is often said that the higher the level at which the primary track crosses the sphincter complex, the greater the possibility of impaired function after fistulotomy, and the weaker the sphincters before surgical intervention, the greater the likelihood of such morbidity. A similar line of thinking argues that the amount of muscle divided at fistulotomy is an important determinant of resultant function. In fact, as with liver resection, it is the amount left behind which is crucial and really quite high fistulas may be laid open with good results.

Traditionally, greater importance has been apportioned to the external than the internal anal sphincter in the context of muscle preservation in fistula surgery. Indeed, the importance of eradication of the presumed aetiological source, the diseased anal gland in the intersphincteric space, led Parks[7] to advocate internal sphincterectomy (excision of that segment of internal sphincter overlying the diseased gland) as an essential part of surgical management. Nowadays, most surgeons divide rather than excise the circular muscle, but the concept of getting rid of the intersphincteric source remains widely held.

To determine the physiological and functional effects of fistula surgery, a prospective study[33] of 37 patients successfully treated for either intersphincteric (15 patients) or trans-sphincteric fistulas was performed. All patients underwent division of the internal anal sphincter and anoderm below the level of the primary track; 15 of the 22 patients with trans-sphincteric fistulas also underwent division of the external sphincter, at least to the level of the dentate line, whereas the remaining seven patients with trans-sphincteric fistulas were successfully treated without external sphincter division. As might be predicted, distal anal canal and maximum resting pressures were reduced to a similar extent in all patients whether the internal alone or both sphincters were divided. The addition of external sphincter division in the 15 patients who underwent fistulotomy of trans-sphincteric tracks did, however, result in significant reductions in distal anal canal and maximum squeeze pressures.

Functional outcome was not related to division of the external sphincter, with an equal incidence of minor disturbances of continence reported by those in whom it had been preserved (53% vs 50%, respectively). Furthermore, the severity of postoperative symptoms was no different between the two groups, being related to reduced postoperative resting pressures, reduced maximum resting pressure and higher thresholds of anal electrosensitivity in the sector of surgery, rather than to postoperative squeeze pressures.

We have demonstrated similar findings in subsequent studies of fistulotomy[34,35] in which a 1 in 3 or 1 in 4 risk of flatus incontinence and mucus leakage or 'skid marks' in the underwear occurs with division of any amount of internal or external sphincter as long as a minimum length of external sphincter is left behind (2 cm as a rule but less in some cases), and in the presence of a normal bowel habit. This forms the basis of our informed consent for fistulotomy.

Total sphincter conservation would be optimal in terms of functional outcome, but the drawback is that no sphincter-preserving method heals the underlying fistula as surely as lay-open. This is important, because although the studies discussed above revealed a relatively high incidence of (minor) functional disturbance, the vast majority of patients were satisfied with their management and tolerated a reduction in function as a reasonable price to pay in order to be rid of chronic anal sepsis. When asked prospectively, patients are frightened by the term 'incontinence' and generally seek to avoid it.[36] It is important, instead, to outline the anticipated functional result and to be descriptive (e.g. wind might escape inadvertently and there might be 'skid marks' in the underwear), avoiding using emotive words such as 'incontinence' and also to acknowledge that patients at different stages of their 'journey' will have different goals and differing willingness to accept a risk of functional impairment to obtain cure.

Principles of fistula surgery

Acute sepsis is an indication for urgent surgical drainage, usually followed by early fistula treatment. However, in cases where a more complex procedure than lay-open is contemplated, acute sepsis should have been eradicated, leaving well-established chronic tracks. A loose seton may be required to achieve adequate drainage of the primary track. Secondary tracks should be either laid open, curetted or drained, according to their position in relation to the levators. Often, authors recommend parenteral antibiotics perioperatively and postoperatively for any of the more complex reconstructive procedures.

In the UK, fistula surgery is usually performed under general anaesthesia, but in North America local or regional anaesthesia is widely employed. There is some advantage of light general anaesthesia in that it is still possible to gauge muscle tone and determine how much muscle might remain were the fistula to be laid open. Similarly, in the UK most anal fistula surgery is performed with the patient in the lithotomy position, although the prone jack-knife position is favoured by some. The operative findings and treatment should be recorded; the St Mark's Hospital fistula operation sheet (**Fig. 17.11**) based on the Parks classification provides an excellent standardised format for documentation.

Surgical treatment – general principles and interpreting the evidence

Lay-open remains the surest way of eliminating an anal fistula. However, the risk of functional impairment, whether to stool (which is rare and can generally be avoided) or to flatus with marking of the underwear (which occurs at a rate of 1 in 3 when muscle is divided) may cause some to hesitate. Others prefer this risk to that of recurrence, particularly when the fistula is already recurrent or longstanding.[37] The multiplicity of techniques designed to preserve sphincter function and at the same time eradicate fistula pathology (the so-called sphincter-preserving procedures), reflects their relative lack of success. A degree of caution and scepticism may be appropriately apportioned when assessing reported results of the various approaches, since:

1. patient populations may be markedly different;
2. fistula classification may be variable;
3. reports of successes may not be tempered by honest reporting of failures;
4. reports of success in terms of fistula cure have historically not always been accompanied by reports of changes in continence;
5. despite the increasing drive for evidence-based medicine, the use of adequately powered prospective randomised trials is perhaps rarely achievable, because of individual fistula (and sphincter) variability and individual surgeon preference and skill;
6. follow-up may be inadequate and MRI confirmation of healing, which can substitute for longer follow up, may also be lacking.

The 'sphincter preserving' procedures do not succeed in permanently eradicating the fistula as often as fistulotomy, but some are also unable to demonstrate that they are truly protective of the patient's continence. This may be due to a degree of injury to the sphincter complex but may also relate to other aspects of the continence mechanism. It is possible to consider these procedures according to the element of fistula pathology to which they are directed. For example, the advancement flap and LIFT procedure disconnect the track from the gut tube (potentially causing a degree of sphincter damage in the process). The glues and plugs fill the space. Stem cells are thought to exert an anti-inflammatory effect but also to facilitate the wound repair process. Video assisted anal fistula treatment (VAAFT) and FiLaC obliterate the luminal aspect of the track to encourage healthy tissue to heal.

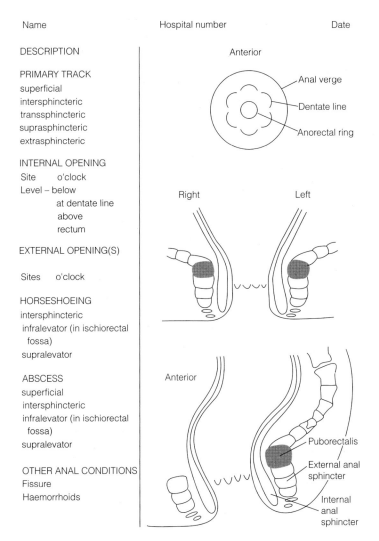

ST. MARK'S HOSPITAL
FISTULA OPERATION NOTES

Name   Hospital number   Date

DESCRIPTION   Anterior

PRIMARY TRACK
superficial
intersphincteric   Anal verge
transsphincteric
suprasphincteric   Dentate line
extrasphincteric
                                                    Anorectal ring

INTERNAL OPENING
Site   o'clock
Level – below   Right   Left
           at dentate line
           above
           rectum

EXTERNAL OPENING(S)

Sites   o'clock

HORSESHOEING
intersphincteric
infralevator (in ischiorectal
     fossa)
supralevator

ABSCESS   Anterior
superficial
intersphincteric
infralevator (in ischiorectal
     fossa)
supralevator   Puborectalis

                                                    External anal
OTHER ANAL CONDITIONS   sphincter
Fissure
Haemorrhoids   Internal
                                                    anal
                                                    sphincter

Figure 17.11 • The St Mark's Hospital fistula operation sheet.
Reproduced with thanks to Mr James P.S. Thomson, Emeritus Consultant Surgeon, St Mark's.

In order to improve outcomes, many techniques include elements thought (but rarely proven) to enhance healing or avoid complications, or to address an additional aspect of pathology. The use of antibiotics, mechanical bowel preparation and 'track preparation' are examples.

Track preparation

Track preparation is an increasingly explicit concept in surgical fistula trials. If one assumes that epithelialisation will prevent healing or that a secondary extension or undrained collection will induce early recurrence, a period of seton drainage followed by thorough debridement of the luminal aspect of the track should improve the chance of success. This question has been considered in a number of studies of seton drainage before transanal advancement flap repair, with some identifying a benefit and others not.[38] A study randomising patients to a full programme of track preparation with evidence of success (which might be measured by resolution of secondary extensions or abscesses, or reduction in inflammatory activity) before definitive surgery is required to answer this question.

Some techniques (such as the plug, LIFT or FiLaC) probably require a particular track anatomy (such as a single, straight, trans-sphincteric track) in order to be successful. In these cases, track preparation involves complete healing of secondary extensions (usually by laying open with seton drainage of the primary track) before the definitive operation can be attempted.

Track preparation has often been omitted in previous reports and the true success rate of some procedures may yet improve, or be found to be closer to that found in publications claiming superior rates.

Fistulotomy

Fistulotomy means laying open and allowing to heal by secondary intention. If fistulotomy is being considered, it is important to be aware of pre-existing bowel habit to help judge how much muscle should be preserved at surgery. In principle, high trans-sphincteric (especially anterior tracks in women) and suprasphincteric tracks should generally not be considered for fistulotomy. Intersphincteric and low trans-sphincteric tracks are probably best treated by this method.

We recommend the surgeon assess the fistula with a probe or a seton right through the fistula to determine whether it can be safely laid open based on the amount of muscle that would remain and a knowledge of the patient's bowel habit and wishes. If a sphincter-preserving procedure is planned, no fistulotomy is performed, since division of the internal sphincter would impose the risk of minor incontinence described above and not benefit the patient, instead compromising advancement flap surgery or a LIFT procedure. Also, 'medialisation' of the external opening is often unsuccessful and leads to bifurcation of the track outside the external anal sphincter with tracks to both new and old external openings – instead, a seton should be left in place. Hydrogen peroxide, the passage of a second probe through the other opening and the use of lachrymal probes may make it easier to traverse the difficult track with a probe. The internal opening is often lower than one assumes; the track may turn caudad in the intersphincteric space, and some tracks narrow at this point like an hour glass and will not allow a Lockhart–Mummery probe to pass but will accept a lachrymal probe.

✓✓ Marsupialisation, i.e. suturing the divided wound edge to the edges of the curetted fibrous track, results in a smaller wound and faster healing.[39,40]

Secondary extensions from the primary track can be dealt with in two ways. The traditional method in the UK is to lay these open widely to allow maximal drainage, which is followed by healing by secondary intention. As long as the external sphincter is intact, the residual scarring after healing

is remarkably little. In the USA, the use of incisions, counter-incisions and the placement of encircling drains is sometimes preferred; these drains are left in for 2–4 weeks, with more rapid healing and less deformity claimed.

Fistulotomy and immediate reconstitution

Parkash et al.[41] reported a series of 120 patients treated by fistulotomy, immediate reconstruction of the divided musculature and primary wound closure. The results were impressive: 88% of wounds had healed by 2 weeks, there was a 4% recurrence rate and all patients were satisfied with the functional outcome. However, 118 of the 120 fistulas were classified as low intersphincteric or simple trans-sphincteric, and the authors acknowledged that similar success would not be expected with more complex fistulas. The technique has been applied to a small cohort of patients with recurrent complex fistulas, not amenable to fistulotomy, with good results in terms of healing, manometric and functional outcomes, and with no report of dehiscence of the reconstituted sphincter.[42] More recently, Roig et al. published parallel case series of rectal advancement flap and fistulectomy with immediate sphincter repair for complex cryptoglandular fistula. In the fistulectomy and sphincter repair group, the new minor incontinence (soiling and flatus incontinence) rate following surgery was around 20% despite similar resting tone pre- and post-surgery.[43]

✓ A randomised trial of 55 patients with non-recurrent complex fistulas comparing fistulotomy combined with immediate sphincter reconstitution and advancement flap yielded equivalent results in terms of healing and functional outcomes.[44] This technique may be particularly useful in those with a pre-existing sphincter injury and continence deficit, in whom continence may improve.[45]

Fistulectomy

The technique of fistulectomy, which excises rather than incises the fistula track, has been criticised on the basis that the greater tissue loss leads to delayed healing.[46]

However, Lewis[47] advocates core-out fistulectomy rather than excision of the track, claiming that:

1. the precise course of the track is more accurately determined by core-out under direct vision, and does not involve the passage of probes along the track and thus creation of false tracks;

2. coring out the primary track reduces the risk of missing secondary tracks, which are seen as transected granulation tissue and which may be followed by the same technique;
3. the relation of the primary track to the external anal sphincter may be correctly ascertained before any sphincter muscle is divided;
4. a complete specimen is available for histology.

Once the track has been cored out, the decision as to whether the tunnel left can be safely laid open is made. For a non-recurrent single trans-sphincteric track, Lewis recommends simple anatomical closure of the cored-out tunnel, with mucosal closure and closure of the holes in the muscles. The wound outside the sphincters is lightly packed.

Of 67 low fistulas treated by Lewis[48] by coring out and laying open the resultant tunnel, there was one recurrence. Of 32 patients with high trans-sphincteric or suprasphincteric fistulas treated by core-out and simple anatomical closure, a temporary colostomy was raised in four and there were three recurrences. In the case of recurrent or more complex fistulas, Lewis recommends the adoption of other sphincter-conserving methods, since excessive scarring and the larger defect created by coring out this tissue make simple anatomical closure inappropriate.

Setons

The loose seton

Setons may be loose, tight or chemical. A thread, loosely tied, is often used as a marker of a fistula track when its exact position and level in relation to the external sphincter is unclear at surgery, but is more apparent when the patient is awake and with the track palpably delineated by the thread. The principal role of the loose seton is to drain acute sepsis, to allow inflammatory changes to settle facilitating safer definitive fistula treatment, or to reduce the risk of abscess formation after the administration of biologics in Crohn's disease.

At one time the loose seton was used with the aim of entire external sphincter preservation. Tracks and extensions outside the sphincters were widely laid open, and in the past the internal sphincter was then divided to the level of the internal opening (or higher if there was a cephalad intersphincteric extension). Subsequently, attempts at internal sphincter conservation were made. In the case of the high posterior trans-sphincteric track, the passage of the primary track across the sphincter complex may sometimes be accurately judged only after division of the so-called anococcygeal ligaments, thereby dislocating the posterior sphincter attachments, but others have proposed counter arguments.[49,50]

The seton, passed along the primary track across the external sphincter, is tied loosely to encircle the denuded voluntary muscle. At outpatient review, if there is evidence of good healing both of the wounds and around the seton, the latter is removed at 2–3 months on the basis that the driving force of the fistula in the intersphincteric space has been removed. Any suspicion of ongoing sepsis requires repeat examination under anaesthesia.

A series of 34 consecutive patients with complex idiopathic trans-sphincteric fistulas treated at St Mark's Hospital between 1977 and 1984 showed that cure (not validated by MRI) of the fistula without recourse to external sphincter division occurred in 44%.[51] Of those in whom the method had been successful, 83% reported full continence compared with only 32% of those in whom the external sphincter had subsequently been divided. Of the 16 patients in whom the technique failed, nine reported some degree of incontinence to formed stool; none of those in whom the external sphincter had been preserved reported any disturbance of sphincter function. Success rates of 67% and 78% have been reported. This technique is of mainly historical interest.

The importance of adequate follow-up to determine long-term outcomes following a particular technique has been exemplified by Buchanan et al.,[52] who reviewed 20 patients treated by this method a minimum of 10 years following surgery. Although in the short term 13 of the 20 healed, by 10 years only four had remained so.

With a loose seton in place, there are several options available: (i) the patient may be happy living with a 'controlled' fistula with a long-term draining seton. Our preference is for a permanent loose seton made of No.1 Ethibond with just one surgeon's knot and the 'whiskers' secured with 2/0 silk, to avoid bulkiness and to give comfort (nylon setons tend to be sharp, Silastic setons have bulky knots); (ii) a sphincter-sparing procedure might be considered; (iii) a fistulotomy may be performed (if appropriate); or (iv) fistulotomy may be combined with the raising of a defunctioning colostomy, time allowed for full healing, before sphincter repair and then restoration of intestinal continuity at a final stage. The decision made must be between the individual patient and the surgeon.

The tight seton

The rationale of the tight or cutting seton is similar to that of the staged fistulotomy technique, in that the divided muscle is not allowed to spring apart but there is supposed to be gradual severance through the sphincter followed by fibrosis. Goldberg and Garcia-Aquilar[53] recommend the use of a tight seton whenever the fistula encircles more than 30% of the sphincter complex and when local sepsis or fibrosis precludes the raising of an advancement flap.

The portion of the track outside the sphincters is laid open, although others in the USA have recommended Penrose drainage of horseshoe extensions. The anoderm and perianal skin overlying that portion of the sphincter encircled by the seton are incised and the intersphincteric space drained by internal sphincterotomy, extended cephalad if necessary to drain any high intersphincteric (intermuscular) extension. Tightening of the seton does not commence until any suppuration has resolved, usually at 3 weeks postoperatively. Tightening is repeated every 2 weeks using a silk tie or Barron band until the seton has cut through.

Goldberg described the use of the cutting seton in 13 patients with trans-sphincteric fistulas between 1988 and 1992, and found that the average time for the seton to cut through was 16 weeks (range 8–36 weeks) with no recurrences at a median follow-up of 24 months (range 4–60 months). This was tempered by a relatively high incidence of functional morbidity: one patient suffered major incontinence, and a further seven patients (54%) complained of minor persistent loss of control to flatus or episodic loss of liquid stool.

The critical aspects of management by the cutting seton must be firstly the elimination of acute sepsis and secondary extensions before sphincter division, and secondly the speed with which the seton cuts through the sphincter. In a series of 24 patients with high trans-sphincteric fistulas, Christensen et al.[54] tightened the seton every second day; 62% of patients reported some degree of incontinence postoperatively, including 29% who wore a pad constantly. The 'snug' Silastic (elastic) seton method, in which the muscle is cut through much more slowly but without the need for tightening, in the treatment of inter- and trans-sphincteric fistulas, was associated with healing in all cases, but with a 25% incidence of continence disturbance in the 16 patients followed up at a median 42 months after the seton had cut through.[55] The rates of sphincter disturbance described are similar to those seen with simple fistulotomy and therefore any benefit over single-stage fistulotomy is unclear. Another consideration is the time taken to heal and, in the case of the tight seton, the discomfort of tightening. As a result, it is difficult to define a clear role for this technique. We consider that the tight seton should not be used with high fistulas. Essentially, the decision to be made is whether or not a fistula can be laid open. If it can, then probably there is no advantage to laying it open slowly. If it cannot, then a tight seton will lead to significant faecal incontinence.

The chemical seton

This method, enjoying a resurgence in India where it is known as *Ksharasootra*, involves weekly reinsertion of a thread along the fistula track. The thread is prepared in a multistage process involving layers of agents derived from plants. Apart from its antibacterial and anti-inflammatory properties, the alkalinity of the thread (about pH 9.5) appears to be the means by which the thread slowly cuts through the tissues at about 1 cm of track every 6 days.

In a randomised trial involving 502 patients,[56] apart from a longer healing time (8 weeks vs 4 weeks), the results of this outpatient treatment were comparable with fistulotomy (incontinence rate 5% vs 9%; recurrence rate at 1 year 4% vs 11%).

Recurrences usually occur for the same reasons as after conventional surgery, such as a missed secondary track or another internal opening, but the economic advantages of such a method in a developing country are obvious. For low fistulas, however, a randomised study from Singapore concluded that the method has no advantage over conventional fistulotomy.[57]

Advancement flaps

Elting[58] described advancement flaps in anal fistula in 1912, supported by two principles: severing the communication with the bowel, and adequate closure of that communication with eradication of all diseased tissue in the anorectal wall. To these, modern surgeons have added adequate flap vascularity and anastomosis of the flap to a site well distal to the site of the (previously excised) internal opening. Modifications have included the use of full-thickness rectal flaps, partial-thickness flaps, curved incisions and rhomboid flaps, with or without closure of the defect in and outside the external sphincter,[59] and distally based flaps (anocutaneous flaps transposed upwards). Some authors argue that the flap should include part if not all of the underlying internal sphincter in order to maintain vascularity, but this may have an impact on continence.[43] Apart from the presence of acute sepsis, a large internal opening (>2.5 cm) is considered a contraindication as the risk of anastomotic breakdown is high,[60] and a heavily scarred, indurated perineum precludes adequate mobilisation.

Several studies have reported excellent results, with cure rates of 90–100% for idiopathic anal fistulas and little in the way of functional morbidity. A review of the technique and its results has been published.[61] The report by Athanasiadis et al.[62] is interesting for several reasons. In the larger series of patients (*n* = 224), internal sphincterotomy was performed aiming to eradicate the presumed source, but this led, as might be expected, to a much higher incidence of significant postoperative continence disorders than when internal sphincterotomy had not been performed. The persistent/recurrent fistula rate was 18% for trans-sphincteric fistulas and 40% for suprasphincteric fistulas. Preservation of the internal sphincter in a subsequent group of 55 patients resulted in a much lower incidence of functional morbidity, but unfortunately fistula persistence/recurrence was not reported. Physiological assessment has revealed that the technique may[59] or may not[63] be associated with preservation of resting and squeeze pressures, and success rates in terms of fistula healing decrease with time.[64]

Smoking has been shown to increase recurrence[65] and Mizrahi et al. found that Crohn's disease was also associated with failure.[66]

We find that advancement flap surgery is facilitated when there is a degree of perineal descent or internal intussusception, both of which can be identified in the outpatient setting. In their absence, we would not usually recommend this technique.

In a large series reported in 2010, Mitalas et al. describe successful healing in around two-thirds of 278 consecutive patients with high trans-sphincteric fistulas operated on in two tertiary referral units in the Netherlands.[38] This probably represents a realistic, high-quality series.

Intersphincteric approaches

In 1993 the senior author reported an intersphincteric approach with reasonable results. The LIFT operation (ligation of the intersphincteric fistula tract) is similar and combines disconnection of the track from the gut with destruction of the culprit intersphincteric gland. An intersphincteric approach is made, with ligation (or transfixion) and division of the track as it traverses the intersphincteric space. The external component is curetted and left open to drain whereas the intersphincteric wound is closed. Initial series of low fistulas demonstrated success rates in excess of 90% and then 80% without impairment of continence, but more complex tracks demonstrated a more modest success rate of 57%, also with preserved continence.

Two systematic reviews have examined the technique[67,68] and both found a pooled healing rate of around 75% with little or no impairment of continence. Some heterogeneity in technique and length of follow-up limits these findings but the technique is cheap and safe. The addition of a bioprosthetic implant in the intersphincteric space does not seem to confer a benefit. Recurrence/failure takes the form either of breakdown of the intersphincteric wound, intersphincteric recurrence of the fistula through the intersphincteric wound or full recurrence through the original trans-sphincteric track. Aside from the latter situation, failure is easier to treat than the primary fistula.[69]

Infill materials – glues and plugs (Table 17.1)

Enthusiastic initial reports have not always stood the test of time.[70] In fact, the literature describing fibrin glue and the fistula plug are remarkably similar, both suggesting initial success rates in the order of 80% which have fallen over the years to around 40%. Both approaches are highly attractive, as they require little surgical skill, but their weakness is their uncertain success rate. They may be used as an adjunct to advancement flap surgery. There are many considerations: biocompatibility; rate of decomposition/integration with host tissues; and how to prepare the host environment (drill/core-out/curette the track or leave it alone, prior identification and drainage/eradication of secondary extensions, and so on).[71]

Fibrin glue

Several reviews have discussed the variable efficacy reported for fibrin glue.[72–74] The 2010 Cochrane review of the surgical management of anal fistula evaluated two randomised trials of fibrin glue (versus fistulotomy and advancement flap repair). Fibrin glue was inferior in both and its place in the surgical armamentarium is questionable. Autologous glues have been largely replaced by commercially available virus-inactivated fibrinogen solution from donor plasma. The glue theoretically fills the track, promoting healing through fibroblast migration and activation and the formation of a collagen meshwork. Curettage to remove granulation tissue and debris is stressed. Difficulty

Table 17.1 • Biomaterials that have been used in the treatment of anal fistula

Autograft	Fibrin glue
	Fibroblasts
	Stem cells
Allograft	Fibrin glue
	Acellular dermal matrix plug
	Stem cells
Xenograft	Intestinal submucosal porcine collagen
	Dermal non-cross-linked porcine collagen
	Dermal cross-linked porcine collagen
Man-made/hybrid	Bovine serum albumin/glutaraldehyde
	Modified synthetic cyanoacrylic surgical glue
	Synthetic bioabsorbable polyglycolide–trimethylene carbonate copolymer
	Basic fibroblast growth factor

with this and complete occlusion of secondary tracks may account for failure. Early absorption or leakage from the fistula will also lead to recurrence and often occurs.[75]

Postoperative MRI, despite clinical healing, has shown much lower true healing rates, in the order of 10–20%.[76]

Bioprosthetic plugs

The anal fistula plug also sprang onto the scene with great optimism, with success rates of 80% reported. Subsequent success rates are very variable and proponents argue that surgical technique may be at fault, issuing consensus statements to try to improve outcome.[77]

> ✓ The plug has been compared with an advancement flap in two randomised trials. One closed prematurely due to an unacceptable failure rate with the plug,[78] while in the other, recurrence with a plug was also higher.[79]

Plug extrusion inevitably leads to failure and is thought to contribute to high recurrence rates in some studies. This may explain the association between a track length of over 4 cm and a three-fold increase in success rate.[80] In this study, the 43% success rate was disappointing, particularly given the small number of plug extrusions and the presence of an experienced plug surgeon at every case. However, the 61% success rate in the group with a long track and the median 2-year follow-up are more encouraging. In other studies, longer-term follow-up and MRI assessment have demonstrated a lower healing rate than was initially clinically apparent.[81,82] The results of the FIAT trial are eagerly awaited.

Newer techniques

VAAFT (video assisted anal fistula treatment)

VAAFT was developed by Meinero and first published in 2006.[83] It involves the introduction of a rigid fistuloscope into the track through the external opening, with saline or glycine irrigation to open the track, which can then be followed. The scope has a working channel which can accommodate forceps, brush or diathermy. The surgeon passes the scope into all accessible tracks and can undertake lavage, curettage and cauterisation. Meinero also undertakes closure of the internal opening with an advancement flap. The procedure has two phases: diagnostic and therapeutic. In evaluating this technique it is important to recognise the value of the two phases separately but in general a 'success

rate' meaning healing of the fistula is described. In fact, the main value of this technique may prove to be the identification and eradication of otherwise occult secondary extensions. VAAFT may represent a form of advanced track preparation before another definitive technique is performed.

Another use may be the reduction of symptoms in complex Crohn's fistulas, a technique currently under evaluation.[83a] In the Crohn's patient, the goal of treatment may be symptom control rather than fistula healing. Again, this requires an alternative method of assessment to that found in most studies of fistula surgery and indeed throughout this chapter.

In terms of a healing rate after VAAFT, the two largest series report healing in around 75% at short-term follow-up which seems to have been maintained at 1 year.[84,85] Complications are minor and the most common is perineal oedema caused by extravasation of irrigation fluid. This raises the question of iatrogenic track formation, which has not yet been widely reported.

FiLaC (fistula tract laser closure)

FiLaC was initially described in 2011 by Wilhelm and uses a radial emitting laser to obliterate the luminal aspect of the fistula to a known depth, throughout its length.[86] The technique was initially combined with closure of the internal opening by advancement flap but this was subsequently abandoned with no change to the success rate noted. The procedure is quick and easy. There is some pain postoperatively and the probes and laser are expensive. Success rates initially ranged from around 70–80%, but Wilhelm's 5-year experience shows a primary healing rate of around 65%.[87] Further assessment, particularly in Crohn's patients and in randomised trials, is required and will help establish the place of this technique.

OTSC (over the scope clip)

OTSC was first published in 2012 by Prosst and Ehni, who describe placement of a Nitinol clip over a denuded area around the internal opening, closing it and disconnecting the track from the gut. The largest series to date was published by Prosst in 2016 and describes a success rate of 79% in primary fistulas.[88] This falls to 26% in recurrent fistulas, 20% in rectovaginal fistulas and 45% in the presence of inflammatory bowel disease, although all these groups were much smaller. Clip migration and elective removal due to pain, soiling or for unexplained patient choice imply that the clip is not quite so well tolerated as the developers claim. One study[89] had very poor results with significant complications but the surgeons were inexperienced in the technique and included mostly very complex patients. The FISCLOSE trial is under way and may answer questions about efficacy and complications.

Stem cells

Adipose-derived mesenchymal stem cells (ASC) have been used in both cryptoglandular and Crohn's anal fistulas. In 2009, Garcia-Olmo reported a randomised phase II trial of fibrin glue with ASCs versus glue alone and subsequently reported long-term follow-up.[90] In the ASC group, 17 of 24 patients' fistulas closed at 8 weeks compared to three of 25 in the glue alone group. Two of the ASC group successes then relapsed at 1 year. In the long-term follow-up study, three were lost to follow-up and five relapsed so that of the original 17 successes, seven remained closed at the end of approximately 40 months' follow-up compared to two of the original three successes in the glue alone group.

✔ In Crohn's disease, the ADMIRE CD group have recently published a multicentre double-blind randomised trial of ASC injection versus placebo.[91] This large study with more than 100 patients in each arm used a combined clinical and radiological outcome measure and found remission in 50% in the treatment arm versus 34% in the placebo arm. Adverse events were modest but did include the development of HLA class I antibodies in a significant proportion of patients, although no immediate ill-effect was seen.

Whilst evidence of long-term success is limited, these studies suggest the potential of this technique. The anti-inflammatory, pro-wound healing action of stem cells may alter the immune environment surrounding the fistulas, encouraging healing. Whether in isolation or to enhance definitive surgical or medical treatment, stem cells are an exciting prospect.

Management of the recurrent fistula

Failure of sphincter-preserving methods and persistent symptoms may make lay-open the most sensible option, although some patients may prefer to live with a long-term loose seton. After fistulotomy many patients are able to lead normal lives with the narrowest of (often fibrotic) anorectal rings, as Milligan and Morgan stated.[32] However, some may request sphincter repair. MRI is a useful way of making sure that there is no covert pathology before embarking on repair. Over a 3-year period at St Mark's Hospital 20 patients underwent sphincteroplasty for incontinence after previous surgery for idiopathic fistulas. A good outcome (Parks' grade 1 or 2 continence score) was obtained in 13 (65%).[92]

It is important to consider the possibility of an extrasphincteric fistula arising from pelvic or abdominal disease or from a presacral dermoid cyst when a high 'blind' track is encountered. Failure to image (usually with MRI) is a major reason for delayed diagnosis. If a track is truly high and blind, this might be because the internal opening has closed, or because surgery has dealt with the primary track and recurrence is because of an overlooked secondary extension. In such cases, the component of the track outside the sphincters should be laid open and curetted. As the resulting wound may be large, it is often wise to make a circular rather than radial incision to avoid sphincter damage. Following granulation tissue with curette and probe must be done extremely carefully if false tracks and iatrogenic openings are to be avoided. If the track peters out before reaching the intersphincteric space, it is safest to stop and come back another day. If the track enters the intersphincteric space but no internal opening can be identified, it is reasonable to assume that the opening has healed or is extremely small; internal sphincterectomy of that quadrant is then justified to try to prevent recurrence.

Key points

- A fistula has a primary track and may have secondary extensions.
- Complete eradication of both will lead to cure.
- All lay-open procedures divide some of the internal sphincter, so patients should be warned of a 1 in 3 chance of inadvertent passage of wind and 'skid marks' in the underwear; 'incontinence' is an unhelpful word.
- Lay-open is the most certain treatment where it is possible and when the risks have been properly explained and accepted.
- Anterior fistulas in women should only rarely be laid open, as the risk of impaired continence is high.
- Advancement flaps are intuitively attractive but practically uncertain.

- Glue is only rarely effective – bioprosthetic plugs fare little better.
- Newer techniques appear regularly. Promising early results need long-term evaluation or MRI confirmation of healing.
- STIR sequence MRI is the gold standard for imaging but several newer techniques are under investigation.
- A permanent, comfortable, loose seton will preserve continence and prevent much (although not all) future abscess formation, but continual discharge means patients need explanation, and a minority find it unacceptable in the long term.
- In the balance between minor soiling with almost certain cure versus potential recurrence with a less than certain technique, many patients allowed the choice will choose the former but preferences vary between patients and within an individual patient's journey.

Recommended videos:

Documentary exploring the management of fistula in ano – https://tinyurl.com/yd26552u

Delormes advancement flap for ano-vaginal fistula – https://tinyurl.com/ycbfcy66

Rectal advancement flap – https://www.youtube.com/watch?v=dqVauLWgZ5k

LIFT –https://www.youtube.com/watch?v=7YXOJzIrKFM

FiLaC –https://www.youtube.com/watch?v=8cT4CV1gkAA

OTSC – https://www.youtube.com/watch?v=ZqPfWvCGL1g

Full references available at **http://expertconsult.inkling.com**

Key references

20. Quah HM, Tang CL, Eu KW, et al. Meta-analysis of randomized clinical trials comparing drainage alone vs primary sphincter-cutting procedures for anorectal abscess-fistula. Int J Colorectal Dis 2006;21(6):602–9. PMID: 16317550.

21. Malik AI, Nelson RL, Tou S. Incision and drainage of perianal abscess with or without treatment of anal fistula. Cochrane Database Syst Rev 2010;7:CD006827. PMID: 20614450.

39. Ho YH, Tan M, Leong AF, et al. Marsupialization of fistulotomy wounds improves healing: a randomized controlled trial. Br J Surg 1998;85(1):105–7. PMID: 9462396.

40. Pescatori M, Ayabaca SM, Cafaro D, et al. Marsupialization of fistulotomy and fistulectomy wounds improves healing and decreases bleeding: a randomized controlled trial. Colorectal Dis 2006;8(1):11–4. PMID: 16519632.

18

Minor anorectal conditions

Pasquale Giordano
Gianpiero Gravante

Haemorrhoids

Anatomy and physiology

Haemorrhoids are vascular arteriovenous plexuses that form two sets of anal cushions in the normal anatomy. These plexuses are located in the upper anal canal above the dentate line (internal haemorrhoidal plexus) and at the anal verge (external haemorrhoidal plexus). The internal haemorrhoidal plexus or internal haemorrhoids, also known as anal cushions, lie above the dentate line and are covered by columnar epithelial cells that have visceral innervation. Anal cushions or internal haemorrhoids are classically described as being in the right anterior, right posterior and left lateral aspect of the anal canal ('4–7–11 o'clock' in the lithotomy position).[1,2]

Newer technologies investigating the rectal and anal canal vasculature as a potential target for the treatment of haemorrhoidal disease have established an average of six haemorrhoidal arteries originating from the superior rectal artery and reaching the haemorrhoidal zone (range 1–8).[3] The internal haemorrhoidal plexus drains to the middle rectal veins and then into the internal iliac vessels.

The internal haemorrhoids complement anal sphincter function in normal physiology by providing fine control over the continence of liquid and gas; however, their abnormal enlargement produces haemorrhoidal disease, corresponding to the common complaints experienced by patients and treated by colorectal surgeons. It has been demonstrated that the anal cushions can contribute upto 20% of the resting anal pressure.[4]

The external haemorrhoidal plexus, also known as external haemorrhoids, lies below the dentate line in the subcutaneous tissue at the anal verge and drains via the inferior rectal veins into the pudendal vessels and then into the internal iliac vein. These haemorrhoids are not normally visible and do not really contribute to the physiology of the anal canal. These vessels are covered by anoderm that is comprised of modified squamous epithelium containing pain fibres, this affecting the way they present and are treated.

The words 'haemorrhoids' and 'haemorrhoidal disease' are not synonymous and should be used specifically to name either the presence of normal arteriovenous plexuses or the disease produced by their engorgement, respectively.

Aetiology and pathogenesis

Haemorrhoidal disease affecting the internal haemorrhoids develops when tissues supporting the anal cushions deteriorate and allow them to slide down into the anal canal,[2] which in turn leads to impaired venous drainage, progressive venous engorgement, local stasis and transudation of fluid. The anal cushions function normally when they are fixed to their proper sites within the anal canal by fibromuscular ligaments, which are the anal remnants of the longitudinal layer of the muscularis propria from the rectum (Treitz's ligaments). When these submucosal fibres fragment, the anal cushions are no longer restrained from engorging excessively with blood, and bleeding and prolapse may result. These fibres may be fragmented by prolonged and repeated downward stress related to straining during

223

defaecation. Veins that traverse the anal sphincter are blocked whereas arterial inflow continues, leading to increasing haemorrhoidal congestion. Once prolapse occurs, further engorgement of these vascular cushions leads to pain and anal spasm that prevents reduction, leading to a vicious cycle of prolapse and congestion of the vascular cushions.

Risk factors for this condition are those that directly or indirectly are associated with excessive straining and/or increased intra-abdominal pressure (i.e. constipation, hard stools, pregnancy).[5] The progressive descent of the internal cushions produces various degrees of prolapse, one of the main symptoms of haemorrhoidal disease, while external haemorrhoidal disease manifests directly with venous engorgement. Defaecation in the squatting position may also aggravate the tendency to prolapse as it increases perineal descent and pressure. The anatomical alterations modify the vascular haemodynamics by decreasing venous reflux (especially in the erect position) and increasing the intravascular venous pressure. Microtrauma elicited during defaecation of hard solid stools produces small lacerations of the vessel wall and, consequently, another important symptom – bleeding.

The venous hypertension of the diseased anal cushions augments the filtration of fluid through the vessel wall (transudate), producing what has been referred to as 'soiling' (although its pathogenesis is not due to anal incontinence) and local itching. Local blood stasis also promotes venous thrombosis, and the sudden onset of venous hypertension stretches the mucosa overlying the cushion and causes the typical severe perianal pain experienced during the attack (thrombosed haemorrhoidal disease).

Classification

The classic staging of haemorrhoidal disease refers to the internal plexus prolapse and is classified into four degrees (Goligher's classification): grade 1 – the anal cushions bleed but do not prolapse; grade 2 – the anal cushions prolapse through the anus on straining but reduce spontaneously; grade 3 – the anal cushions prolapse through the anus on straining or exertion and require manual replacement into the anal canal; and grade 4 – the anal cushions are constantly prolapsed. This classification is therefore a clinical classification based on the actual symptoms rather than size or appearance of haemorrhoids.

Symptoms and diagnosis

The most frequent symptom of haemorrhoidal disease is bleeding, normally reported as bright red.[6] Bleeding is usually self-limiting, although in patients on anticoagulation or with a predisposing bleeding diathesis it can be more abundant. Other symptoms include prolapse (**Fig. 18.1**), mucous discharge, itching and feeling of a lump. Thrombosed haemorrhoid from the internal plexus normally presents as a very large and painful prolapsed pile. This non-reducible haemorrhoid should not be called 'external haemorrhoids'. Thrombosis of external haemorrhoids is also responsible for acute anal pain irrespective of bowel movements.[6] Contrary to thrombosed haemorrhoids from the internal plexus, thrombosed haemorrhoids from the external plexus will present as a relatively small and well-defined nodule at the anal verge. This very painful condition is also known as perianal haematoma. External haemorrhoids should not be confused with anal skin tags that are always present and not normally painful.

Haemorrhoidal disease can be diagnosed by history and examination (including inspection of the anal canal). Fresh bleeding not associated with any other anal symptoms and without any other colorectal alarm symptoms (i.e. change in bowel habit, abdominal pain) or without family history of colorectal neoplasia should be investigated with a flexible sigmoidoscope. Anaemia or right-sided abdominal pain/palpable mass should be evaluated by a complete colonic examination (either a colonoscopy or computed tomography [CT] virtual colonography).

Management

Therapeutic strategies normally depend on the severity of symptoms and the amount of haemorrhoidal tissue prolapsing beyond the anal verge (Goligher classification; see Table 18.1).[7]

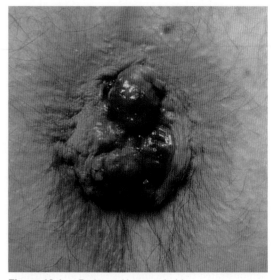

Figure 18.1 • Prolapsed haemorrhoids

Table 18.1 • Level of evidence for the treatment of haemorrhoids according to the severity of prolapse

	Level of evidence			
	I	II	III	IV
First-degree		Dietary changes and flavonoids	Rubber-band banding Sclerotherapy Infrared coagulation	
Second-degree	Rubber-band ligation	HAL/THD	Stapled haemorrhoidopexy	
Third-degree	Stapled haemorrhoidopexy	Haemorrhoidectomy	HAL/THD Rubber-band ligation	
Fourth-degree		Haemorrhoidectomy	Stapled haemorrhoidopexy, HAL/THD with haemorrhoidopexy	
Single external cushion			Haemorrhoidectomy (Ultracision,LigaSure)	

HAL, haemorrhoidal arterial ligation; THD, transanal haemorrhoidal dearterialisation.

First-degree

Dietary changes

If the piles are not prolapsing, non-operative methods should be attempted first (grade II evidence). The primary problems of constipation and straining at stool need to be addressed. In some patients, improving bowel action with laxatives in the form of fibre may help to control the symptoms.[8,9]

Phlebotonics

Phlebotonics consist of plant extracts (i.e. flavonoids) and synthetic compounds (i.e. calcium dobesilate) which improve venous tone, stabilise capillary permeability and increase lymphatic drainage.[10] There are several available phlebotonics, but Daflon 500® (Les Laboratoires Servier, France) is by far the best evaluated in the medical literature, and is widely used in Europe and the Far East.[11] Its pharmacological properties include noradrenalin-mediated venous contraction, reduction in blood extravasation from capillaries and inhibition of prostaglandin (PGE_2, PGF_2)-mediated inflammatory response.[12] Phlebotonics, although currently not available in the UK, improve pruritus, bleeding and leakage, but not pain.[10]

Other forms of treatment that can give more immediate symptomatic relief include rubber-band ligation, injection sclerotherapy and infrared coagulation (grade III evidence). Only cases refractory to non-operative methods should undergo these more invasive treatments.[7] Topical applications are popular with many patients, who testify to relief from bleeding and pain. There are, however, no clinical trials to demonstrate any benefit from such applications.

✅✅ Dietary changes, fibre[8,9] and phlebotonics[10,11] help control symptoms in first-degree haemorrhoidal disease. Invasive treatments should be reserved for refractory cases.

Second-degree

Rubber-band ligation

Rubber-band ligation is the technique of choice for second-degree haemorrhoidal disease (grade I evidence),[7] for which it is effective in 68% of patients at 5 years follow-up, with a 2–5% risk of secondary haemorrhage. Rubber bands are applied in an outpatient clinic or at the end of an endoscopic examination at the apex of the haemorrhoidal tissues just above the dentate line, taking care to avoiding catching the dentate line. The strangulated tissue then becomes necrotic and sloughs off in a few days, after which the wound fibroses, resulting in fixation of the mucosa akin to forming new suspensory ligaments for the anal cushions. The haemorrhoidal tissue is thus prevented from engorging and prolapsing.

✅✅ Rubber-band ligation is the treatment of choice for second-degree haemorrhoidal disease when compared with excisional haemorrhoidectomy. In this group it achieved similar results without the side-effects of surgery. Surgery should be reserved for recurrent or third-degree haemorrhoids.[13]

Anal pain, although uncommon, is a well-known sequel of rubber-band ligation; however, the procedure is relatively painless if correctly performed above the dentate line. The use of local anaesthetic infiltration prior to the rubber-band ligation decreases the amount of post-procedure pain experienced.[14] Some patients may still experience tenesmus for a day or two that is partially relieved by oral analgesia. Up to three haemorrhoids can be banded on the same occasion, although at the expense of greater discomfort. Rubber-band ligation can easily be repeated and often is offered as a course rather than one-off treatment; approximately 4 weeks is the usual interval between each session.[7]

Sclerotherapy

Injection sclerotherapy is an alternative technique used for the treatment of second-degree haemorrhoids, providing at least some temporary symptomatic relief in 69% of patients.[7] Sclerosant agents used include phenol (5%) in almond oil or sodium tetradecyl sulphate. These are injected into the submucosa around the pedicle of the pile, at the level of the anorectal ring, and cause local inflammation leading to reduced blood flow into the haemorrhoids. The sclerosant also causes fibrosis, which draws minor prolapse back into the anal canal.

> ✔ Inadvertently deep injections can cause perirectal fibrosis, prostatitis, infection and urethral irritation. Rare but major complications such as impotence, fatal necrotising fasciitis and abdominal compartment syndrome following sclerotherapy have been reported.[7]

Other treatments

Various other methods have been abandoned over the years. Infrared photocoagulation produced less pain compared to rubber-band ligation and sclerotherapy, but required an additional device.[15] Cryotherapy results in unpleasant and foul smelling discharge and, if not performed properly, can destroy the internal anal sphincter producing anal stenosis and incontinence. Anal stretch, based on the belief that haemorrhoidal disease derives from a narrowing of the lower canal, is not performed any more due to the concerns of damage to the internal anal sphincter and subsequent impairment to anal sphincter function.

Third-degree

Traditionally, third-degree haemorrhoidal disease was removed by excisional haemorrhoidectomy. Haemorrhoidectomy as first described by Milligan and Morgan consists of the excision of the diseased anal cushions. Since then numerous variations to the technique have been described. It can be conducted under local or general anaesthesia; excision of haemorrhoidal cushions can be conducted with scissors,[16] diathermy, laser, vessel-sealing technology

(Ligasure), ultrasonic technology (Harmonic Scalpel)[17] or radiofrequency devices;[18] mucosal wounds can be closed (Ferguson, Parks) or left open (Milligan–Morgan). Open and closed haemorrhoidectomies produce similar results for postoperative pain, complications and hospital stay.[19] The comparison of Ligasure versus diathermy haemorrhoidectomy showed lower postoperative pain and urinary retention rate, shorter operative time, hospital stay and return to work for Ligasure haemorrhoidectomy.[20–22] Similar advantages were found for Harmonic Scalpel versus conventional haemorrhoidectomy with regard to postoperative pain and return to work.[23]

Nowadays, two new procedures have been added to the surgical armamentarium for the treatment of symptomatic haemorrhoids, namely stapled haemorrhoidopexy and haemorrhoidal arterial ligation, also known as transanal haemorrhoidal dearterialisation (HAL/THD).

Stapled haemorrhoidopexy

Conventional haemorrhoidectomy deals with the symptoms alone by excising the anal cushions once they bleed or are painful. It does not act on the pathophysiological mechanism that produced the haemorrhoidal disease, the descent of the mucosal anal cushions. In 1998 a transanal circular stapling instrument was used to treat haemorrhoidal disease. The technique consisted of circumferential mucosectomy and mucosal lifting (haemorrhoidopexy), and aimed not to excise the 'diseased' haemorrhoidal cushions but rather to reconstitute the normal anatomy and physiology of the haemorrhoidal plexus.[24] Once reduced, the engorged haemorrhoidal tissue will decongest and shrink. It is thought that the stapling device restores the normal anatomy of the anal canal and enables the haemorrhoidal cushions to perform their role in continence, as opposed to haemorrhoidectomy techniques that only excise excess tissue.

Since its introduction numerous studies have assessed the short- and long-term efficacy of stapled haemorrhoidopexy, and thus far this technique has produced the largest amount of evidence-based analyses comparing it to classic and modern haemorrhoidectomies. Stapled haemorrhoidopexy produced better results compared to traditional haemorrhoidectomies with regard to early postoperative outcomes such as postoperative pain, bleeding and length of hospital stay.[25–28]

> ✔✔ Short-term outcomes are significantly improved in stapled haemorrhoidopexy compared to techniques of traditional haemorrhoidectomy.[25–28]

Comparison of stapled haemorrhoidopexy to Ligasure haemorrhoidectomy produced similar early postoperative results for pain, bleeding, urinary retention, difficulty to defaecate, anal fissure, stenosis, incontinence, return to normal activities and hospital stay.[29–34] Stapled haemorrhoidopexy is associated with increased recurrence of haemorrhoidal prolapse and anal skin tags when compared to classic haemorrhoidectomy on long-term follow-up.[24,27,28,35,36]

> ✅✅ Stapled haemorrhoidopexy loses its early postoperative advantage when compared to Ligasure haemorrhoidectomy. Furthermore, recurrence is higher compared to classic haemorrhoidectomies at long-term follow-up.[35]

An additional feature of stapled haemorrhoidopexy is the potential to produce significant serious morbidity and even mortality in the immediate postoperative period. These complications, albeit rare and reported mostly as case reports, seriously endanger the patient's life for what is the treatment of an otherwise benign disease and are often heralded by abdominal pain, urinary retention and fever.[37–39] It is believed that such complications derive from a full-thickness (or near full-thickness) staple line and resulting anastomotic leakage. Furthermore, distressing new symptoms such as tenesmus are probably related to the mucosal stimulation of the staple metallic foreign bodies which sometimes require a second operation for their removal.[40]

Haemorrhoidal arterial ligation/transanal haemorrhoidal dearterialisation

This non-excisional technique is based on the occlusion of the haemorrhoidal arterial flow that feeds the haemorrhoidal plexus by Doppler-guided identification and ligation of the terminal branches of the superior rectal artery using a specially designed proctoscope. The reduction in blood flow to the haemorrhoids leads to shrinkage of the anal cushions. Although the sensitive anoderm below the dentate line is avoided to minimise postoperative pain, this is still present in 18.5% of patients.[3] After 1-year follow-up, recurrence was present in 4.8% for third-degree and 26.7% for fourth-degree haemorrhoidal disease, although the addition of a mucosal plication (mucopexy) seemed to further decrease such occurrence in fourth-degree patients.[3]

> ✅✅ Both HAL/THD and stapled haemorrhoidopexy produce equal results in terms of duration of the operation, postoperative complications and recurrence rates, but postoperative pain is significantly less after HAL/THD.[41]

Fourth-degree

Haemorrhoidectomy is the main treatment for fourth-degree haemorrhoids although some authors have suggested that THD may also have a role in the treatment of advanced haemorrhoidal disease.[42-44] In general, newer technologies significantly reduce postoperative pain and speed up postoperative recovery and return to work at the expenses of increased costs due to the disposable devices and possible increased recurrence rate.

Postoperative problems

Common problems that occur after haemorrhoidectomy include urinary retention, transient incontinence to flatus and faecal impaction.

Postoperative pain

Despite the numerous treatments that over the decades have been proposed for the surgical treatment of haemorrhoids, the essential problems encountered remain similar. Whichever technique is used, pain may still be significant in some patients in the postoperative period. Some authors have described post-haemorrhoidectomy pain as being akin to passing pieces of sharp glass fragments, such that many patients would rather suffer the discomfort of large prolapsing haemorrhoids for years than submit to surgery. Pain is multifactorial, spasm of the internal sphincter as well as the actual skin wound with its exposed nerves being the most significant factors.

Numerous meta-analyses have evaluated the effects of various adjuncts to oral analgesics (non-steroidal anti-inflammatory drugs, paracetamol and opiates) to control postoperative pain. Local anaesthetic infiltration (pudendal nerve block) has been shown to significantly improve immediate postoperative pain.[45] Glyceryl trinitrate is thought to decrease muscle spasm and increase anodermal blood flow in the first 2 postoperative weeks following haemorrhoidectomy; it improves pain, healing and resumption of daily activities at the expense of an increased incidence of headaches.[46] Similar results were also achieved with local calcium channel blockers and botulinum toxin A.[47] The effects of oral and topical metronidazole on postoperative pain have been assessed in numerous comparative studies with contrasting results.[48–53]

> ✅✅ Local anaesthetics,[45] glyceryl trinitrate (GTN)[46] and calcium channel blockers and botulinum toxin are useful postoperative adjuncts for postoperative pain.[47]

Postoperative haemorrhage

A less frequent problem is postoperative haemorrhage. Bleeding in the immediate postoperative period is usually due to inadequate intraoperative haemostasis. Submucosal adrenaline (epinephrine) injection has been shown to be effective for addressing bleeding after excisional haemorrhoidectomy.[54] Secondary bleeding is more often a result of postoperative infection and it affects approximately 5% of patients undergoing haemorrhoidectomy. The advocated treatment is antibiotics. Following stapled haemorrhoidopexy, bleeding may follow the rare staple-line dehiscence.

Anal stenosis

Post-haemorrhoidectomy anal stricture is an uncommon occurrence seen in only 3.7% of haemorrhoidectomies,[55] and is a complication of technical failure to leave sufficient mucocutaneous skin bridges. The stricture usually presents 6 weeks postoperatively and is treated with anal dilatation and stool softener.

Thrombosed haemorrhoids

Prolapsed thrombosed internal haemorrhoids (**Fig. 18.2**) and perianal haematoma are best managed conservatively. The course of these conditions is self-limiting and normally symptoms resolve within a couple of weeks. Laxatives, stool softeners, sitz baths, ice packs, oral and topical analgesia are often helpful. Perianal haematomas presenting very early may be considered for surgical excision or drainage. Very rarely prolapsed thrombosed internal haemorrhoids with a gangrenous component may also require excision (**Fig. 18.3**).

Conclusions

Anal cushions are normal structures contributing to the mechanism of continence. They may become abnormal resulting in symptomatic haemorrhoids following straining and other factors. First- and second-degree haemorrhoidal disease often responds

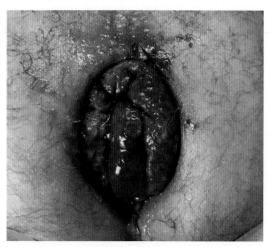

Figure 18.2 • Thrombosed prolapsed internal haemorrhoids.

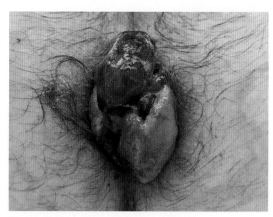

Figure 18.3 • Gangrenous haemorrhoids.

to conservative measures and can be managed without surgery; however, surgical intervention should be considered for large prolapsing piles.

Anal fissure

An anal fissure is an ulceration of the squamous epithelium of the anal canal distal to the dentate line. It is a common complaint encountered in the colorectal clinic. Medical treatment is simple but is frequently not followed by patients and is not successful in a significant proportion of cases. Surgical management has become less used recently due to the application of botulinum toxin in current practice.

Aetiology

Two main factors contribute to the formation of posterior anal fissures. First, hard faeces contribute by increasing the local trauma on the anal mucosa, although 25% of fissures present in patients without constipation.[56] Second, affected patients frequently present with internal anal sphincter hypertonia which, in turn, enhances the traumatic effect of the hard faeces and provokes a relative tissue ischaemia with decreased blood supply to the anal mucosa. The internal anal sphincter alone appears to be responsible for the hypertonia.[57] Hypertonia of the internal anal sphincter is caused by the decreased production of nitric oxide, a substance that normally relaxes the muscle. This results in the high mean resting anal pressures frequently seen in affected patients.

After the initial tear, a vicious cycle of non-healing and repeated trauma leads to development of chronic deep fissures. In this cycle, local pain increases sphincter reflex contraction, which in turns worsens the effects of hard stools and local tissue ischaemia. This mechanism can explain the achievement of high healing rates with therapies able to reduce the sphincter hypertonia and improve the local blood flow.[58]

Although this mechanism is valid for most patients, other factors have to be considered in elderly patients or postpartum patients where anal fissure has been reported in the presence of normal or hypotonic internal sphincters.[59]

Classification

Anal fissures are classified according to their duration into acute or chronic, their morphological appearance into 'superficial' or 'deep' fissures, and according to their location into posterior (80–90%), anterior (2.5–10%), or in unusual positions. Furthermore, primary anal fissures are not caused by underlying chronic disease whereas secondary anal fissures are associated with other diseases such as chronic inflammatory bowel disease, human immunodeficiency virus, tuberculosis, syphilis and some neoplasms.[59] Secondary fissures are usually multiple or located in unusual positions.

Anal fissures are considered to be acute if they have been present for less than 6 weeks, are superficial and have well-demarcated edges. They are considered chronic if they have been present for more than 6 weeks and have keratinous edges, if there is a sentinel tag and hypertrophied anal papilla and if the fibres of the internal anal sphincter are visible in the base of the fissure (**Fig. 18.4**).[59]

Superficial fissures, as the name implies, involve only the superficial mucocutaneous layers of the anal canal, presenting with a superficial separation of the anoderm with sharp edges. The base of the fissure does not reach the internal anal sphincter. The vast majority of superficial fissures will heal spontaneously within days or within a few weeks of appropriate conservative treatment. Deep anal fissures are recognised by the characteristic deep, wide, pear-shaped ulcer, often with visible fibres of the internal anal sphincter and minimal granulation tissue at the base. Other features of a chronic anal fissure include the distinctive triad of indurated ulcer edges, a distal skin tag (sentinel pile) and a proximal hypertrophic anal papilla. Deep fissures often persist and either tend not to heal without intervention or recur regularly.

Posterior anal fissure presents in the posterior triangular space, also called space of Brick or triangle of Minor. The space is formed by the peculiar architectural arrangement of the sphincter mechanism in the posterior midline, where there is a 'Y'-shaped deficiency of the fibres of the external sphincter.[60] This space is an area where traumatic factors act most and where high resting anal pressures and reduced local perfusion are found. Furthermore, branches of the inferior rectal artery at the posterior commissure are less dense in the subanodermal space and within the internal anal sphincter in the posterior midline.[61] In contrast, anterior anal fissures are more frequent in women and are usually associated with occult external anal sphincter injuries and impaired sphincter function. Such pathogenetic mechanisms have important implications and exclude treatments such as lateral sphincterotomy or botulinum toxin injection.[62]

> ✓ Anterior fissures have aetiopathogenetic mechanisms different from those located posteriorly. High sphincter pressures seem less responsible for these fissures and therefore treatments not acting on the anal pressures, such as anal flaps, should be preferred.

Symptoms and diagnosis

Pain is usually the predominant symptom in anal fissures, with or without the presence of fresh bleeding. The pain classically presents during defaecation and is described as excruciating and sharp, like 'a knife cutting', which lasts for several minutes or the entire day. Anal fissures can be visualised by gentle parting of the buttocks with eversion of the anal verge. Superficial anal fissures will show as a linear tear, while deeper fissures may expose the white transverse fibres of the internal anal sphincter. Chronic fissures may also have fibrotic edges and are commonly associated with external skin tag, called a 'sentinel skin tag', and occasionally a hypertrophic anal papilla at the level of the dentate line. Intra-anal examination should not be attempted in the clinic due to the severe pain. If the clinical suspicion of a secondary pathology is high, digital rectal and proctoscopic examinations

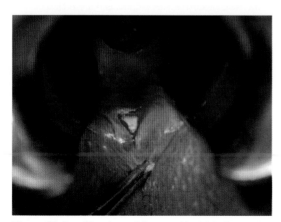

Figure 18.4 • Chronic anal fissure with visible fibres of the internal anal sphincter and sentinel skin tag.

should be performed under regional or general anaesthesia.

Differential diagnoses include all causes of secondary fissures, anal cancers and intersphincteric abscesses. Where in doubt, biopsy and appropriate histological examination and/or cultures are indispensable.

Management

The current treatment of anal fissures in the UK is summarised into the recommendations of the ACPGBI (Association of Coloproctology of Great Britain and Ireland) statement. This relies on a stepwise approach from conservative to progressively more invasive treatments, taking into consideration particular cases such as women following vaginal deliveries or men with previous proctological surgery.[56]

Initial treatment – conservative measures

When managing anal fissures, the logical strategy is to treat factors that influence the persistence of the fissure. Any abnormal pattern of defaecation (hard constipated stools) needs to be addressed by appropriate dietary advice and medication (increasing liquid intake, stool softeners and topical analgesics). Patients with relatively normal bowel function but excessive straining at defaecation might benefit from anorectal biofeedback to correct it. All these treatments are non-specific, and aim at softening the stools and facilitating regular bowel movements; these alone result in healing anal fissures in almost 50% of cases.[63]

Glyceryl trinitrate

If non-specific conservative treatment fails, specific medical treatments can be offered to reversibly decrease the hypertonic sphincter spasm and improve local tissue ischaemia. These are used with a stepwise approach, from the least to the most invasive. Glyceryl trinitrate (GTN) and diltiazem are two local creams most commonly used that help to relax the internal anal sphincter. Botulinum toxin, recently introduced, acts by blocking the release of the acetylcholine neurotransmitter. These approaches, also called 'chemical sphincterotomy' (as opposed to the surgical sphincterotomy), are effective when associated with the modification of the predisposing factors (hard stools, constipation, straining).

> ✔✔ GTN is better than placebo in healing anal fissure. Diltiazem and botulinum toxin are equivalent to GTN in efficacy with fewer adverse events. Medical therapy is not as effective as surgical sphincterotomy; however, it is not associated with the risk of incontinence in any of the randomised controlled trials reported.[64]

GTN acts by relaxing the internal anal sphincter musculature through the local donation of nitric oxide. It has been shown to produce fissure healing in 68% of patients after 8 weeks of treatment, but late recurrence is in the range of 50% of those initially cured.[64] However, almost half of these could be successfully treated by a second topical course.

> ✔ Topical 0.4% GTN cream (Rectogesic 4 mg/g rectal ointment) is licensed in the UK for the relief of pain associated with chronic anal fissure in adults for a maximum of 8 weeks,[65] generally applied twice daily. The cost per 30 g is approx. £57.75 (NHS electronic drug tariff; January 2013). This is the first drug to be used in patients with anal fissure who require medical treatment. The cost of the 0.2% formulation is about £34.80 per 30 g). Topical 0.2% GTN ointment does not currently have a UK licence for treating chronic anal fissures.

No cases of permanent faecal incontinence have been described. The major drawback to the use of GTN local cream is the occurrence of significant headaches, which has been reported in 25% of patients.[56] This can be sufficient to reduce compliance to the treatment including definitive withdrawal from it in 3.3% of cases.[66]

Diltiazem

Diltiazem is a calcium channel blocker and vasodilator, which increases blood flow to smooth muscles and relaxes muscle tone. In a recent meta-analysis that compared diltiazem to GTN, the former was equally effective but was associated with a lower incidence of side-effects, headache and recurrence.[67] No cases of permanent incontinence were reported.

> ✔ Although the ACPGBI[56] recommends topical diltiazem as first-line treatment in the management of anal fissure (twice daily for 8 weeks), according to the NICE guidelines this product is not licensed in the UK for treating chronic anal fissure.[68] The NHS price for 2% diltiazem cream is £73.83 per 30g tube and the NHS price for 2% diltiazem ointment is £163.07 per 30g tube.

Botulinum toxin

Botulinum toxin normally binds to presynaptic cholinergic nerve terminals and inhibits the release of acetylcholine at the neuromuscular junction. This leads to relaxation of the anal sphincter for 2–3 months, an effect that appears to be independent of the technique, site of injection or the dose used (median 23 U, range 10–100 U).[69] In a meta-analysis of six randomised controlled trials, botulinum toxin was as effective as GTN for the management of chronic fissures (healing rate 76%) but is associated with lower complication rates, especially headaches.[69] Temporary incontinence is present in 5–10% of cases. The main drawback is related to its higher costs (£200 for 100U), not including costs of administration (general or regional anaesthesia in a hospital operating theatre), which limit its use to refractory cases.[56] To decrease costs, patients can be grouped on the same list and one vial can be used for four patients.[56]

Surgical treatments
Anal dilatation
Anal dilatation was first described in 1838 by Lord in the treatment of haemorrhoids. Lord's original eight-finger dilatation was abandoned in favour of a more gentle four-finger stretch for 4 minutes and more recently a standardised dilatation procedure using a Parks retractor opened to 4.8 cm. Although anal dilatation resulted in successful healing of anal fissures comparable to lateral internal sphincterotomy, both the internal and external sphincters can be irregularly disrupted with a higher risk of incontinence than sphincterotomy. This treatment has therefore only an historical role and is definitely abandoned in modern practice.[70]

Lateral anal sphincterotomy
Lateral sphincterotomy involves the division of the internal anal sphincter to restore a normal anal sphincter tone from the initial hypertonia. It can be performed either as an open or closed procedure with little difference in terms of fissure persistence or risk of incontinence.[64] The optimal amount of sphincter to be divided is a matter of discussion, and additional factors have to be considered such as age of the patient, sex, previous vaginal deliveries or operations involving the anal canal. Theoretically, 30% of the sphincter muscle fibres should be divided, which does not correspond anatomically to 30% of the sphincter length. As a rule of thumb, in a tailored sphincterotomy the internal sphincter is divided up to the highest point of the fissure only (in the past sphincterotomy was done with division of the internal sphincter up to the level of the dentate line). This more conservative approach seems to decrease the impairment of continence. Healing rates are in the range of 85%.[56] In a pooled analysis of 4512 patients, flatus incontinence was present in 9%, soiling in 6% and incontinence to solid stool in 0.83%.[71]

Compared to all other treatments for anal fissure, lateral sphincterotomy produces the highest healing rates but also a significant risk of incontinence.[72]

Fissurectomy
Surgical removal of the fissure (fissurectomy) has shown promising results. Fissurectomy includes excision of the fibrotic edge of the fissure, curettage of its base and excision of the sentinel tag and/or anal papilla if present.[56] Success has been reported in 67% of patients when associated with botulinum toxin injections,[73] 100% when associated with advancement flap anoplasty, with 0--7% de novo incontinence.[74] Recurrence after fissurectomy was 11.6% at 5 years follow-up,[75] and nil when associated with other treatments (isosorbide dinitrate, botulinum toxin injections, skin flap anoplasty).[73,74,76,77]

Anal advancement flap
Anal fissures without anal hypertonia (low pressure sphincter) pose a peculiar challenge for the colorectal surgeon.[62] Common therapies that decrease the sphincter tone cannot be used in this situation because they would not resolve the fissure and actually produce or exacerbate incontinence. Patients with low resting sphincter pressures may be helped by anal cutaneous advancement flaps (anoplasty),[78] with or without fissurectomy.[79] The literature on this matter is quite mixed as various types of flaps exist (island, V-Y, rotational) and are frequently associated with other procedures (botulinum toxin, fissurectomy).[79,80] Because anal flaps decrease local pain, therefore helping relaxation of the sphincter complex, they have also been proposed with good results for the treatment of all chronic fissures (not just low-pressure ones).[81,82]

Patients with recurrence after lateral sphincterotomy require anal manometry and ultrasound to identify patients with low resting anal pressures from patients with persistently raised resting pressures, therefore guiding treatment towards a repeat lateral sphincterotomy in the opposite lateral quadrant or an advancement flap anoplasty.

Conclusion

Anal fissure is a common anorectal complaint. Over the years lateral sphincterotomy has been progressively abandoned due to the well-known risks of incontinence and substituted by medical treatments, which are effective in most patients. Stepwise standardised approaches have been recommended by national societies, but the local delivery of this therapy is frequently influenced by additional factors, including costs. An important distinction is between fissures presenting with high anal sphincter pressures or low pressures, as the latter contraindicates the use of most common therapies aimed at reducing anal hypertonia and may require the use of anorectal advancement flaps to decrease local pain and promote tissue healing.

Pruritus ani

Pruritus ani is a frequent symptom. It is sometimes managed by dermatologists, but it is not uncommon for the colorectal surgeon to have referrals in the outpatient clinic. The surgical assessment is mostly based on excluding associated and sometimes more sinister causes which might require an operation.

Aetiology and pathogenesis

There are numerous direct causes of perianal itch (Box 18.1). Clinically, however, idiopathic pruritus ani is most usually associated with a minor degree of faecal incontinence. The object of history taking and examination is to find the likely cause of faecal leakage. This may be due to local pathology permitting stool to leak to the outside or to difficulty with thorough anal cleansing, or to anal sphincter dysfunction or other contributory causes such as irritative foods and, importantly, a high-fibre diet. In addition, application of inappropriate topical creams and even excessive cleansing may further aggravate the situation.

Box 18.1 • Secondary causes of pruritis ani

Neoplasia
- Rectal adenoma
- Rectal adenocarcinoma
- Anal squamous cell carcinoma
- Malignant melanoma
- Bowen's disease
- Extramammary Paget's disease

Benign anorectal conditions
- Haemorrhoids
- Fistula-in-ano
- Anal fissure
- Rectal prolapse
- Anal sphincter injury or dysfunction
- Faecal incontinence
- Radiation proctitis
- Ulcerative colitis

Infections
- Condyloma acuminatum
- Herpes simplex virus
- Threadworm
- Candida albicans
- Syphilis
- Lymphogranuloma venereum

Dermatological
- Neurogenic dermatitis
- Contact dermatitis
- Lichen simplex
- Lichen planus
- Lichen atrophicus

Diagnosis

The diagnosis of causes of minor anal leakage is most often revealed by good history taking and physical examination. Physical examination should include any evidence of skin disease elsewhere. The perineum and underclothes should be carefully inspected for any evidence of soilage.

Digital examination may reveal anal sphincter dysfunction or other reasons for the pruritus. Wiping with moist gauze may confirm staining and thus anal leakage. Repeat examination after straining may be required to reveal a rectal prolapse. Endoscopy may be required in certain cases. Skin lesions may need to be biopsied and examined for fungus or other dermatological problems.

Another cause of pruritus ani is *Enterobius* or threadworm. Placing a piece of adhesive tape on the anus and then transferring to a microscopy slide may reveal these. The presence of ova is indicative of infection.

Treatment

Treatment is dependent on the primary pathology. Advice should be cautious before any surgical intervention, as cure is not certain. In primary pruritus ani, the aims of treatment are the reduction of leakage, maintenance of good personal hygiene and the prevention of further injury to the perianal skin. Reducing flatulence by lowering dietary fibre and adding probiotics may decrease soiling. Loose stools may also be solidified with antimotility medications. Small amounts of loose stool trapped within the anus may leak out and cause irritation later in the day, long after the perineum had been cleaned.

Cleansing of the perineum using water with drying by gentle dabbing is preferred to vigorous rubbing with toilet paper. An anti-itch powder and the use of antihistamine medication may be useful to break the vicious cycle of itching and scratching. Loose underwear made of non-allergenic material may decrease the chance of contact dermatitis.

The desire to scratch may be due to fresh leakage and immediate flushing with water may obviate the desire to scratch, which otherwise may be well-nigh irresistible. Short-term use of a hydrocortisone cream may help to break the cycle, but steroid use should not be prolonged.

In a study by Lysy et al.[83] topical capsaicin was shown to be effective for idiopathic pruritus ani: 44 patients were randomised to topical capsaicin 0.006% or placebo (menthol 1%) and crossover was carried out after 4 weeks. Of these patients, 31 experienced relief with capsaicin but none with menthol.

In patients with refractory pruritus ani, anal tattooing with methylene blue destroys the nerve endings around the anus, leading to hypoaesthesia of perianal skin and can give relief from the annoying itch.[84]

Conclusion

Pruritus ani remains a difficult problem to manage. Treatment is aimed at stopping anal leakage, whether from faecal soiling or flatulence. Avoiding a high-fibre diet helps. Good personal hygiene remains an important aspect of treatment and prevention of further irritation to the perianal skin.

Pilonidal sinus

The word 'pilonidal' is derived from the Latin words *pilus* meaning hair and *nidus* meaning nest, due to trapped hair found within the sinus. It usually affects hirsute young adults, males twice as often as females.[85]

Aetiology

Pilonidal sinus is an acquired disease resulting from a foreign body reaction to extruded hair in the skin. Keratin plugs and other debris may contribute further to the inflammation. This theory arose from the observation of pilonidal sinus appearing in the hands of a barber.[86] Bascom postulated that the disease arose from infection of hair follicles in the natal cleft, which may have been occluded by keratin.[87] The infected hair follicle theory is supported by epidemiological findings that the age of presentation starts after puberty, affecting young adults. Obesity is another risk factor. Hormonal changes at puberty and obesity are closely linked to an increased incidence of infected pilosebaceous glands. Whether the cause is exclusive to either theory or a combination of both is unclear.

However, most authors agree that propagation of the inflammation to a chronic sinus is related to a foreign body reaction from a non-healing abscess. Loose hairs from the region tend to gather toward the natal cleft due to the anatomy and suction of the buttocks on movement. These hairs migrate into the sinus, tip first, and get trapped, aggravating the inflammatory process.

Clinical manifestation

Pilonidal disease often presents as an acute abscess in the midline of the sacrococcygeal region. Following incision and drainage, many patients still develop a pilonidal sinus with a primary tract epithelialised and forming a small pit in the midline of the natal cleft. Some patients also develop secondary tracts, which persist as discharging sinuses lined by granulation tissue.

Hence, patients often present either in the acute abscess stage or with an off-midline discharging sinus. When they present with a chronic pilonidal sinus, it is common to note midline pits in the natal cleft that correspond to the healed primary tracts. In such cases, the pilonidal sinus will be situated slightly cephalad to the primary pit, 1–3 cm lateral to the midline, over the underlying sacrum.

If no primary pits are seen or if the sinus drains either lateral to the sacrum or appears caudal to the primary pits, other diagnoses should be considered. It is very unusual to find multiple sinuses that open into both buttocks simultaneously. In such a case, the differential diagnosis would include hydradenitis suppurativa, complex anal fistula, osteomyelitis with draining sinuses to the skin, as well as infective conditions, such as tuberculosis or actinomycosis.

Treatment

Pilonidal abscess

Simple incision and drainage is the treatment for pilonidal abscesses when diagnosed, with up to 58% of patients having complete healing.[88] Meticulous skin care and good hygiene avoid skin maceration and regular hair shaving prevents hair from penetrating the healing scar. Such diligent wound care will further lower recurrence rates. As such, whichever surgical technique is used, careful attention to skin hygiene and hair exfoliation cannot be overemphasised.

Chronic pilonidal sinus

A chronic pilonidal sinus is a pilonidal sinus appearing after treatment of an acute pilonidal abscess. The term is also used for patients who have a discharging sinus at first presentation with or without an abscess. The surgical management of a chronic pilonidal sinus aims to obliterate the epithelialised sinus tract and heal the wound.

Outpatient options

Simple outpatient options include phenol injection and excision or lay-open of the chronic tract. Phenol destroys the epithelium in the tract and sterilises the wound. An injection of 1–2 mL of 80% phenol is given into the tract, with great care taken to protect the surrounding skin with paraffin or other ointments. The surrounding hair is shaved off and wound dressing performed daily. The phenol injection can be repeated every 4–6 weeks till the wound has healed. This simple technique has the advantage of minimal time away from work, with a variable healing rate of 59–95%. However, the side-effects include skin necrosis and abscess formation in up to 22% of patients. Some authors have advocated a reduced strength of 40% phenol, with a reduced complication rate of 12% and a healing rate of 77%.[89]

Alternatively, the sinus tract can be laid open under local anaesthesia and dressed in the outpatient setting. Some authors have advocated using fibrin sealant or regular wound brushing to reduce the wound healing time or recurrence rate. However, whatever modifications are used, the recurrence rate is generally low, from 10% to 18%, with the added advantage of minimal complications or time away from work.

Surgical options

Once a surgeon decides to perform a more complex procedure, the options increase but the best method remains debatable. The principles of the operation are to eradicate the sinus tract, ensure complete healing of the overlying skin and prevent recurrence. The options include laying the wound open to heal by secondary intention or primary closure of the surgical wound. The techniques including primary closure are further categorised into midline closure or off-midline closure.

Lay-open methods include simple excision of subcutaneous tract (sinectomy), wide excision down to sacral periostium and marsupialisation of the wound.

> ✔✔ Lay-open methods involving wide radical excisions are associated with long healing times, limited excisions with shorter times (sinusotomy/sinectomy).[90]

Conversely, many have adopted primary closure techniques because the time to wound healing and return to work is shorter. Theoretically, off-midline closure should be favoured over midline techniques, there being fewer recurrences with off-midline closure (1.4% vs 10.3% for midline closure) and wound infections (6.3% vs 10.4% for midline closure).[91] The theory behind off-midline techniques is that the natal cleft is an anatomical trough, which loose hairs tend to gravitate toward. Negative pressure in the natal cleft produced by movement of the buttocks on sitting and walking also creates a suction effect attracting the tips of loose hair towards the natal cleft. Any wound in the midline will preferentially gather loose hairs in the wound, predisposing midline wounds to recurrence. Techniques of off-midline closure change the natal cleft contour and disperse suction pressure over a wider area, thereby reducing the likelihood of loose hair implanting in the healing wound.

> ✔✔ A meta-analysis confirmed that recurrence rates are lower but healing times slower after open healing compared to primary closure techniques. For primary closure recurrence is lower and healing time faster after off-midline compared to midline closure techniques.[91]

Drainage following primary closure seems to have no role in the prevention of postoperative infections or recurrences.[92] Use of a gentamicin collagen sponge after surgical excision of sacrococcygeal pilonidal sinus disease showed no influence on wound healing and recurrence rate, but a trend towards a reduced incidence of surgical site infections.[93]

Various techniques of closure have been proposed over the years for the treatment of pilonidal sinus. In the Bascom operation an incision is made lateral to the midline to curette the deep cavity free of loose hairs and granulation tissue, together with excision of the primary midline pits using small stab incisions of about 7 mm. The midline incisions are closed primarily and the lateral wound left to heal by secondary intention.[87] Some authors close the lateral wound over a drain to reduce the healing time, with good results. Another popular technique is the Karydakis procedure where a 'semilateral' 'D-shaped' incision is made incorporating the sinus tract down to the presacral fascia:[94] the defect is convex on one side and straight on the other (next to the midline) (**Fig. 18.5a**). The flap of tissue on the straight wound side is mobilised down to the fascia to allow the flap to be brought over to the convex wound edge and sutured down in layers (**Fig. 18.5b**). Karydakis reported a recurrence rate of only 1%, with an 8.5% wound complication rate.

Recurrent pilonidal sinus

Even with proper technique and meticulous wound care, a small group of patients develop recurrent pilonidal disease. In such cases, the local tissue scarring usually precludes the techniques mentioned above and rotational flap procedures are

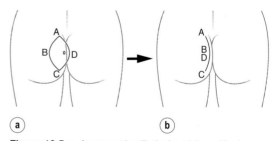

Figure 18.5 • Asymmetric elliptical excision with closure of the cavity with Karydakis flap.
Modified from Balì Ì et al. Effectiveness of Limberg and Karydakis flap. Clinics (Sao Paulo) 2015;70(5):350–5.

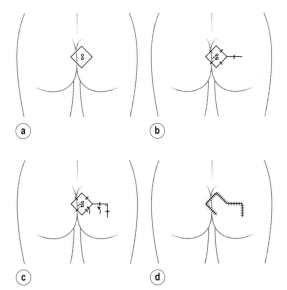

Figure 18.6 • Modified Limberg flap for recurrent pilonidal sinus showing **(a)** off-midline rhomboid-shaped incision incorporating sinus tracts; **(b)** lateral extension of incision of length equal to the side of the rhomboid incision; **(c)** caudal extension perpendicular to lateral incision; and **(d)** securing rotated flap with sutures.

recommended. Z-plasty, modified Z-plasty, gluteus maximus myocutaneous flap, V–Y fasciocutaneous flap, rhomboid fasciocutaneous flap (Limberg/Dufourmentel) (**Fig. 18.6**), and asymmetric elliptical excision with closure of the cavity with Karydakis flap have all been described. The principles involved in this surgery are complete excision of the recurrent pilonidal sinus and scar tissue, mobilisation of a flap of adjacent healthy tissue down to fascia (at least) and tension-free repair of the flap. A review of the various rotational flap techniques showed no individual superiority.

> ✔ Both off-midline closure and flaps are superior compared to midline closures,[95] and rhomboid flap (Limberg) seems superior to Karydakis procedure in terms of infection rates and wound dehiscences.[96] Off-midline procedures are preferred for primary pilonidal sinus because they are simpler to perform, while flaps are preferable for recurrent disease in view of the significant amount of scarring already present.[95]

Conclusion

Pilonidal sinus disease can present as an acute abscess, a chronic pilonidal sinus or recurrent disease. Acute abscesses should be treated with a simple incision and drainage. In chronic pilonidal sinus, open delayed healing reduces the chances of recurrence over primary closures. If primary closure is preferred, off-midline techniques are superior to midline closures. In recurrent disease, a rotational flap procedure is the preferred method of treatment.

Anal stenosis

Anal stenosis is an abnormal narrowing of the anal canal with physical obstruction at that level. This is in contrast to anal canal spasm secondary to painful lesions or functional abnormalities where examination shows a supple and fully compliant anus.

Aetiology

The commonest cause is surgery with excessive mucocutaneous excision, usually but not only following haemorrhoidectomy. Other causes are listed in Box 18.2. Recurrent anal fissures, perianal abscesses with repeated surgical procedures and excessive excision of perianal skin in Bowen's or Paget's disease may present with anal canal stenosis.

Box 18.2 • Aetiology of anal stenosis

Congenital
- Imperforate anus
- Anal atresia

Acquired
- Irradiation
- Lacerations
- Following surgery of anal canal/low rectum (commonly anastomotic failure)

Neoplastic
- Perianal or anal cancers
- Leukaemia
- Bowen's disease
- Paget's disease

Inflammatory
- Crohn's disease
- Tuberculosis
- Amoebiasis
- Lymphogranuloma venereum
- Actinomycosis

Other
- Chronic anal fissure
- Ischaemic

Clinical presentation

A history of constipation, decreasing stool calibre, difficulty in voiding with the need to strain excessively, and tenesmus are usually the first symptoms of anal stenosis. Bleeding may occur from traumatic defaecation or digitation. Scarring from previous anal surgery may be obvious, if digitation is possible. The stenosis may be mild to moderate and the level of the stenosis relative to the dentate line as well as the length of the stenosis must be noted. Anatomical findings may not correlate well with the magnitude of the obstructive symptoms.

Treatment

A biopsy may be essential if there is no history of previous surgery or anal trauma. Treatment of anal stenosis depends on the severity and level of stenosis within the anal canal, as well as when it has arisen in relation to any prior anal operation. Anal stenosis below the dentate line is often related to previous anal surgery, such as excisional haemorrhoidectomy, or to inflammatory conditions, such as Crohn's disease. Anal stenosis above the dentate line may be secondary to stapled haemorrhoidopexy or low anterior resection with partial staple-line dehiscence or infection.

Prevention

The key to treatment lies in its prevention with good surgical judgement. Excessive removal of the anoderm during haemorrhoidectomy is often the cause of significant anal stenosis. Preserving a 'mucocutaneous skin bridge' of anoderm at least 1 cm wide between wounds and limiting the distal extent of tissue resection to the anal verge may minimise anal stenosis. However, preserving anodermal 'bridges' is crucial to all anal surgery and not haemorrhoidectomy alone.

Anal dilatation

Mild stenosis (tight anal canal but permitting the passage of the index finger) may be treated occasionally with bulk laxatives, but the recurrence rate is high. After initial manual dilatation, many surgeons have recommended regular dilatation with the patient's own finger or an appropriately sized anal dilator (e.g. St Mark's anal dilator or Hagar dilators) to maintain the anal diameter. Good functional results may be achieved in this manner for mild cases, particularly if a post-surgical stenosis is caught early. The patient should be guided to pass the dilator beyond the anal stricture twice daily for 2 months, but regular anal dilatation may not work if the scarring has already matured at the time of diagnosis. Further forceful dilatation at this stage may worsen the fibrosis and lead to more serious stenosis.

> ✅ Four-finger manual dilatation performed under anaesthesia should never be performed and is always unnecessary. The uncontrolled manner of anal tearing can lead to excessive anal sphincter damage and subsequent faecal incontinence.

A very scarred and stenotic anus, or narrowing associated with Crohn's disease, may occasionally be self-maintained using Hagar dilators after initial Hagar graded dilatation under general anaesthesia if the patient is not keen on more complicated surgery. However, a worsening of scarring with time is inevitable. The principles of surgical treatment are outlined in Box 18.3.

Sphincterotomy

In the past some surgeons believed that a hypertrophied internal anal sphincter could cause anal stenosis and hence recommended anal sphincterotomy. However, there are no studies to verify this. These patients with so-called 'anal stenosis' actually have anismus or dyssynergic defaecation. Anecdotal experience of sphincterotomy showing benefit is likely due to reduction of anal pressure in the short term. In the longer term, it could theoretically lead to faecal incontinence, though this is as yet unproven. These patients are better treated with biofeedback, a form of re-training of the various muscles involved to provide an appropriate coordination of defaecation. Injection of botulin toxin may also help.

Stricturoplasty

Severe anal stenosis, with inability to pass the index finger through the stenosis, will usually require surgical intervention. In cases of anal stenosis proximal to the dentate line, as in stapled haemorrhoidopexy, stricturoplasty has proved to be a simple and reliable method of treatment. The stricture along the anastomosis is palpated and two to four vertical incisions are made over the scar with a small narrow proctoscope. This incision is deepened

Box 18.3 • Principles of surgical treatment for anal stenosis

- Stool bulking
- Anal dilatation
- Examination under anaesthesia with graded Hagar's dilator followed by postoperative self-maintenance
- Removal of cutaneous scarring
- Stricturoplasty for anal stenosis proximal to dentate line (worst cases may need an abdominal pull-through operation)
- Skin advancement (inwards)
- Mucosal advancement (outwards)
- Colostomy in desperate cases

until the entire thickness of the scar is incised without cutting the muscle layer of the rectal wall. The mucosa is approximated transversely with sutures and not left to heal by secondary intention. Two (anterior and posterior midline) or four (at 3, 6, 9, 12 o'clock positions) incisions across the stenosis can be performed based on the degree of stenosis. Special care must be taken not to cause full-thickness perforation to prevent septic and bleeding consequences. Adequacy of stricturoplasty is assessed by digital examination showing a supple and distensible anorectal wall at the level of the previous stenosis.

Flap procedures

Mucosal advancement flap (above to down)

This involves the advancement of anal mucosa into the stenotic area by way of a vertical incision made in the stenotic area perpendicular to the dentate line in the lateral position. An excision of the scar tissue allows widening of the stenosis. The incision is then undermined for about 2cm and closed in a transverse manner, stitching the mucosal edge down onto the skin edge of the anoderm.

Y–V advancement flap (outside to in)

Originally described by Penn in 1948, a Y incision is made, with the vertical limb of the Y in the anal canal above the proximal level of the stenosis. The 'V' of the Y is drawn on the lateral perianal skin. The skin is incised and a V-shaped flap is raised; the length-to-breadth ratio must be less than three. After excision of the underlying scar tissue in the anal canal the flap can be mobilised into the anal canal and stitched into place. This may be done bilaterally with good results and provides relief in 85–92% of cases. Tip necrosis occurs in 10–25% of cases and stenosis may recur.[97]

V–Y advancement flap (outside to in)

Unlike the Y–V advancement flap, the V–Y flap has the advantage of bringing a wider piece of skin into the stenosis to keep it open. The V is drawn with the wide base parallel to the dentate line about 2cm long. A similar length-to-base ratio as in the Y–V flap should be maintained. Marking the skin flap is followed by its mobilisation such that it may move without tension into the anal canal. Sufficient subcutaneous tissue must be mobilised with the flap, which derives its blood supply from the perforating vessels arising within the fat. The skin is then closed behind the flap to produce the limb of the Y. A treatment success rate of 96% has been reported with this flap.

Island advancement flap (outside to in)

First described in 1986, the island flap may be constructed in various shapes (e.g. diamond, house or U-shaped).[98] The flap is mobilised from its lateral margins together with the subcutaneous fat after the scar tissue in the stenotic area has been excised. A lateral sphincterotomy may or may not be performed. A broad skin flap (up to 50% of the circumference) may be brought into the entire length of the anal canal and simultaneously allow for closure of the donor site. Improvement of symptoms may be as high as 91% at 3 years of follow-up; 18–50% suffer minor wound separation.[99]

Conclusion

The best form of treatment for anal stenosis remains prevention. Gentle and regular anal dilatation can help mild stenosis but recurrent or severe cases require surgery. High stenosis above the dentate line is probably best treated by transanal stricturoplasty, or in the worst cases, an abdominal pull-through operation.

Sexually transmitted diseases

Sexually transmitted diseases (STDs) may present to colorectal surgeons. Signs and symptoms include diarrhoea, rectal bleeding, tenesmus and ulcerative or fistulous lesions of the rectum, anus and perineum. All healthcare providers should be aware that high-risk behaviours, including unprotected sex, multiple partners and illicit drug use, can increase transmission of STDs as well as human immunodeficiency virus (HIV).[100] The presence of more than one infecting organism is not uncommon.

The commonest organisms causing STDs of the anorectum present in three symptom categories: suppurative, ulcerative and fistulous disease (Table 18.2). The diseases presented in

Table 18.2 • Anorectal STDs categorised by predominant presentation

STDs with proctitis	STDs with ulcers	STDs with fistulas
Gonorrhea	AIDS-associated anal ulcers	Lymphogranuloma venereum
Chlamydia	Lymphogranuloma venereum	Complex Bushke–Lowenstein tumours
Herpes simplex virus	Primary syphilis – chancre	
Syphilis	Chancroid	
	Granuloma inguinale	
	Herpes simplex virus	

AIDS, acquired immune deficiency syndrome; STD, sexually transmitted disease.

Table 18.3 are categorised by aetiological agent. Medications are suggested, but clinicians should consult full prescribing information and request specialist advice before using them.

Human papillomavirus and anal warts

Human papillomaviruses (HPVs) are small DNA viruses that cause benign and malignant changes to the epithelium of the anorectum and genitalia. Infections may remain subclinical or be active and induce benign, hyperproliferative lesions of the epithelia, called warts, papillomas or condylomata.

The α-papillomavirus group of HPV types are those that typically infect the anogenital tract. These HPVs are further classified into non-oncogenic or low-risk (LR) types, such as HPV-6 and HPV-11, and potentially oncogenic or high-risk (HR) viruses, including HPV-16, HPV-18, HPV-51 and HPV-53. Lesions induced by the oncogenic types can progress to high-grade dysplasias and cancers. In contrast, the LR HPV-6 and HPV-11 are rarely found in anogenital cancers.[101]

The natural host tissue for the infection cycle of all HPVs is the squamous epithelium lining of body openings. A band of rapidly cycling and dividing keratinocytes called the transformation zone establishes a squamo-columnar junction at each body opening.[101] Transmission occurs most commonly at sexual contact with infected individuals, although perianal and genital involvement can occur without anal intercourse at skin-to-skin or skin-to-mucosa contact.

Table 18.3 • Sexually transmitted organisms that affect the anorectum

Organism	Symptoms	Anoscopy/proctoscopy	Laboratory	Treatment
Viral				
HIV	Pain unrelated to defaecation	Broad-based ulcers proximal to dentate line	Serology	HAART, debridement, unroofing cavities, intralesional steroid injection
Herpes simplex virus (HSV)	Anorectal pain, pruritus, rectal bleeding	Perianal erythema, vesicles, ulcers, diffusely inflamed and friable rectal mucosa	Cytological examination of scrapings or viral culture of vesicle fluid PCR	Aciclovir *or* Famciclovir *or* Valaciclovir
Human papillomavirus (condylomata acuminatum)	Pruritus, bleeding, discharge, pain	Perianal warts	Excisional biopsy to determine serotype	Topical agents, excision or destruction
Molluscum contagiosum	Painless skin lesions	Flattened, round, umbilicated lesion	Excisional biopsy and staining for molluscum bodies	Expectant, excision or destruction
Bacterial				
Chlamydia trachomatis	Tenesmus, perianal pain	Friable, often ulcerated mucosa	Tissue culture, nucleic acid amplification, serological antibody titres	Azithromycin *or* Doxycycline
Lymphogranuloma venereum (LGV)	Systemic symptoms, inguinal adenopathy, anogenital ulceration	Friable ulcerated rectal mucosa	LGV serotyping with nucleic acid amplification, confirmation at specialty laboratories	Doxycycline *or* Erythromycin
Haemophilus ducreyi (chancroid)	Anal pain	Anorectal abscesses and ulcers	Culture, Gram stain with 'school of fish' pattern, PCR	Azithromycin *or* Ceftriaxone *or* Ciprofloxacin *or* Erythromycin
Neisseria gonorrhoeae (gonorrhoea)	Rectal discharge	Proctitis, mucopurulent discharge	Culture of discharge on Thayer–Martin or Modified New York City agar	Ceftriaxone *plus* Treatment for *Chlamydia* if chlamydial infection is not ruled out

Table 18.3 • Sexually transmitted organisms that affect the anorectum—cont'd

Organism	Symptoms	Anoscopy/ proctoscopy	Laboratory	Treatment
Calymmatobacterium granulomatis (granuloma inguinale)	Perianal mass, ulceration	Hard, shiny perianal masses	Smear or biopsy of mass or ulceration	Doxycycline *or* Azithromycin *or* Ciprofloxicin *or* Erythromycin *or* Trimethoprim– sulfamethoxazole until all lesions have healed
Treponema pallidum (syphilis)	**Primary syphilis** Painful anal chancre, inguinal lymphadenopathy, lesions infected with spirochetes **Secondary syphilis** Condyloma lata, foul discharge, lesions infected with spirochetes **Tertiary syphilis** Rectal gumma, tabes dorsalis, severe perianal pain, paralysis of anal sphincters	See text	Dark-field microscopy of ulcer scrapings, immunostaining from biopsy, serology	Benzathine penicillin G

HAART, highly active antiretroviral therapy; PCR, polymerase chain reaction.

Infection can be clinically silent or result in bleeding, pruritus, pain, wetness and/or the feeling of a lump. The lesions can range in appearance from a single, pinkish-white lesion, to multiple large cauliflower-like masses (**Fig. 18.7**). Diagnosis is primarily made on physical examination; anoscopy is necessary for complete evaluation because involvement within the anal canal can occur. Because associated genital lesions are common, patients with anal condyloma should undergo thorough physical examination, including a vaginal examination and cervical smear in women. Anal canal lesions that are missed on simple visual inspection with anoscopy can be detected with 5% aqueous acetic acid; regions of active HPV mucosal infection briefly turn cloudy white ('aceto-whitening'), as does anal intraepithelial neoplasia. Lesions that are confused with anal condylomata include condyloma lata (syphilis), molluscum contagiosum and hypertrophied anal papillae. Histopathology will confirm the diagnosis.

Treatment

The goal of treatment is to destroy all visible disease while minimising morbidity. Because only gross lesions are treated, virus will remain in adjacent epithelium and can lead to recurrence. For small (1–3 mm) external and accessible lesions on the perianal skin, a topical patient-applied agent such as imiquimod, cidofovir or green-tea extract (sinecatechins) is first-line therapy, although all have shown substantial failure and recurrence rates. Patient-applied topical therapies are approved for external lesions only. If one type of topical therapy fails, another may be initiated.[102,103]

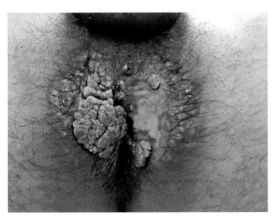

Figure 18.7 • Anal warts. On patient's left side is the area of previous surgical excision.

Lesions inside the anal canal require provider-administered therapies including trichloracetic acid, cryotherapy and surgery.[102,103] Tangential excision or fulguration of small internal and external lesions (smaller than 5mm) can be performed in the outpatient setting with local anaesthetic after a circumferential anal block. Larger and broad-based lesions, which would require excision of a substantial portion of perianal skin, are treated by electrodessication, usually with a spinal anaesthetic, local anaesthetic, deep sedation or a combination thereof. The superficial-most layer of the condyloma is fulgurated with the cautery tip until it takes on a grey–white appearance. This is followed by curettage or simply abrading the fulgurated tissue with forceps or gauze. Treatment is repeated until the condylomata are completely removed without burning into the deep dermis. Pedunculated warts can be transected at their base. Tissue from HIV-positive patients, those with history of intraepithelial neoplasia as well as larger, flat, recurrent warts or suspicious lesions should always be sent for histopathology.

> ✓ Compared to patient-applied and provider-applied therapies, surgical excision has the greatest success in treating anal condyloma, with recurrence rates between 4% and 29%.[104]

Laser destruction has been advocated as less painful and associated with fewer recurrences than other destructive techniques, but no prospective, randomised data support these claims. A risk of laser is the problem of aerosolised viral particles in the plume and medical providers developing condylomata in their respiratory tract after using a laser to treat warts has been reported.

Buschke–Lowenstein tumour: giant anal condyloma

Buschke and Lowenstein described giant condyloma accuminata (GCA) in 1925. It is associated with low-risk HPV serotypes 6 and 11, but it does have histological differences from ordinary anal condyloma. These condylomata have a propensity for perianal fistula formation, infection and malignant transformation (in situ or invasive squamous cell cancer).[105] Wide local excision with a 1cm margin is the treatment of choice and local tissue flaps or skin grafting may be required. Temporary diversion may be needed for hygiene and wound healing. Abdominoperineal excision has been used for GCA if the anal sphincters are involved. Chemoradiation is an option, especially in those who are poor surgical candidates or when

clear surgical margins are not attainable, but results in decreased cure rates compared to surgery.[106]

Other STDs affecting the anorectum

Herpes simplex (HSV) is a DNA virus of the Herpesviridae family that includes varicella zoster, Epstein–Barr and cytomegalovirus. HSV-1 is usually associated with oral, labial or ocular lesions, but with increasing oral–genital contact the rate of HSV-1 genital infections has increased and accounts for up to 13% of anorectal herpes infections. HSV-2 is more typically responsible for anogenital infections from direct anogenital contact, accounting for almost 90% of such infections (**Fig. 18.8**).

Molluscum contagiosum is caused by a virus of the pox virus family and transmitted by direct contact. It presents with painless discrete 2–6mm skin-coloured papules with central umbilication. Multiple lesions are common; however, immunocompromised patients can develop a severe form with hundreds of skin lesions. While it is generally a self-limiting disease, treatment can be used to prevent spread and for cosmetic purposes. Various treatments including curettage, cryotherapy, trichloracetic acid and electrocautery are used but none has proven superior in trials.

Chlamydia trachomatis is the most frequently reported bacterial STD in Western countries. It is an obligate intracellular bacterium that is sexually transmitted and can cause infections that resemble gonorrhoea. Anorectal transmission occurs primarily through anoreceptive intercourse. Clinical syndromes resulting from chlamydial infection include cervicitis, pelvic inflammatory disease (PID), urethritis and proctitis. Small vesicles that become ulcerated are the initial signs of infection at the site of inoculation. Areas of necrosis occur within the lymph nodes, which can then form abscesses, or a large matted mass with overlying

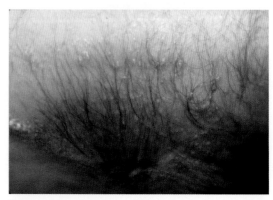

Figure 18.8 • Herpetic vesicles.
Courtesy of L. Gottesman, MD.

erythema, mimicking syphilis. After resolution of these an anogenitorectal syndrome occurs, with signs of systemic infection (fevers, myalgia) and a more aggressive infection involving the perianal, anal and rectal areas resulting in ulceration, rectal pain, discharge, bleeding and severe proctitis. On sigmoidoscopy, there is a severe, non-specific granular proctitis with mucosal erythema, friability and ulceration. Biopsies of the mucosa are consistent with infectious proctitis, including crypt abscesses, infectious granulomas and giant cells, and can be difficult to distinguish from Crohn's disease.[107] Diagnosis is by culture, microimmunofluorescent antibody titres or polymerase chain reaction.

Long-term chronic inflammation from LGV serotypes results in stricture, fistulas, lymphoedema and in women can lead to the development of rectovaginal fistulas. Sexual contacts from the past 60 days should be treated, and patients should refrain from sexual activity for 7 days after completion of treatment with doxycycline.

Chancroid, caused by *Haemophilus ducreyi*, is a Gram-negative coccobacillus that is a frequent cause of painful anogenital ulcerations in underdeveloped countries, but is uncommon in the USA and Western Europe.

Neisseria gonorrhoeae is a Gram-negative intracellular diplococcus. Symptoms of anorectal involvement include pruritus ani, bloody or mucoid discharge, tenesmus and anorectal pain. Mucopurulent discharge in combination with proctitis is the characteristic physical finding in gonococcal proctitis. On anoscopy, there is a thick, yellow mucopurulent discharge that can be expressed from anal crypts when pressure is applied. Even when the anal canal is spared, one may still see perianal erythema. A single intramuscular dose of ceftriaxone plus treatment for chlamydia (i.e. azithromycin or doxycycline) is first-line therapy.

Syphilis is a mucocutaneous STD caused by the spirochete *Treponema pallidum*. It can present in one of several progressive stages: primary (chancre or proctitis), secondary (condyloma lata) or tertiary (with involvement of the nervous and vascular systems). Anal syphilis occurs during anal receptive intercourse. The primary stage begins within 2–10 weeks of exposure with the appearance of an anal ulcer called a chancre. This is a raised, 1–2cm lesion that begins as a small papule that progresses into an indurated, clean-based ulcer without exudates. Anal ulcers are frequently painful (in contrast to genital ulcers), they may be single or multiple, and can be located on the perianal skin, in the anal canal or in the distal rectum. Differentiation from idiopathic anal fissure may be difficult; however, chancres are usually eccentrically located (off the midline), multiple and, if opposite each other, are known as 'kissing ulcers'. Painless but prominent lymphadenopathy is also common. If secondary bacterial infection occurs, patients can experience worsening anorectal pain. Rectal mucosal involvement results in tenesmus, rectal discharge or bleeding, though proctitis may occur with or without chancres.[108]

Untreated lesions usually heal in 2–4 weeks. If primary syphilis is untreated, haematogenous spread occurs 4–10 weeks after the primary lesions and leads to secondary syphilis. This presents with systemic symptoms including fever, malaise, arthralgia, weight loss, sore throat and headache, and as a non-pruritic macular rash on the trunk, limbs, palms and/or soles. Condyloma lata, a grey or whitish wart-like lesion teeming with spirochetes, may be found near the initial chancre. These lesions are moister and smoother than anal condyloma from HPV, are pruritic and have a foul discharge. Mucosal patches or ulcerations may appear in the rectum.[109] Tertiary syphilis is rare and presents with classic neurological and vascular symptoms.

Treponema pallidum cannot be cultured. Serology, specific immunofluorescent staining or dark-field microscopy of scrapings from chancres or lymph nodes help with the diagnosis. Treatment is with penicillin.

Key points

- Haemorrhoidal disease is common but other more significant diseases must be excluded before ascribing symptoms to haemorrhoids. Treatment by rubber-band ligation or submucosal injection is appropriate in early stages. Consideration should be given either to transanal haemorrhoidal artery ligation, stapled haemorrhoidopexy or excisional haemorrhoidectomy for more severe degrees of prolapsing piles, depending on the degree present and the expertise available.

- Most anal fissures derive from an increased anal sphincter tone and treatment is based on a stepwise approach from non-invasive treatments to lateral sphincterotomy in refractory cases. Low-pressure fissures may need flap closure to control pain and achieve remission.

- Pruritus ani may result from many anorectal or dermatological conditions and remains a difficult problem to manage and treat. Reduction of anal leakage, reduction in fibre consumption and good personal hygiene remain important aspects of treatment.

- Treatment of pilonidal sinus depends upon presentation as well as patient preferences in terms of healing time, time off work and recurrence rates. Incision and drainage is the preferred treatment for acute presentation. Open wound surgery is associated with fewer recurrences but longer healing times compared to wound closures. Off-midline wound closure is preferred to midline if primary wound closure is performed. Flap techniques of reconstruction should be employed in recurrent cases due to the significant amount of scarring.
- Anal stenosis has many aetiologies but the commonest is a result of anal surgery. Treatments range from anal dilatation to flap procedures.
- Although STDs are best managed by an STD service, a high index of suspicion and knowledge of most common lesions is required because they might still present to the colorectal surgeon. Obtaining an appropriate sexual history and physical examination is important because these diseases are usually associated and present with other infections such as hepatitis and HIV. Patients and partners should be involved in the process.

▶ Recommended videos:

- THD – https://tinyurl.com/y7y3jnyp
- Stapled haemorrhoidopexy –https://tinyurl.com/pfrkhqv

🌐 Full references available at http://expertconsult.inkling.com

Key references

8. Alonso-Coello P, Mills E, Heels-Ansdell D, et al. Fiber for the treatment of haemorrhoids complications: a systematic review and meta-analysis. Am J Gastroenterol 2006;101:181–8. PMID: 16405552.

9. Alonso-Coello P, Guyatt G, Heels-Ansdell D, et al. Laxatives for the treatment of haemorrhoids. Cochrane Database Syst Rev 2005: CD004649. PMID: 16235372.

Two meta-analyses that show decreased symptoms with the use of fibre for the conservative treatment of haemorrhoids.

10. Perera N, Liolitsa D, Iype S, et al. Phlebotonics for haemorrhoids. Cochrane Database Syst Rev 2012: CD004322. PMID: 22895941.

Cochrane meta-analysis showing significant positive effects of phlebotonics on numerous haemorrhoidal symptoms.

11. Ho YH, Tan M, Seow-Choen F. Micronized purified flavonidic fraction compared favorably with rubber band ligation and fiber alone in the management of bleeding haemorrhoids: randomized controlled trial. Dis Colon Rectum 2000;43:66–9. PMID: 10813126.

A randomised study comparing ispaghula husk alone, rubber-band ligation plus ispaghula husk, or micronised purified flavonidic fraction plus ispaghula husk.

13. Shanmugam V, Thaha MA, Rabindranath KS, et al. Rubber band ligation versus excisional haemorrhoidectomy for haemorrhoids. Cochrane Database Syst Rev 2005: CD005034. PMID: 16034963.

Grade 2 haemorrhoids should be treated with rubber-band ligation while surgery is reserved for grade 3 haemorrhoids or recurrent haemorrhoids after rubber-band ligation.

25. Lan P, Wu X, Zhou X, et al. The safety and efficacy of stapled hemorrhoidectomy in the treatment of haemorrhoids: a systematic review and meta-analysis of ten randomized control trials. Int J Colorectal Dis 2006;21:172–8. PMID: 15971065.

26. Sutherland LM, Burchard AK, Matsuda K, et al. A systematic review of stapled hemorrhoidectomy. Arch Surg 2002;137:1395–406. discussion 1407. PMID: 12470107.

27. Laughlan K, Jayne DG, Jackson D, et al. Stapled haemorrhoidopexy compared to Milligan–Morgan and Ferguson haemorrhoidectomy: a systematic review. Int J Colorectal Dis 2009;24:335–44. PMID: 19037647.

28. Shao WJ, Li GC, Zhang ZH, et al. Systematic review and meta-analysis of randomized controlled trials comparing stapled haemorrhoidopexy with conventional haemorrhoidectomy. Br J Surg 2008;95:147–60. PMID: 18176936.

Four meta-analyses and systematic reviews comparing stapled haemorrhoidopexy with Milligan–Morgan haemorrhoidectomy. RCTs included were average level II evidence with variability among studies.

35. Jayaraman S, Colquhoun PH, Malthaner RA. Stapled versus conventional surgery for haemorrhoids. Cochrane Database Syst Rev 2006: CD005393. PMID: 17054255.

Cochrane meta-analysis comparing stapled haemorrhoidectomy versus conventional haemorrhoidectomy. The former is associated with higher risk of recurrence or symptoms of prolapse than excisional haemorrhoidectomy.

41. Sajid MS, Parampalli U, Whitehouse P, et al. A systematic review comparing transanal haemorrhoidal de-arterialisation to stapled haemorrhoidopexy in the management of haemorrhoidal disease. Tech Coloproctol 2012;16:1–8. PMID: 22183450.

This meta-analysis compared HAL/THD versus stapled haemorrhoidopexy. Both procedures produced equal results in terms of duration of the operation, postoperative complications and recurrence rates, but postoperative pain was significantly less in the THD/HAL group.

45. Sammour T, Barazanchi AW, Hill AG; PROSPECT group (Collaborators). Evidence-based management of pain after excisional haemorrhoidectomy surgery: a PROSPECT review update. World J Surg 2017;41(2):603–14. PMID: 27766395.

Pudendal nerve block is recommended for all patients. Combinations of oral analgesics, topical lignocaine and glyceryl trinitrate, laxatives and oral metronidazole are recommended postoperatively.

46. Liu JW, Lin CC, Kiu KT, et al. Effect of glyceryl trinitrate ointment on pain control after hemorrhoidectomy: a meta-analysis of randomized controlled trials. World J Surg 2016;40:215–24. PMID: 26578318.

Glyceryl trinitrate is useful in the early postoperative period to control pain.

47. Siddiqui MR, Abraham-Igwe C, Shangumanandan A, et al. A literature review on the role of chemical sphincterotomy after Milligan–Morgan hemorrhoidectomy. Int J Colorectal Dis 2011;26:685–92. PMID: 21212965.

Diltiazem and botulinum toxin are also effective measures to control postoperative pain.

64. Nelson RL, Thomas K, Morgan J, et al. Non surgical therapy for anal fissure. Cochrane Database Syst Rev 2012: CD003431. PMID: 22895929.

Seventeen agents were used and most studies referred to glyceryl trinitrate, diltiazem and botulinum toxin. Medical therapy is less effective than lateral sphincterotomy but reports no risk of permanent incontinence. The former is also associated with a higher rate of recurrence.

90. Enriquez-Navascues JM, Emparanza JI, Alkorta M, et al. Meta-analysis of randomized controlled trials comparing different techniques with primary closure for chronic pilonidal sinus. Tech Coloproctol 2014;18:863–72. PMID: 24845110.

Systematic review comparing (1) open wide excision versus open limited excision (sinusectomy) or unroofing (sinotomy); (2) midline closure (conventional and tension-free) versus off-midline; (3) advancing versus rotation flaps; and (4) sinusectomy/sinotomy versus primary closure.

91. Al-Khamis A, McCallum I, King PM, et al. Healing by primary versus secondary intention after surgical treatment for pilonidal sinus. Cochrane Database Syst Rev 2010: CD006213. PMID: 20091589.

When closure of pilonidal sinuses was the desired surgical option, off-midline closure should be the standard management as it led to faster healing times and fewer recurrences compared to midline wounds.

Index

NB: Page numbers followed by *f* indicate figures, *t* indicate tables and *b* indicate boxes.

T